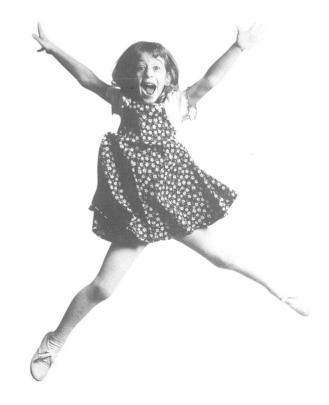

natural health bible stay well, live longer the natural health bible stay well, live longer the natural health bible stay well, live longer the natural health bible stay well, live longer the **Lisha Simester** stay well, live longer **the natural health bible** stay well, live longer the natural health bible stay well, live longer the natural health bible stay well, live longer the natural health bible stay well, live longer the natural health bible stay well, live longer the natural health bible stay well, live longer the natural health bible stay well, live longer the natural health bible stay well, live longer the natural health bible stay well, live longer the natural health bible stay well, live longer the natural health bible stay well, live longer the natural health bible stay well, live longer the natural health bible stay well, live longer the natural health bible stay well, live longer the natural health bible stay well, live longer the natural health bible stay well, live longer the natural health bible stay well, live longer the natural health bible stay well, live longer the natural health bible stay **quadrille** longer the natural heal

To my partner on this journey, Peter Simester with love.

Publishing Director: Anne Furniss
Creative Director: Mary Evans
Art Director: Françoise Dietrich
Editor & Project Manager: Lewis Esson
Art Editor: Rachel Gibson
Assistant Editor: Emma Noble
Production: Julie Hadingham

First published in 2001 by
Quadrille Publishing Limited,
Alhambra House,
27-31 Charing Cross Road,
London WC2H OLS

Reprinted in 2002 (twice), 2003, 2005
10 9 8 7 6 5

Cataloguing in Publication Data: a catalogue record for
this book is available from the British Library

ISBN 1 902757 66 1

Printed and bound in Singapore

Medical advisor:
Dr David Smallbone MB., ChB, LRCP, MRCS, MFHom, FCOH

Specialist consultants and contributors:
Patrick Holford BSc. Dip ION
Celia and Brian Wright
Pierre Jean Cousin MBACC, GCRCH
Eddie and Debbie Shapiro
Jennifer Dodd, ITEC, Dip. SPA
Caroline Turner RSA, ACE
Catharine Christof ITEC, ISTM
Dominique Radclyffe
Jerome Burne

contents

introduction

Modern medicine is in crisis. While advances continue to be incredible, the errors and incompetence occurring on a daily level make submission to a doctor or a hospital a potentially dangerous process – a kind of roulette wheel. We no longer have the old blind faith that doctors have all the solutions to our health problems and can give an accurate diagnosis every time. We have awakened to the fact that 'orthodox ' medicine does not always hold the key to perfect health and that hospitals are not always sanctuaries of healing and miracle cures. While most of us accept that current advances in medical and surgical skills are staggering, they are not always without side effects, risks and failures.

The discovery and regular use of antibiotics and vaccinations have wiped away many diseases that used to ravage the population with uncontrollable epidemics. Yet in their wake have emerged stronger and more deadly bacteria and viruses – 'superbugs' that are able to resist and overpower even the strongest drugs. At the same time the second half of the last century has seen more people travelling around the world than ever before. Air travel circulates people and germs at sound barrier breaking speeds and at no other time in history have our immune systems been so sorely challenged by changing environmental conditions and time zones. The world is not a safer or healthier place, in spite of the amazing scientific and technological feats achieved.

The information revolution ensures we are far better educated about our minds and bodies than generations before us. Yet so many of us have lost touch with the simple folk knowledge about ourselves and our relationship with the natural world of which we are but a part. More and more people are waking up to the fact that there is a lot we can do to prevent illness in the first place. Today it is far better and safer to stay well. There are so many paths we can take to create and maintain optimum health. It is up to each of us to discover a health regime that fits our unique disposition, type and needs. Most of us now understand how vital a healthy immune system or nervous system is to our health. We can not possibly keep fit unless these systems are in good working order. In fact all the systems of the body/mind/spirit are equally important to our well-being and good health. We now understand each of us is in the front line when it comes to our own health – that the way we treat our body and mind each day determines our state of health and well-being in the short and the long term. Most of us in the developed world will live to a ripe age of 70 plus – a lot longer than our ancestors. We can affect the quality of life we experience in the advancing years. Do we spend our golden years struggling with degenerative diseases and ill health or do we live our days out in a state of wholeness and well-being, confident in our ability to adapt to the stresses of time, wear and tear and the normal aging process? If we learn to take better care of ourselves earlier we can prevent many of the illnesses so common today. We have the power – it is just a question of recognizing and using it, of really tuning into our bodies and minds and objectively assessing our condition, our type, and what habits we have which might be contributing to any negative lifestyle patterns that disturb the natural balance. It is possible to achieve a high level of well-being and vitality by creating an individual health programme tailored to our very own needs and temperament. The choices we make play the largest role in the state of our health.

In this book we seek to explore the rich, varied and fascinating world of life-enhancing options from which we can choose to enhance the health of our bodies, minds and souls. We are not cataloguing health problems and cures in this volume, but rather emphasizing the joys of, and route to, positive natural good health. Here we are celebrating the many available paths to a more holistic, and therefore more vital, healthy life. Put simply, the purpose of The Natural Health Bible is to present many of the best options from which to choose and create a personal plan for positive well-being – increasing good sound health and improving the quality of life.

In calling this book a 'bible', we in no way mean to suggest this is the last word, or the most inclusive/exclusive work on the vast subject of the natural health field. This book is the reflection of a personal journey to wholeness which is, and will remain, ongoing as long as I live. In that sense it is a personal bible. Each of the subjects within this volume could be a huge book on their own. For lack of space we have only been able to touch briefly upon many areas of natural health and well-being that warrant more in-depth exploration. We have set out to present the widest possible selection of options and possibilities from which you may be stimulated to begin to create your own individual programme for lasting well-being.

the natural body

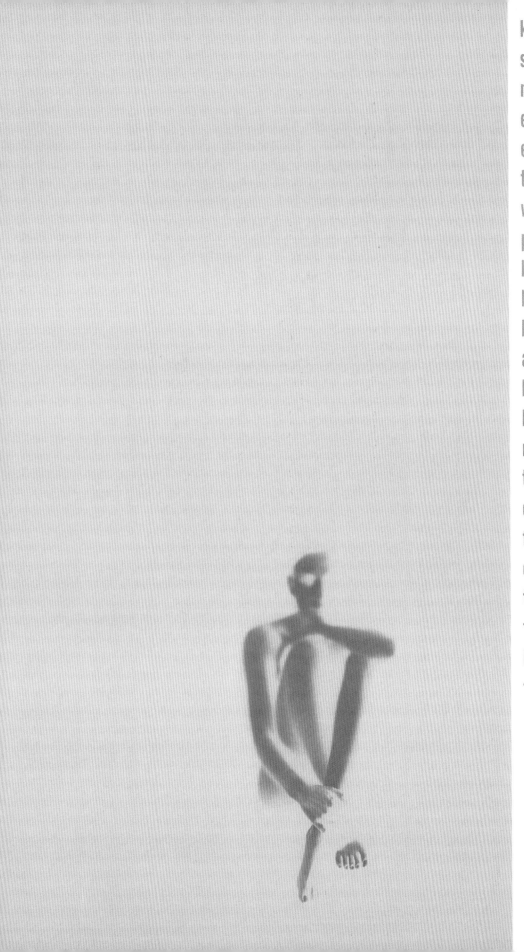

the healthy body

know your body type

Your body has many more things in common with those of everyone else than differences. In spite of the fact that your physiological structure is the same as every other person's, the diverse expression of the human form seems infinite. Basically our physical differences are things like height, weight, colouring, size of features, the finer smaller details of our physiology. But we all have one head, one nose, two eyes, etc.

As you look at the people around you and get past the small differences, huge variations and many similarities, you notice people seem to fall into 'body types', like tall and thin or short and stocky. Students and teachers of physiology have been attempting to identify and understand the major differences in body types. Different cultures have different approaches to classifying our diversity. Chinese and Indian medical systems have been classifying and filing types according to holistic elemental typing for thousands of years. Invariably, those attempting this sort of classification seemed to find that there were strong links between body type and personality and emotional traits.

One of the systems we use in the Western world was developed in the 1940s by an American psychologist, W.H. Sheldon, although physicians from Hippocrates onwards had attempted to classify 'body types'. Sheldon called his system somatotyping, in which he observed very recognizable, distinct, identifiable body types. He thought we have tendencies toward one type but we might also have some characteristics of one or both of the other types. Sheldon believed we are all an individual unique mixture of the three somatotypes. Sheldon's body types are cast by body structure not including height. You can be any combination of the three types no matter what your height. You inherit your body type and basically there is not much you can do to alter the fact that you are 7 feet tall and naturally lean or 4 foot 6 inches and naturally round.

Recognizing and accepting your body type is important to your well-being and, in some cases, your life direction. If you are a short endomorph you would be wise to give up your dream of super-model stardom and set your sights on a more realistic goal. However, it is important to remember most of us are a rich mix of the three types.

Mesomorph

Muscular build, classic wide body and shoulders, small waist, narrow hips. Naturally athletic bodies. Aggressive, dynamic, competitive, courageous and domineering personalities who need to win. Action men and women who like to take risks, have adventures and participate in sports and exercise.

Endomorph

Large, round body, heavily built, possibly fat, short plump neck, legs and arms thickly set. Easygoing, tolerant, slow, relaxed and sociable. A rather complacent personality.

Ectomorph

Tall and narrow, with a very thin angular body in which the muscle is lean rather than well developed. Nervous, sensitive individuals, smart and fussy, quick-witted, alert and defensive.

the ayurvedic types

VATA, PITTA, KAPHA

At the heart of Ayurvedic medicine (see pages 262–263) is the concept of seeking harmony by balancing the 'doshas' or bodily humours. The three doshas are contained in every cell of the body, as they govern the three principles necessary to the maintenance of life. Kapha controls the physical structure and fluid balance of the body; Vata governs motion and movement throughout the body; and Pitta manages digestion and metabolism.

All three are equally important to our mental and physical well-being, but all three are not present in equal proportions within us. It is our unique blend of doshas that creates our individual constitutional or body type ('prakriti', the Ayurvedic term for body types, is the Sanskrit word for 'nature'). We are a blend of all three doshas – but that blend is completely unique – a blueprint for our own innate characteristics and qualities – and knowing that blend can help us understand how to live appropriately for our unique nature and its needs.

What may feel natural in terms of diet and exercise for you is different from what feels 'natural' for your partner, best friend or sister! By exploring the three doshas and identifying our dominant dosha we can have a better idea of how to address our individuality so as to enhance, promote and maintain our best health.

Vata

Vata governs motion and movement, so Vata types are full of vital energy and lead a creative and active life. Vatas usually have dry, coarse skin and hair and a fast metabolism – they are slim with little body fat. They are restless with lots of ideas and are very perceptive – Vatas are capable of intuitive leaps. They move quickly and their lifestyle can be variable and erratic; they strongly dislike routine. They may suffer from insomnia.

A person strong in balanced Vata will sleep well, think clearly and experience balanced and well-regulated bodily functions.

Unbalanced Vata

Underweight. Their teeth decay easily and their skin tends to be overly rough and dry. They may have very bad circulation and often feel cold; they suffer from excess energy, which manifests itself in nail-biting, jumpiness and occasional insomnia. Their thought patterns are erratic, they are sometimes impatient with friends and their memory is poor. They have a tendency to be rash and to make hasty decisions. They are prone to nervous exhaustion.

Pitta

Pittas are of medium height and frame but slender. Their skin is soft and lustrous but they may have freckles or birthmarks and so should avoid getting too much sun. They have straight hair, tending towards oiliness, usually fair and often prematurely greying. Pittas have sharp teeth, good eyesight and a highly developed sense of smell, and may even have a distinctive, but not unpleasant, smell themselves. Their appetite is good and they enjoy food.

A person strong in balanced pitta is intelligent, direct, ambitious and assertive, and an impassioned speaker.

Unbalanced Pitta

A tendency to overheat: they should stay out of the sun, away from explosive situations and avoid spicy foods! Fevers and sweating may be a problem. Their hair may thin or grey easily. They can suffer poor digestion, possibly irritable bowel syndrome; also inflammatory conditions – acid indigestion, gout and skin disorders. Often poor vision.

Kapha

Kapha is the dependable force within you that builds cells, strengthens bones and fights disease. Kapha people have well-developed bodies but tend to gain weight because of a slow metabolism. They have a vital, almost elemental strength and a steady sexual appetite. They are good-looking: their hair is thick and lustrous and their eyes are big. They move slowly and calmly and see no reason to rush; they don't like change.

People strong in balanced Kapha are courageous, loyal and caring. They should avoid cold, damp weather, oversleeping and rich, heavy foods.

Unbalanced Kapha
Unhealthy weight gain. They have a flabby physique and weak muscles. They may suffer a loss of sexual desire, perhaps frigidity or impotence. They are sluggish, constantly tired and their digestion is poor. They are possessive and jealous. They may suffer from excess congestion, mucus and fluid retention.

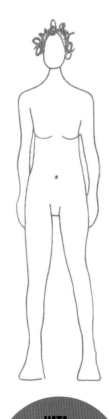

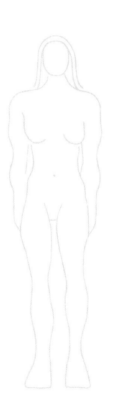

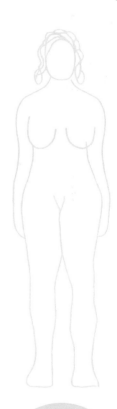

VATA (ECTOMORPH)
Slim, dark, quick wit, nervous energy, light sleeper

PITTA (MESOMORPH)
Moderate build, fair, active, leader, ambitious

KAPHA (ENDOMORPH)
Firm, heavy-boned, likes routine, good appetite

which type are you?

To help you determine what your particular dosha mix might be, answer the three questionnaires that follow – one for each type. Score zero for 'never' answers, 3 for 'sometimes' and 6 for 'often', then add up your total for each type. In most cases one dosha will have an obviously higher score – this will be your dominant dosha and you are a single-dosha type. If no single dosha dominates, you are probably a two-dosha type (most people are) and you must consider the traits of both. If all three scores are more are less equal, then you are that great rarity, a three-dosha type.

No = 0
In between = 3
Yes = 6

pitta

You have a medium build and strength.

You have red, blond or light-brown hair.

Your skin is fair or ruddy.

You have freckles or get them easily in the sun.

You get sharp hunger pangs and cannot skip meals.

You get thirsty easily.

You can feel quite uncomfortable in hot weather.

You like to avoid the sun.

You tend to perspire easily.

Hot and spicy foods do not appeal to you.

You quite like cold foods and cool refreshing drinks.

You have a strong appetite and can eat a lot at one time.

You tend to regular bowel movements.

You see yourself as quite efficient.

You are very precise and orderly.

You have a tendency to be quite a perfectionist.

You can be quite strong-minded and forceful in your manner.

You can lose your temper easily.

You tend to be impatient or easily irritable.

You are usually too hot rather than too cold.

You are considered stubborn by the people who know you well.

You can be very determined when you want something.

You are quite critical of yourself and of other people.

kapha

You are well built, with a large, solid body.

You tend to gain weight easily.

You lose weight slowly.

You have good stamina with a steady level of energy.

You are a slow eater.

You can feel heavy after eating, especially after heavy foods.

You have a slow digestion.

You store fat easily and have a tendency to a full plump body.

You are slow and deliberate in your movements.

You are naturally calm.

You are not quick-tempered and your feathers are not easily ruffled.

You have an easygoing, placid disposition.

You need at least eight hours of sleep a night.

You tend to oversleep and are slow to get going in the morning.

You are a very deep sleeper.

You are naturally relaxed and cannot be rushed easily.

You are a slow learner but once you learn something you really retain it.

You have a good memory.

You are quite methodical in your approach to learning.

You are quite methodical in your actions.

You don't like damp cold weather.

You have a tendency to sinus problems, excess mucus and chronic congestion.

Since there are broad similarities between the somatotype and the Ayurvedic types, we have decided to use the Ayurvedic system to provide you with a quick guide to help you find information appropriate to your body type in various parts of the book. So, once you have established which Ayurvedic type(s) you are, you can go to the coloured boxes appropriate to your type(s), say, the Kapha box in the Healthy Eating chapter on page 49 to find broad guidelines on diet.

vata

You have quite a thin build.

You don't gain weight easily.

Your hands and feet tend to be cold.

Your skin can be very dry, particularly in winter.

Your eating habits are irregular.

Your sleeping habits are not very regular.

You often have difficulty falling asleep, and then sleep lightly.

You have a very active mind.

You have a restless mind with a good imagination.

You learn quickly but can forget quite quickly.

Your movements can be very quick.

You tend to walk very quickly.

You worry easily and frequently become anxious.

You can find it difficult to make decisions.

You speak quickly.

Friends consider you talkative.

You are easily excited.

You are very active and your energy comes in bursts.

You have a tendency to wind and constipation.

You are quite an emotional person and your moods change easily.

You are usually enthusiastic and positive.

You are most uncomfortable in cold weather.

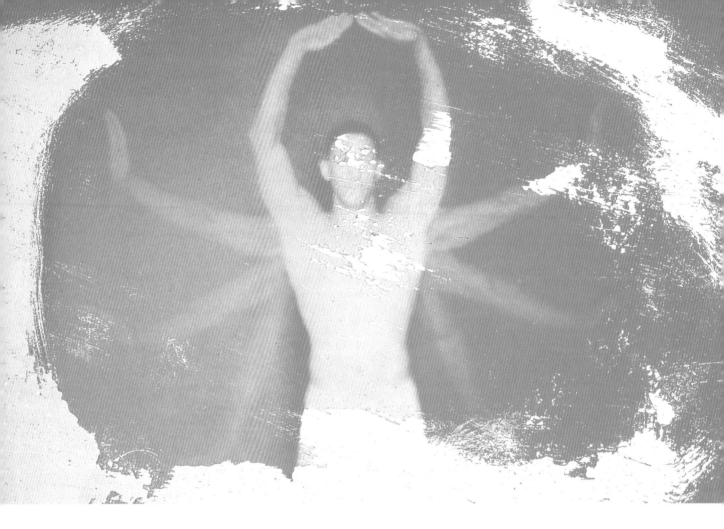

body basics

Of all our bodily functions, breathing is possibly the one we take most for granted. Without thinking about it, every moment of the day we are either breathing in oxygen-rich air and, hopefully, breathing out wastes and toxins in the form of carbon dioxide. We are mostly quite unconscious of this basic instinct that is so necessary to our health and well-being – indeed, to our very survival!

Most people, particularly in the West, do not breathe fully and are undermining their chances for optimum health. Your body does not function at its best when you are not actually breathing to full capacity. Your energy reserves may be lowered, and chronic fatigue, allergies, colds and many more health problems may result from habitually breathing too shallow, too fast, or too long.

breathing into being

'You can live two months without food and two weeks without water, but you can only live a few minutes without air.'

HUNG YI-HSIANG, TAOIST MASTER

The supreme importance of breathing in maintaining true well-being is increasingly recognized by health professionals and holistic practitioners alike. You might find it very surprising to discover the power of good breathing to stimulate the healing energies within the body. Paying more attention to our breathing patterns during times of physical illness or psychological stress can be completely empowering and supportive, conscious breathing and applied breathing exercises done at the right time can truly offer us help and hope during our greatest trials. For example, breathing exercises are among the most important ways in which a woman can take control over her labour and facilitate an easier, more pain-free childbirth.

Learning how to breathe properly is an important part of everyone's education. This is a long-accepted basic good health tip in many Eastern traditions, particularly those of India and China. The increasing popularity of Indian yoga in the West is largely due to the practical and clear health teachings of pranayama, the art and science of breathing, practised alongside the physical postures in yoga.

According to yoga philosophy, this subtle energy or life-force in the air is called prana. Pranayama, the art/science of breathing, is mastered by a series of breathing exercises that teach you how to be conscious of your breath. You can learn to use your breath properly in any good yoga class (see pages 168–181). Here in the West, because we are not properly taught breathing techniques, many people just develop bad habits out of ignorance combined with laziness. We breathe too fast or too shallowly and thus we retain too much stale air in our lungs, because we begin to breathe in again before we have completed breathing out.

Research into breathing by Dr Robin Monro, director of the Yoga Biomedical Trust, based at London's Royal Homoeopathic Hospital, has shown that people who are very tense and suffering from stress problems tend to breathe too shallowly, using only the upper part of the chest and not using the very important diaphragm. Such shallow breathing can lead to rapid breathing and hyperventilation, from which many stressed people may suffer and which only makes their condition worse.

To breathe correctly you must use your nose and not your mouth. The nose is designed to cleanse and warm the air before it reaches your lungs. Breathing through the mouth means an increase in the risk of infection. In correct breathing, when you breathe in, the lungs expand, the rib cage moves upward and outward and the diaphragm moves downward pushing out the lower ribs and abdomen.

Deep breathing and using the respiratory system fully is particularly difficult for women who have been conditioned to 'tuck those tummies in' since adolescence and have worn all sorts of attire like girdles, pantyhose, cinch belts and Lycra ever since.

The habit of sucking in the stomach is difficult to reverse and is responsible for a lot of collective shallow breathing. Too many people use only the upper narrow part of the lungs rather than the bottom part which has greater capacity.

Respiration begins when we breathe air through the nose and then the larynx, trachea and bronchi, which clean, moisten and warm the air to prepare it for ready absorption into the bloodstream through the lungs. Here the air is pulled into a network of expanding and contracting air sacs. This is where blood and air meet. Blood enters the lungs through an artery and flows around the air sacs in capillaries. Here oxygen is taken in and carbon dioxide expelled. The blood then carries the oxygen through the pulmonary vein to the heart, and the respiratory system carries the carbon dioxide out of the body when we exhale.

Too much carbon dioxide is toxic, but we always need to have a little amount in the body to help regulate body chemistry and the function of the internal breathing mechanism. It is when the oxygen from the air meets and mixes with the glucose in the blood that vital energy is released and circulated.

Does the respiratory system have an important part to play in preventing illness in the first place and if it does, what part does it play? Qigong (see page 183) is the Chinese equivalent of India's pranayama; it also means 'energy control' and 'breathing exercise', has been a formal branch of Chinese medicine for over 2,000 years and is regarded as a science. The Chinese believe the body's supply of vital energy is created by correct breathing and that all our vital functions, from blood pressure to hormone secretions, are regulated by our breathing and therefore the respiratory system plays the central role in our well-being and our longevity.

Asthma

It is estimated around 3 million people in the UK suffer from asthma and around 2,000 die every year from fatal attacks. Too many people, including doctors, know too little about this condition, how to prevent it and what to do in case of a serious attack.

World-wide, asthma is on the increase and no one knows why or what causes it. Some people attribute their asthma to food allergies or a natural inclination to sinus problems like hayfever. Others connect their stressful life situations or challenging environmental conditions with the source of the problem. Whatever the root cause of your asthma this condition can be considerably helped by changing your lifestyle. Positive diet and exercise changes (including some regular relaxation and breathing exercises) are sometimes all that is needed to begin to turn this problem around. Sufferers do not react to the same allergens in the same way.

Many who suffer asthma in childhood grow out of it, but some people suffer it all through their lives. They can expect at any time – and often quite out of the blue – attacks of breathlessness and wheezing. A serious attack is very frightening. What starts out as a nasty, irritated cough can escalate to the muscles in the bronchial

tubes contracting involuntarily and squeezing the tubes too tight, causing the sufferer literally to fight for breath.

You are probably under a doctor's care if you are an asthma sufferer. If you use an inhaler follow your doctor's instructions. Try to work with the health professionals in your life to make the necessary adjustments to promote more balance and well being in your life. Yoga is one of the best health programmes for helping asthma conditions naturally. There are many simple things that asthma sufferers can do to help their own condition and prevent other members of the family from developing the condition.

The following is a list of a few natural hints for preventing or coping with asthma.

- Cut down and in some cases, cut dairy and wheat products out of your diet.
- Try to stay away from the food allergens or pollens and grasses that really irritate you.
- You could be sensitive to a number of airborne allergens including dust, animal hair, mites, mould, feathers, cigarette smoke or certain perfumes or petrochemicals. Try to keep your immediate environment clear of these kind of substances.
- Use natural fibres and floors rather than lots of heavy carpets, rugs and curtains in your home.
- Keep your rooms well ventilated and your central heating on low.

Exercise is an excellent and effective way to strengthen the lungs and the entire respiratory system, and to increase confidence, which is important when fighting this condition. Breathing exercises are particularly effective – slow deep breathing is just one of many that can help. Many asthma sufferers have reported tremendous benefits from yoga therapy and from swimming, which also brilliantly exercises the lungs. Some people believe yoga therapy has played an important part in curing their condition and there are studies now in process at Dr Monro's Yoga Therapy Centre, Royal London Homoeopathic Hospital, 60 Great Ormond Street, London WC1N 3HR.

SIMPLE BREATHING EXERCISE 1

Slowly inhale and exhale through the nose. With each inhalation, bring the air down to the diaphragm, allowing the abdomen to expand with each inhalation; and contract with each exhalation, gently pulling in the abdomen.

SIMPLE BREATHING EXERCISE 2

To get in touch with the natural action of the diaphragm and abdomen in deep breathing, lie down on your back, relaxing your body, with your feet about a foot apart. Place your hands palms down on each side of your abdomen and follow your breath from your nose down through your chest to your abdomen and then back. As you inhale, allow the chest and then the abdomen to expand and as you exhale, allow the gentle contraction of first the abdomen and then the chest.

BREATHING FOR WEIGHT LOSS

Sounds too good to be true... but oxygen depletion is common among many people, particularly smokers and those in cities and polluted environments generally. Most of us shallow-breathe into the upper chest, so the cells do not receive the full replenishment of oxygen. This can hamper attempts to lose weight and affect energy levels. Try breathing fully into the lungs using the diaphragm (see above).

nurturing systems

We are consciously aware when eating that we are stimulating the digestive process but we often do not take it to the next level and contemplate how what we digest can either nurture or harm us. Being conscious that what we eat nurtures us in the same way we nurture our children, or creatures in our care, is a way of keeping in our consciousness the thought that what we eat can be either healthy or detrimental. It is a very self-empowering decision-making process that we go through many, many times every day. How conscious are we of the power we have to enhance our well-being by the simple process of awareness of what we put into our mouths?

To feed and nourish your body and mind, the food that you eat and the drinks that you drink journey through the entire digestive system before assimilation and nourishment can take place. Digestion begins in the mouth, where chewing food stimulates the production of saliva, which contains an enzyme that makes food easier to swallow, and begins to break it down into a usable and mobile material to nourish and meet the body's nutritional needs. This is why you have teeth and why chewing your food well is so important.

In simple terms, food is chewed and ground into a mush in the mouth by mixing with the saliva you produce by chewing. In the mouth, an enzyme, ptyalin, is released to begin breaking down some starches into sugar. From the throat, food passes into a narrow channel about 25 cm (10 inches) long, called the oesophagus, which carries it into the stomach.

The stomach is an amazing muscular sac that stores and breaks down the food we eat by producing some of the important enzymes required for the digestive process to move on to assimilation, nourishment and elimination. One of the most powerful digestive juices kills bacteria. Hydrochloric acid is secreted by the stomach to break down and dissolve food further, which leads to the production of other digestive enzymes, like pepsin, necessary for the digestion of protein.

You can see why the walls of the stomach are thick with a mucous lining for protection. How else could your stomach survive the daily onslaught of chemical combinations you ingest and produce? Heartburn, indigestion and eventually ulcers are the result of too much acid in the stomach. An excess of acid is the result of wrong eating and mixing of foods. Eating too much protein and mixing proteins and carbohydrates together in large quantities, for instance, place strains on the digestive system.

In order for protein to be digested, hydrochloric acid is required. However, when large quantities of carbohydrates are eaten, the stomach does not release sufficient amounts of hydrochloric acid, so that when proteins and carbohydrates are eaten at the same time a certain amount of stress is placed on the stomach and a delay in digesting protein means the meat stays in the stomach longer than is either necessary or healthy.

This is one of the big food-combining secrets. Experts around the world are finding some agreement in the art and science of food combining (see page 83). It's probably quite difficult for you to believe that egg or hamburger and chips, or steak and baked potato, don't digest well together, but that is apparently the case. It is far better to eat vegetables with your meat, not starch, and not eat too much meat. Generally food, except fruits and vegetables, remains in your stomach for 3 to 4 hours, where it mixes with the digestive enzymes and is broken down further. It takes under 2 hours to digest fruits and vegetables, while proteins, starches and fats take considerably longer. Fatty red meat, for instance can take up to 6 hours to complete its process in the stomach.

This is why fruit is considered the healthiest and easiest food on your digestive system. Because of the high water content of fruits, they also act as cleansers as well as carriers of easily absorbed nutrients. The toxins that accumulate in your body create acidity. Your body requires and retains water when there is an acid build-up and a need to neutralize your acid level. This can lead to a cycle of bloating and overweight.

On leaving the stomach, food enters the duodenum, the first part of the small intestines, where partially digested food receives digestive juices from the gallbladder and the pancreas, further preparing and breaking it down for the journey through the intestinal system, where nutrients are made absorbable. The pancreas, a gland behind the stomach, produces digestive juices and the gallbladder in the liver produces bile, along with the intestine's own secretions which are all alkaline and able to balance the stomach acids, further breaking down food into absorbable nutrients.

As food enters the small intestines, many more enzymes are produced to make it possible to absorb the nutrients into the bloodstream through capillaries that run along the surface of the small intestine. Before this can happen, proteins must transform into smaller units, such as peptides and occasionally amino acids, while carbohydrates must change into simple sugars and fats into tiny units. This is the least that is necessary for absorption to succeed.

Your small intestine is about 6 metres (20 feet) long. The intestinal walls are covered by countless tiny soft hair-like projections called villi, which separate waste materials from the nourishing protein (building blocks), sugar and fat your body needs to thrive. These protruding villi act as a filter, separating nutrients from toxins and waste. It is important to reduce the risk of blockage and damage to your villi by

COMFORT EATING

A common habit for many of us to slip into when we are upset, unhappy or stressed is to eat for comfort. This can become a serious issue for some, where eating disorders take over because emotions cannot be expressed and they are sometimes completely suffocated by their eating habits. Lesser degrees of comfort eating include stuffing on snack foods and sweet foods when troubled. To avoid this eat foods rich in serotonin, which is the feel-good factor number-one chemical. Such foods include lean meat, tofu, pumpkin and sesame seeds, and almonds. Ensure your levels of serotonin remain constant by supplementing with 5-HTP daily.

cutting out of your diet, or at least cutting down considerably, the things known to irritate the stomach and intestines. These are:

- overeating
- gluten in wheat (bread and pasta)
- excess sugar
- fried foods
- alcohol
- tea and coffee
- carbonated drinks (sodas and colas)
- strong spices
- excess salt
- any overprocessed foods, junk foods and fast foods

Excessive proteins, carbohydrates and fats the stomach and small intestines have failed to absorb may be stored in the heaviest organ of the body, the liver. This important organ is amazingly diverse and multi-talented. Perhaps because its functions are so numerous it is described in Chinese medicine as the 'minister of planning', organizing and storing nutrients for future use. The liver releases glucose into the blood and tissues, in order to meet our energy needs, and it also produces the bile stored in the gallbladder to help facilitate the digestive process in the duodenum. The liver also stores vitamins, particularly some of the B vitamins that help red blood cells mature.

One of its other most important functions is to remove toxic waste substances from the blood. This is why too much alcohol places such stress on the liver. The accumulation of toxins from too much fermentation takes its toll over time! Only drink alcohol in moderation, or not at all, if you value your liver.

Bathed in digestive juices, chewed up and churned about, food takes a four-to-eight-hours' journey through the small intestines, riding the waves of a rippling movement called peristalsis, while the villi stir up the materials, sorting nutrients out and absorbing them into the blood and lymph systems. The last phase of the digestion process takes place in the large intestine over a period of ten to twelve hours. The remainder of the food solution loses much of its water content here, sheds some more nutrients and feeds the healthy bacteria that live in the intestine, so that by the time the remnant food is ready to be excreted, most of its goodness has been removed.

Recent research concludes most ulcers are linked to the presence of a bacterium called *H (Helicabacter) Pylori* and can be treated with simple antibiotics. This has been one of the biggest breakthroughs in the understanding and treatment of ulcers in years! The same bacterium is also now being linked to early stomach cancer.

Some simple guidelines for a healthy digestive system include:

- 'Graze don't gorge' is one of the health catch-phrases of the moment. Overeating places a lot of strain on the body systems.
- Remember that the digestive system needs the right foods at the right times to function efficiently.
- Through eating a wide and varied diet, high in fresh raw fruits, vegetables and whole grains, i.e. fibre, you can prevent many of the disabling diseases that are the result of poor diet, the root of an unhealthy lifestyle.
- Consult your doctor or a nutritionist if you believe you need to make major changes in your diet or if you have any chronic condition which you believe is linked to your digestive system.

Chocolate

Just because it's so yummy and pleasurable to eat doesn't mean that chocolate isn't good for you. In fact, you're enhancing your health and well-being by eating (not too refined) chocolate regularly and in moderation.

- The cocoa bean is native to Latin America and was used by the Aztecs to treat depression and poor sex drive.
- The cocoa bean and cocoa are abundant in antioxidants called polyphenols, also found in red wine, which are believed to reduce the risk of strokes and heart disease. They have also been shown to provide protection against cancer and to slow the ageing process!
- Eat organic chocolate with at least 65–70 per cent cocoa bean and one that is low in sugar for the healthiest results. Dark chocolate is more nutritious and richer in minerals.
- Cocoa beans have been used as an aphrodisiac for centuries. They contain phenylethylamine (PEA), a natural amphetamine we release when in love and which make us feel euphoric.
- Just smelling chocolate can lift our spirits and help to protect us against disease. Smelling chocolate causes us to increase the levels of an antibody called immunoglobulin, which protects against colds and slows down brainwaves – which helps us to feel calm.
- Chocolate is a natural relaxant as it contains valeric acid.
- Because chocolate contains a stimulant, theobromine, which is a caffeine-like substance, it could help us to feel more alert. Theobromine doesn't have the damaging side-effects of caffeine.
- Chocolate may help to increase lifespan due to the antioxidants it contains. See Laughter and Chocolate on pages 206–207.

FOODS TO SOOTHE AN IRRITATED STOMACH OR INTESTINE

Oatmeal
Milk
Rice pudding
White cabbage juice
Banana
Melons
Camomile tea
Slippery elm
Aloe vera juice
Live yoghurt (necessary to eat if you are taking antibiotics to replace the healthy bacteria the antibiotics destroy along with the infection!)

CARBOHYDRATE CRAVINGS

Getting hungry at odd times of the day and night? This probably means your blood sugar level is low. Avoid this by eating regular small amounts of foods that slowly release sugar (see page 43). Ensure you also have enough vitamin B3, magnesium and chromium.

the heart

In an average lifetime, the human heart beats around 2.5 billion times, about one hundred thousand times every day, and around seventy times every minute. Our heart is the central pump within our body, the centre of a system that circulates about 7 litres (6 quarts) of blood through over 96 thousand miles of blood vessels. All the organs of the body need a continuous flow of blood to function properly. The heart's circulatory system transports oxygen and nutrients to the tissues through its supply of fresh blood and then takes away the waste and carbon dioxide.

Those 7 litres (6 quarts) of blood circulate around our body between three to five thousand times every day and are made up of over twenty-four trillion cells. Every second, seven million new blood cells are produced. By the end of an average lifetime the heart will have pumped 50 million gallons of blood around the body. The heart, a mighty machine capable of such fantastic feats, generating and sustaining our lives, is, in fact, a muscle the size of a fist and weighing less than 500 g (1 pound)!

The heart is actually a double pump, with two chambers in each pump – one sends blood around the body taking oxygen to the tissues; the other sends blood to the lungs to pick up the vital oxygen supply. The arteries and veins carry the blood and oxygen, connecting the different organs and their functions. Our heartbeat is the sound of the two ventricles contracting, and the valves between the atria and ventricles closing, sending blood to the lungs and to the tissues. The closing of the valves in the big blood vessels (leading to the lungs and the body) after each pulse of blood has rushed past them causes the second half of the heartbeat.

Heart disease is perhaps one of the greatest health challenges facing us today. The UK has one of the highest rates of heart disease in the world; every day nearly a thousand people in this country suffer a heart attack. According to the British Heart Foundation, 'A heart attack is caused by the blockage of one of the small coronary arteries that lie on the surface of the heart... While a narrowed coronary artery can cause intermittent angina pains, a totally blocked artery will cause a heart attack.'

One of the main causes of heart disease is the clogging up of the arteries with fatty deposits of cholesterol. This furring up of the arteries is usually the result of eating too much saturated fat (the kind found in meat and dairy products). Our bodies also produce cholesterol, occasionally too much – its self-regulating system being subverted by too much saturated fat in the system (see pages 40–41). In any case, adjusting our diets to reduce the amount of all fatty foods is a step in the right direction. Coronary heart disease has many causes; smoking and high blood pressure are also recognized as major risk factors.

In the early 1990s, the *British Medical Journal* reported on research from St

FOR A HEALTHY HEART, CUT DOWN ON:

Animal fat
Dairy products
Sugar
Salt
Refined (white) flour
    products
Fried foods
Alcohol
Cigarettes

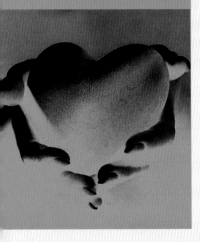

Bartholomew's hospital, London (who checked 47,000 people). By eating half a tablespoon less salt a day, one person in six could be saved from suffering heart disease and the number of people needing medication for high blood pressure would be halved. Researchers found that salt has such a powerful effect on blood pressure that 40,000 premature deaths a year could be prevented by reducing the average British salt intake! Don't forget that processed foods have a very high salt content and reducing these too could double the numbers of prevented premature deaths.

Oily fish such as salmon, herring, sardines and mackerel contain an essential fatty acid, EPA, which has the effect of thinning the blood and reducing the amount of fat in it, which considerably helps reduce the risk of heart disease. See pages 41–42.

The alarming increase of heart disease in recent decades has been proven to be linked to diet and lifestyle. Today it is obvious that degenerative diseases are related to the foods we eat, the cigarettes we smoke, the extra weight we carry and the lack of exercise in our daily lives. The reason we require tens of thousands of heart bypass operations every year in the UK alone is that we eat too much of the kind of food that clogs rather than cleanses our bodies. Eating too much animal fat adds to the build-up of fatty deposits in the walls of arteries throughout the body. These deposits dangerously block the flow of blood.

Exercise is very important in maintaining a healthy heart and preventing coronary degeneration. The heart is a muscle and, like any muscle, you must use it or lose it. It's vital to do some form of energetic exercise every day. A brisk walk, swimming or dancing all provide an excellent full body workout (see pages 129–165).

Heart health tips

- Avoid saturated fatty meats, like beef, pork and lamb; choose the leanest cuts, cutting off any excess fat. Eat more lean meats like chicken (without skin) and fish.
- Grill, steam or bake food instead of frying it. Don't add fat.
- Avoid full-fat dairy products; choose skimmed milk and a low-fat spread or a margarine that is high in polyunsaturates.
- Reduce your intake of sugar, salt, processed foods and alcohol.
- Eat one of the oily fish, like salmon, herring, sardines and mackerel, at least three times a week. Grill, bake or steam it.
- Eat foods rich in the essential fatty acid EPA (again found in oily fish like herring, sardines, salmon and mackerel and fish oils). It helps reduce the level of fat in the blood and thins the blood.
- Increase your intake of fibre-rich foods, like wholemeal bread, oats and beans.
- Dramatically cut down on biscuits, cakes, crisps and all confectionery.
- Eat more fresh vegetables and fruit on a daily basis.
- Take more regular exercise.

FOODS TO REDUCE CHOLESTEROL THAT SHOULD BE INCLUDED IN YOUR DAILY DIET:

Avocados
Olive oil
Oatmeal
Garlic and onions
Oily fish, sardines,
   salmon, mackerel
Dark green and orange
   vegetables
Sunflower seeds

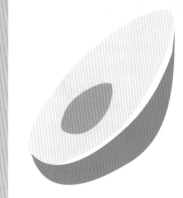

- Give up smoking! Smoking a packet of cigarettes a day gives you twice the risk of heart disease and five times the risk of a stroke.
- Reduce your stress levels – learn how to relax! Excessive stress increases the risk of high blood pressure and stroke.

Heart disease

Every year there are around 170,000 deaths attributed to arterial disease, where the arteries become blocked by the build-up of fatty deposits, a dangerous plaque that causes circulatory problems and heart conditions in one in four adults over the age of 45!

For people in the high-risk category there is a natural, non-surgical treatment that is safe and effective, chelation therapy. Patients are placed on a drip of vitamins, minerals and amino acids in therapeutic doses, often over a number of weeks. This treatment improves the condition of the heart, arteries and circulatory system in eight out of ten patients. This is mainly a private treatment, but some health authorities are looking at it because it is so much cheaper than surgery.

Some people are naturally at risk because of hereditary factors, but most people exacerbate their potential for heart disease by unhealthy habits and lifestyle. A diet high in saturated fats, alcohol, salt and sugar, and low in vegetables and fruits, will definitely increase your chances of developing heart disease. The simple lifestyle changes you could make to reduce your risk of heart disease considerably are:

1 Reduce your intake of alcohol or give it up altogether.
2 Stop smoking.
3 Eat a healthy diet.
4 Exercise regularly.
5 Lose weight if you are overweight.

12 aids for keeping your heart healthy

The following 12 nutrients, either obtained from foods or taken as supplements, will help reduce your risk of getting coronary heart disease or dangerously high cholesterol and, for those already suffering, the following can be beneficial in conjunction with their current treatment.

1 Omega-3 and -6 fats Eating three portions of oily fish per week is recommended to obtain the required levels of omega-3 and -6 fatty acids. Those with a heart condition should ensure they do get three portions a week, others can exist on slightly less. The best sources are sardines, pilchards, herring, mackerel, salmon, trout, anchovies, kippers and fresh tuna. Linseeds (flax seeds) and their oils are also good. See pages 41–42.

2 Vitamins A, C, E These three highly beneficial antioxidant vitamins all have the ability to prevent deposits sticking to artery walls, including fats, and can help to prevent damage to the arterial lining caused by free radicals. Best sources of A are fish oil, egg yolk, liver; C is richest in citrus fruits, kiwis, strawberries, red peppers, peas; E in avocados, chickpeas, almonds, tuna, sunflower oil and muesli. See more on pages 94–98.

3 Selenium This is a valuable antioxidant mineral which works with vitamin E to produce the prostaglandins which are needed for normal growth. It is found in lentils, wholemeal bread, sardines and Brazil nuts (see page 104).

4 Allicin Information provided by the British Heart Foundation states that allicin, which is found most abundantly in garlic and also to a lesser degree in onions and leeks, may help in preventing blood clots from forming in coronary arteries and it is known to have blood-thinning properties.

5 Folic acid Folic acid helps reduce the risk of cardiovascular disease associated with levels of homocysteine in the blood. Folic acid can be found predominantly in green leafy vegetables, mushrooms, pulses, nuts, fruits and root vegetables (see page 96).

6 Co-enzyme Q10 Co-enzyme Q10 is an antioxidant and is also a vital energy-releasing component and cardiac muscle strengthener. Co-Q10 can be found in lean meat. Levels of Co-Q10 in the system lessen due to old age, stress and illness. See more on page 117.

7 Flavonoids Flavonoids inhibit the action of platelets, which are the blood cells that join to form blood clots. Flavonoids can be found in fruit and vegetables, especially apples and onions. They are antioxidants which also help the absorption and action of vitamin C.

8 Monounsaturated fatty acids These lower the levels of potentially harmful LDL cholesterol and maintain the necessary levels of beneficial HDL cholesterol (see pages 40–41). They can be found in rapeseed, walnut and groundnut oils, and avocados. Olive oil is another useful source and extra-virgin olive oil also contains protective antioxidants. See more on page 40.

9 Vitamin B6 This vitamin is essential for the production of healthy blood. B6 can be found in fish, pulses, nuts, chicken and potatoes (see pages 95–96).

10 Phytoestrogens These are currently under investigation as their health-giving properties seem prolific and include the ability to fight coronary heart disease. They reduce excess cholesterol, are rich in essential vitamins and minerals. They are found in soya, watermelon, onions, garlic, broccoli and even in tea.

11 Lycopene This is a carotenoid noted for its use in reducing the risk of coronary heart disease. It is fat-soluble and is therefore more efficiently absorbed when eaten with oil. It can be found in any tomato product and raw tomatoes (see page 55).

12 Beta-carotene This is another carotenoid which makes fruit brightly coloured. It helps to prevent the build-up of toxins in the arteries as well as having many other health-giving properties. It is found in spinach, tomatoes, cabbage, broccoli, peas, carrots and sweet potatoes (see page 94).

ASPIRIN

A report published in the *British Medical Journal* on 30th June 2000 refutes the claim that a daily aspirin helps reduce stroke. It now appears there is a risk of developing bleeding in the stomach due to the blood-thinning properties of aspirin. More research is needed in this area, but it seems those most likely to be prescribed aspirin, that is those with high blood pressure, are the ones most at risk of stomach bleeding. Even in low doses, bleeding occurred in people with high blood pressure. It can be a more effective prescription for those with low blood pressure, but the risks could still outweigh the benefits and therefore other ways should be found of reducing blood pressure in those with high blood pressure.

the holistic back

BEATING BACK PAIN

- **Think muscle! It is more likely to be muscle than spinal problems that cause your back pain. Exercises that strengthen muscles should be done regularly.**
- **Healthy eating helps to remove toxins from your system that may otherwise cause harm to your spine.**
- **Learn relaxation techniques that will help you to combat stress.**
- **Improve your posture. Learn techniques and retrain yourself to eradicate bad habits.**
- **Learn to breathe correctly to increase the levels of oxygen being taken into your system. Not only will this help in de-stressing generally, it will aid in the elimination of toxins from your system, also combating stress.**

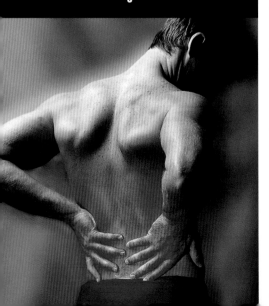

Research in 1998 revealed that 16 million people in the UK, i.e. 40 per cent of adults, experienced back pain which continued for more than one day. For 8 million people, that pain lasted more than four weeks and 2.5 million people suffered back pain every day of the year. It therefore makes sense to ensure you do not join the unhappy throng of sufferers by treating your back respectfully and ensuring you maintain strength and suppleness throughout life.

Back problems can affect anyone. One in three 16–24-year-olds had back pain last year. It is most common in middle age, nearly half of people between 45 and 64 experienced some back pain. Young people usually experience short acute back pain and older people chronic pain. One in four people over 65 had back pain for the whole year.

Manual workers are at higher risk than white collar workers. Occupations that can cause back pain without involving injury are: driving, driving a train, work involving intensive use of telephones without headsets (a survey of London office workers showed half using a phone and a computer for at least two hours a day report neck pain and 31 per cent report lower back pain), supermarket cashiers (57 per cent experience lower back pain in a year).

Back pain is rarely 'cured' by surgery or treatment of the spine itself. Dr Art Brownstein, in his book *Healing Back Pain Naturally*, suggests most back pain is caused by problems in the muscles. When the back muscles are in a state of imbalance, they may be tense, tight, weak, untoned and therefore unable to support the spine. The back muscles, as they influence almost every major muscle group in the body, can cause a knock-on effect of pain through the body when injured, and this can create dramatic problems throughout the body – not just in the back. There may be other causes of back pain – structural injury because of accidents or habitual poor posture, for example, but it is the muscles that transmit pain messages to the brain as they are directly connected to nerves.

Many do not recognize how damaging stress and tension can be to the back. Tension will cause muscles to stiffen. Even if undergoing treatment for injuries sustained to the back, if you are emotionally distraught and tense, the back will not heal. Healing just cannot take place in tight muscles. If you have had a diagnosis of pinched nerves, disc problems or any other condition, you can be sure, according to Dr Brownstein, that the problem began in the muscles and not in the spinal column.

The only way to a back-problem-free existence is to reclaim full use and mobility of the back by ensuring the muscles are toned and healthy, and that you do not suffer from excessive stresses. Shutting out the powerful message of pain by using pain killers and relievers denies you the wisdom of the message. Ways to release endorphins and encephalins, which are the body's natural painkillers, include exercise, laughter, deep relaxation and stress management techniques. Learn stretching techniques that work the back muscles and learn how to relax them with breathing exercises and exercise generally.

Stretching is a very important and powerful way of relieving muscular pain. The muscles can be retrained to be resilient and elastic and loose, as they should be. Stretching is probably the single most important physical activity you can do to ensure that your back will be healthy for years to come. When you stretch, you release stored-up tension in your muscles, releasing knots, tightness, spasms and pain.

Any negative, angry, distressing thoughts you have travel via powerful electrical impulses through the nerves to every part of your body including the muscles of the back. Learn ways of relaxing that are powerful enough to really induce a feeling of peace that is long-term. Practice makes perfect, and retraining will take time and patience. However the effects of stretching, stress management and deep breathing will be felt immediately. With practice and retraining of the muscles they will 'learn' to remain relaxed and not tighten or tense up unnaturally, even if this has been habitual for many years. You only need practise the techniques for a few moments each day really to help your back and your whole body/mind for that matter.

Diet is also very important in keeping your back healthy. Generally a well-balanced and healthy diet is vital. Other parts of the body must be well maintained, too, in order to take stress out of the back. If the leg muscles are weak this will place stress on the back when walking, for example. Walking, jogging and cycling are all simple exercises that develop general muscular strength in the legs.

Abdominal muscles are essential as the abdomen holds up the body and so supports the back. Doing sit-ups is a good way to build strength in these muscles. Start low, just doing 5 a day, and don't do fast jerky repetitions. Always keep movements slow as this will enhance the action of the abdominal muscles. Build to no more than 50 per day. Crunches place less stress on the back and are done with bent knees, so would be advisable if there are back problems.

NATURAL REMEDIES FOR THE BACK

- **Vitamin C helps to repair damaged tissue. Adults can take between 2 and 4 g daily.**
- **Cramp bark in tea, capsule or tablet form acts as antispasmodic and muscle relaxant so is helpful for a back that is knotted up and painful. Take 2 to 3 times a day.**
- **Bromelain, an enzyme found in pineapples, can help ameliorate inflammation in the back.**
- **Valerian in the form of tea, capsule or tablet, with its muscle-relaxant and natural tranquillizing properties, acts as a natural pain killer and can aid restful sleep.**
- **Camomile in tea, capsule or tablet form helps to calm the mind, acts as a tranquillizer and is mildly relaxant to the muscles. In cases where insomnia is a result of back pain, camomile tea, for example, should be drunk about one hour before bed to aid restful sleep.**
- **St John's wort in capsules, tablets, as dried bulk for teas and as an extract is notably useful for treating mild depression and SAD, and is also valuable in the treatment of chronic pain. It is not to be taken by anyone on prescription antidepressants.**
- **Other vitamins and minerals that can help include: boron, selenium and vitamin B complex, which helps to build strong bones; vitamin E also helps repair damaged tissue.**

bones of the matter

Osteoporosis is a common medical condition linked to the ageing process, where the level of bone density begins to fall as the rate of bone loss accelerates. Osteoporosis is a thinning of the bones, making them more fragile and vulnerable to breaks and fractures. More women develop this degenerative, depressing condition earlier than men: almost one in three women will suffer. An even more alarming statistic reported by Dr Margaret Rees in the UK magazine, *Medicine & You*, shows 'that more women die from hip fracture than from cancers of the cervix, womb and breast combined'.

Unless you take steps to prevent this debilitating and life-threatening condition, osteoporosis could gradually affect you. Women become much more vulnerable to bone loss after the menopause because the ovaries are no longer producing the hormones that help your body maintain the balance of bone loss with new bone formation.

All through life your bones replace lost bone with new bone formation, although unfortunately this process does slow down as we age. There are two main types of cells in your bone: osteoblasts, which make new bone, and osteoclasts, which eat away areas of old bone. When their activity is equal and balanced, you are in the healthy state of homeostasis; when all your nutrients, hormones, enzymes, pH factor and other elements in parts of your body's internal balance get upset, the osteoclasts become relatively more active so more bone is lost than is replaced. Sometimes intense bone loss is the result of a sedentary lifestyle or immobility, which will greatly accelerate bone loss at any age in either sex. So exercise, particularly weight-bearing exercise, is also important in maintaining this state of homeostasis or balance.

How to prevent osteoporosis

1   It is vital to ensure you eat good-quality fresh produce every day, concentrating on fruit and vegetables as the main components of your diet. Your vitamin and mineral balance is essential in preventing osteoporosis. For instance, it is not only your bones that need calcium, so does your blood. If you have too little calcium in your body, your blood takes it from your bones to keep its levels normal.

2   Maintaining or increasing bone density is encouraged by a regular weight-bearing exercise programme. Exercise helps keep the bones strong and improves tone. Weight-bearing exercises are essential for building strong bones and to improve tone, strength, flexibility, stability and balance in the musculature.

SQUATTING

Squatting is excellent for the pelvic, sacral and lower spine, and also for strengthening your leg and hip muscles. This is a natural pose to adopt and is one that many Eastern cultures can attain with ease. Children find squatting effortless and easy. Anthropologically, when we gathered from the land we may have worked in this pose. Birthing in some countries is undertaken in squat pose.

This gives your skeleton the best and strongest support, while helping to prevent the falls which can lead to more serious bone problems if osteoporosis does start to develop. We have to look at the loss of normal everyday exercise over the last 50 years, as cars and home entertainment have taken over.

3   Reduce the stress and anxiety in your life! When you are stressed or distressed your adrenal glands produce adrenaline, the fight-or-flight hormone. Too much stress stimulates too much adrenaline, which can be a disaster for your skeletal system, as adrenaline is capable of dissolving bone! Give up or reduce your intake of coffee as it stimulates the adrenal glands to secrete adrenaline. Also, stress increases the need for magnesium and vitamin C, both of which are needed for good bone structure.

4   Avoid fast foods and drugs that upset the body's chemistry and natural state of balance. Refined processed foods, coffee, tea, colas, sugar, salt, alcohol, antacids and drugs all upset the delicate balance in the body which will affect your body's ability to absorb and use the nutrients it needs when it needs them.

5   Osteoporosis is known to occur more frequently in very thin women. Be careful not to over-diet or to lose too much bulk. At the menopause, fuller-figured women have more oestrogen in their systems as the natural steroids in fat also produce oestrogen – so even though the ovaries may stop, a fatter body keeps the oestrogen flowing much longer.

6   Keep your endocrine system in healthy balance as much as you can. The parathyroid gland naturally produces a hormone called calcitonin, which plays an important role in normal bone function by slowing down the cells that eat away at old bone. Salmon is a good food source for stimulating calcitonin levels.

Dr Nancy Appleton, in her book *Healthy Bones,* places the endocrine system balance high on the list of preventative approaches to osteoporosis. She writes, 'The endocrine glands, which are scattered throughout the body, secrete hormones into the bloodstream and help regulate the body chemistry. Each of these glands – the adrenals, pancreas, thyroid, parathyroid, pituitary and gonads – plays an important part in maintaining homeostasis. Whenever we upset our body chemistries, a chain reaction occurs among these guardians of homeostasis. As they try to bring balance back to the bloodstream they often pull calcium and other minerals from the bones. When this happens repeatedly over years of upset bone chemistry, osteoporosis is a likely result.' Good bone formation in puberty is crucial for bone health in later life.

the endocrine system

One of the newer branches of physiology, endocrinology was developed in the last century. The endocrine system is a system of glands that secrete hormones, chemical messengers, directly into the bloodstream; these travel around the body stimulating specific and separate effects. In 1905 an English physiologist, E. H. Starling, coined the word 'hormone', derived from the Greek 'to excite', to describe these minute and mighty messengers that govern all the important functions in the body.

The endocrine glands are associated with the brain and central nervous system, as well as the circulatory, digestive and reproductive systems. Their subtle effect is so powerful that they actually govern the nature and efficiency of our entire body chemistry. They are the main chemical regulators of the body's metabolism. The healthy functioning of the endocrine system is vital to the body's health and well-being.

The connection between brain and body is increasingly recognized in orthodox medical circles. Researchers are studying the relationship of mind and body in a new science that looks at the interaction between psychology and the central nervous, immune and endocrine (hormone) systems. Medical science is discovering that the human brain is not just the seat of consciousness but also a gland, perhaps the most prolific gland in the human body. 'Secreted by the brain, the immune system and the nerve cells, are neuropeptides – hormones that act as chemical messengers – carrying emotions from the mind to the body and back again. They create an intricate and elaborate two-way communication system that links the emotions with all areas of the body.' according to Debbie Shapiro in her book *Your Body Speaks Your Mind*.

To get a general 'overview' reading of the efficiency of your glandular system and body chemistry check out your blood sugar levels and the calcium-phosphorus ratio. Your blood sugar level should be 100 milligrams of blood sugar per 100 cubic centimetres of blood. Blood sugar levels affect the level of calcium-phosphorus in the blood. You may not also realize that your blood cholesterol level is more closely linked to your glandular activity than your diet.

Hormones can determine whether your body is functioning properly or not, and should be considered when searching out root causes for serious imbalances. Endocrine secretions are so powerful that only a minute amount may be required at any one time. Hormone therapy is highly individual and must be undertaken with an expert's guidance.

THE GLANDS

- **BUILD-UP GLANDS**
  Islets of Langerhans of the pancreas
  Posterior pituitary
  Parathyroid and
  Adrenal cortex
  Ovaries

- **BREAK-DOWN GLANDS**
  Thyroid
  Anterior pituitary
  Adrenal medulla
  Testes

These two sets of glands balance each other out when functioning in a healthy state. Experts believe the root cause of many, possibly most, degenerative diseases is persistent imbalance in the glandular system. To look at possible glandular imbalances, consult your doctor and request extensive blood analysis, blood pressure readings and urine tests.

the immune system

Do you ever wonder why some people never catch infections even though they are exposed again and again, while others seem prone to catching every single one? It all comes down to the immune system. The body's self-protection system is essential for fighting invading bacteria, viruses and any other foreign substances that could prove destructive. We are constantly exposed to millions of bacteria, but very few lead to infection. Without a healthily functioning immune system you simply couldn't survive.

The immune system is totally bound up in the lymph and the lymphatic system. The body's cells are surrounded by a fluid, lymph, that slowly moves through a network of tubes covering much of the body, which makes up the lymphatic system. In the course of blood circulation, the pressure causes excess fluid naturally to leak through the blood vessels and capillaries. This lymph fluid contains plasma (the basic carrier stuff of blood), white blood cells, water and protein. The lymphatic system drains the excess of this escaping fluid, picking out bacteria and other nasties.

The lymphatic system is a second circulatory system and almost as extensive. Its first function is to catch the escaping lymph and return it through the thoracic duct in the chest to the circulatory system. Its second and hugely important function is to manufacture white blood cells, which move easily between the two systems and are your body's first line of defence against invading germs. The lymph nodes, located in the neck, armpits, chest, groin and pelvic area, make the white blood cells that destroy bacteria. The lymph nodes act like filters, sorting out the foreign invaders, as well as factories producing our natural weapon against disease. The tonsils and adenoids are large lymph nodes. White blood cells are the army within. Also made in the spleen and in the bone marrow, they organize and mount your resistance to infection and therefore play a vital role in keeping you fit and well. Those immune cells destined to become the highly important invader-killing T-cells are carried to the thymus gland, located close to the heart, where they mature.

Not having a pump like the heart, lymph fluid moves more slowly and is greatly helped along by muscular movement throughout your body. This is yet another good reason to exercise and to explore various natural therapies, like aromatherapy, which have an excellent effect on your lymphatic/immune system.

It's interesting to consider the body/mind relationship here. There is growing evidence of a link between the immune system and emotional state. Studies show how deep grief can dramatically reduce the immune system, as can other extreme emotional trauma, stress or crises. On the other side of the coin, laughter has been found to boost immune function considerably, so get your sense of humour in shape if you are going to achieve optimum health and keep it! See Laughter and Chocolate, page 206.

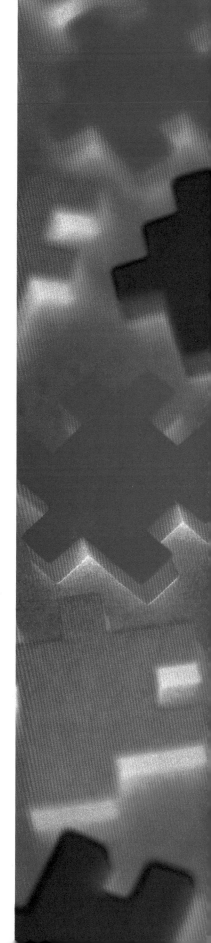

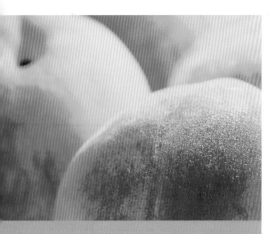

skin

The skin is such an incredible organ of the body. As well as serving to protect us and help regulate our fluid levels and temperature, it also breathes in air and excretes unwanted material. The skin is covered in tiny pores that open and close to allow such processes to take place, as well as nerve endings that carry the direct messages about the joys and pains of the outer world inside to our internal one. The skin is the conduit of delicious sensual sensations that promote all sorts of feel-good actions in our mind and our body.

Skin consists of layers. The outer layer that you can see – the epidermis – itself has different layers: the top, horny level sheds dead cells that constantly flake and fall off; the bottom basal level produces new cells that push upwards as they divide, moving toward the skin's surface. If this layer of skin gets damaged it will heal without scarring. The inner layer, or dermis, is rich in blood vessels, sweat glands, nerves, elastic fibres and layers of collagen, which provide support, keeping the skin firm and supple.

The body breathes not only through the nose, mouth and lungs, the respiratory system, but also through the skin. The skin is covered in countless tiny pores which take in from the atmosphere around and eliminate anything not wanted. If the pores are clogged with creams that do not allow the skin to breathe, then the natural shedding process can be inhibited. Dead skin cells will then build up on the top layer and the skin will become dull and lifeless.

Notice the silky smoothness of a baby's skin. Over time, your skin is bound to suffer some of the effects of stress and the pressures of environmental pollution, cigarette smoke, too much alcohol, sweets and other 'junk food', lack of exercise or sleep or just plain tender loving care. To minimize time's wear and tear on your skin there are a few simple rules to follow.

1   Keep your skin clean. Make skin cleansing a regular part of your morning and evening health rituals. Not easily seen by the naked eye, your skin easily accumulates dirt, grime, old make-up, sweat, dead cells and oil, which will lead to a bacteria build-up and developing skin problems. A clean skin is not a good host to poor skin conditions.

SKIN FACTS

- Our skin covers up to 2 square metres (21 square feet) and weighs up to 3.2 kg (7 lb).

- One square centimetre of skin has about 100 sweat glands, 10 hairs, 15 sebaceous glands and 1 metre (3 feet) of blood vessels.

- Each day we get rid of about 4 per cent of our entire complement of skin cells.

- The thickness of our skin varies in different parts of the body. On the palms and soles it could be more than 4 mm (⅙ inch) thick and on the face only about 0.1 mm.

- Skin reflects health habits. Clear healthy skin indicates a healthy lifestyle. Sallow, dull skin indicates lack of self-care and an unhealthy lifestyle.

2 Protect and nourish your skin with regular application of moisturizing cream. To help conserve the skin's own natural moisture, it is essential to moisturize your skin regularly. Daily lubrication will help protect your skin against bad weather, environmental hazards, prevent the deterioration of the skin's layers and help keep it soft and smooth.

3 Gentle exfoliation about once a week can help to alleviate a build-up of dead skin cells. Pimpling and spotting can often be attributed to dead skin cell build-up. Notice how weekly full-body exfoliation can help to alleviate this and give you a smoother, clearer and unblemished skin. It also has great health-giving benefits in that the skin is free and can breathe.

4 Try to buy body products, bath and shower products, and skin creams that are natural and not burdened with chemicals. Not only will you be helping your skin and your whole self, you will also be doing something towards helping the environment in which we live. Everything that you flush away down the sink goes towards potentially damaging the environment. Your skin deserves the best, and natural products will help keep you looking and feeling healthier.

Using deodorants

Antiperspirants and deodorants, although seemingly essential in our society are potentially damaging to the body. As the armpits are full of lymph nodes, it is important to keep them clean and clear of chemicals. The chemicals and alcohol used in many deodorizing products travel directly into the blood system through the lymph nodes and capillaries in the armpits. The fact that some also inhibit sweating makes them doubly harmful, as sweating is an essential part of the elimination process. Sweating is the body's way of keeping cool in the heat, and of eliminating toxins; when sweating is suppressed, toxins remain in the body and travel back into the system through the lymph and blood stream.

Try using mineral deodorant stones instead. These do not inhibit sweating, last for six months and are thus much cheaper. Check your diet. If you are 'smelly', you are probably eating a diet rich in unhealthy fast foods, drinking too much alcohol, stressed, or even possibly ill. Toxins need to come out. Try switching a coffee or two a day for just plain water. Soon you will find you are less smelly and need deodorizing less! Eating healthy food also helps in general elimination of toxins, as well as keeping you healthy.

HEALTHY SKIN GUIDELINES

- The number one tip is never to go out without sunscreen. Even winter sun in the Northern hemisphere can be damaging to the skin, not just those hot days of summer spent on beaches. Use creams with UVB and UVA protection at all times.

- Cleanse thoroughly but not excessively. Over-cleansing can remove natural oils from the skin that are essential to keep it looking and feeling fresh, and can also lead to premature ageing.

- Read the labels on products. Different areas of your face and neck and body have different needs. The skin around the eyes, for example, is much thinner than that on the cheeks and also has no oil glands. So it may be wise to use different lotions in different areas.

- Avoid products that are heavily perfumed, riddled with chemicals or contain a lot of alcohol. Try always to use the most natural products you can find. For example, using products with high-quality pure essential oils will work much more favourably for your skin than heavily perfumed alternatives. Take time to seek out what feels right for you.

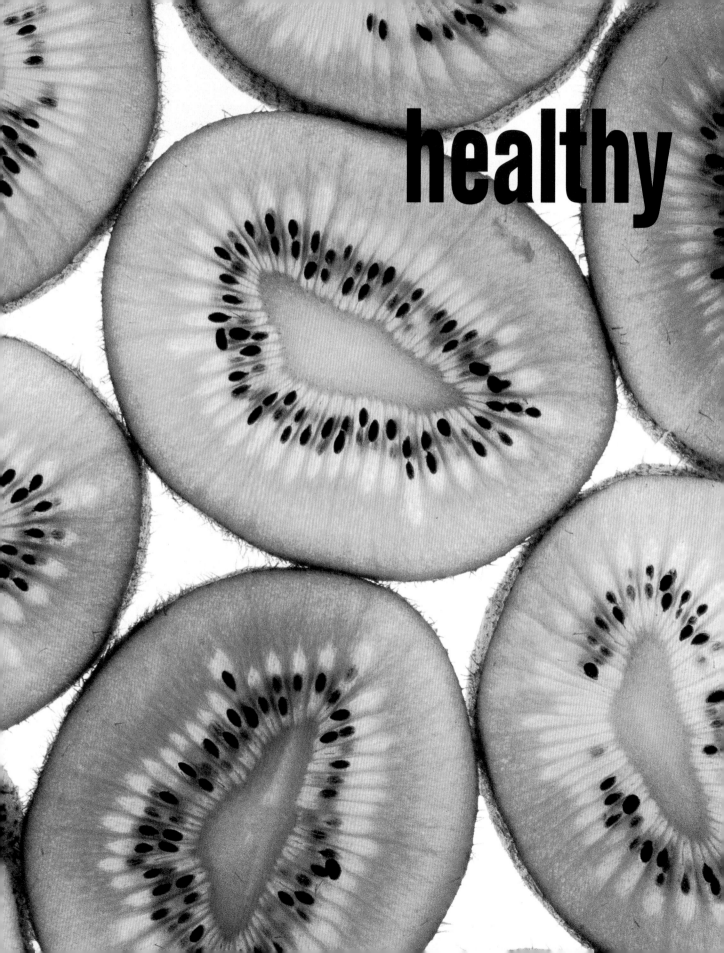

healthy

eating

As well as being one of life's greatest pleasures, eating well is the most important contribution that we can make to our ongoing health and well-being. It's easy to take our eating habits for granted; our tastes have been with us for a long time. At some point, though, it dawns on most of us that our chosen diet and lifestyle hold the key to the state of our body and our mind. We need to realize that the front line in the battle for the health of our whole being lies in our diet – in what we choose to put in our bodies and, just as importantly, what we choose *not* to eat or drink.

Most people would agree a well body is one that is free of serious imbalances, excesses, toxins and dysfunction, and certainly free from degenerative disease. To reach a level of whole health and well-being you need simply to realize that you have the ability to achieve a balanced body and mind, by reviewing your dietary habits and lifestyle honestly and implementing a few simple changes to redress the balance.

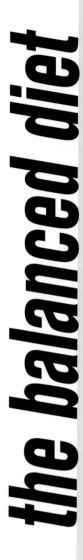

laying the foundation

Medical and nutritional experts around the world are more or less in agreement on what constitutes a healthy balanced diet. The consensus is that we should eat more fresh fruits and vegetables, more whole-grain bread, pasta and cereals, more lean meat and fish, and less red meat and fatty foods, less refined flour and sugar products like cakes and biscuits, less white bread, junk foods, salt, carbonated drinks and alcohol. All the nutrients you need are to be found in a balanced diet like this.

OUR BODIES' BASIC NEEDS:

Carbohydrates

These provide energy and other nutrients. There are two kinds: simple carbohydrates, which are sugars, and complex carbohydrates, which are the starchy foods like vegetables and grains. Although sugars are an excellent source of quick energy, it is far healthier to get most of our energy from complex carbohydrates, as they have few health drawbacks and come in forms that bring lots of other nutrients and benefits.

Fats

These are another good source of energy and fat-soluble vitamins A, D, E and K (see pages 94–8). Some fat in the body is essential for maintaining body heat, protecting vital organs and providing cell wall structure. See The Fat Crisis overleaf for much more.

Proteins

Necessary for the growth, maintenance and repair of body tissue, proteins help the building of cells, hormones and enzymes by providing the amino acids that are the 'building blocks' of life. Among meat-eaters and lacto-vegetarians, most proteins in the diet come from animal products, but vegetables contain adequate proteins too. However, most vegetable proteins don't contain a full complement of the essential amino acids the body needs. (Only one food contains all eight essential amino acids, the egg.) In a good balanced diet, rich in a wide variety of vegetables and whole grains, this is not a problem though, as each type of food contains a different range of amino acids and these complement each other.

Proteins are also an important energy source, but your body may not need as much as you think. Too much can create a toxic reaction in the digestive system and the body as a whole; over time, this can cause havoc. More and more serious illnesses may be linked to consuming too much meat – particularly red meat.

Fibre

As well as providing the bulk that facilitates the passage of foods through the system, fibre in sufficient quantities may also help prevent several intestinal problems, including bowel cancer. Derived from plant cell walls, fibre is classified as 'insoluble fibre', which is cellulose, and 'soluble fibre', mainly pectin, which is important in helping reduce blood cholesterol levels and stabilizing blood sugar. A diet rich in fruit, vegetables and grains will ensure you get adequate fibre.

Vitamins and minerals

These are the substances, required in fairly small amounts (apart from the bone- and tooth-building minerals such as calcium), that are essential for the body's processes to function correctly. For a full discussion, see pages 91–105.

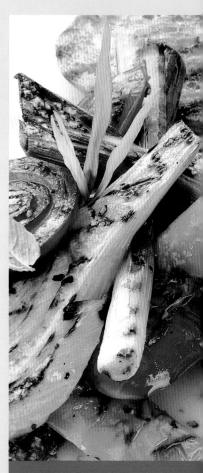

THE IDEAL BALANCE OF NUTRIENTS IN THE DIET

Nutritionists recommend that we get a minimum of 60 per cent of our calories from carbohydrates, up to 10 per cent from proteins and a maximum of 30 per cent in the form of fat.

Perhaps because of its obvious correlation with body weight, the one message about healthy diet that seems to have got into the public consciousness is that high fat intake is bad. Unfortunately, all too often it has produced a general fear of fat that is not only unnecessary but dangerous. There are several different types of fat and only two are really harmful, while others are not simply highly beneficial in moderate quantities, but essential for our well-being.

THE DIFFERENT TYPES OF FAT

All the fats and oils we eat are a combination of what are termed 'saturated' and 'unsaturated' fats. The fat in most foods is a mix, but usually either saturates or unsaturates predominate.

Saturated fats

These are the fats that naturally go hard when left at room temperature. Most animal fats, including those in poultry and dairy products, are predominantly saturated. Saturates are implicated in high blood cholesterol levels, the furring of the arteries and coronary heart disease. They are, therefore, considered the type of fat you need to keep in check and even reduce in your diet.

Unsaturated fats

These are generally the fats that are naturally liquid at room temperature. The oils from vegetables, nuts and seeds are predominantly unsaturated. Unsaturated fats have the effect of reducing the bad (LDL) cholesterol in the blood (see below).

There are two main categories of unsaturated fats: monounsaturated fats, at their highest in olive, groundnut and rapeseed oils; and polyunsaturated fats, at their highest in corn, sunflower, safflower and fish oils. Monounsaturates seem doubly healthy in that not only do they help reduce bad cholesterol but they can help maintain or even boost levels of good (HDL) cholesterol.

Cholesterol

This white crystalline organic compound is found in most animal and vegetable tissue and is essential for many metabolic functions. The body makes its own cholesterol and normally regulates levels in the blood, no matter how much we consume. It has been established, however, that when the diet is high in both damaged cholesterol and saturated fats, then blood cholesterol levels rise.

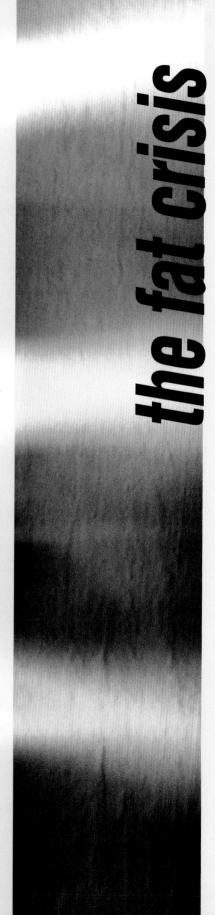

the fat crisis

Cholesterol is a constituent of lipoproteins, which carry fats in the blood: low-density lipoprotein-cholesterol (LDL-cholesterol); in excess, forms deposits on the artery walls, leading to cardiovascular disease; on the other hand, high-density lipoprotein-cholesterol (HDL-cholesterol) acts as a scavenger, helping clean the blood of fats and cholesterol. Sex and stress hormones are made from cholesterol.

Trans fats

For decades, people all over the world have been replacing butter with margarine, believing they were making a healthier choice. Experts still maintain it is essential to keep a tight rein on the intake of saturated fatty acids to avoid the risk of heart disease, and that favouring cooking oils and spreads that are high in monounsaturates and polyunsaturates is much healthier. To complicate matters somewhat, recent research has shown that not all fats, margarines and spreads made from vegetable oils are necessarily healthier. The reason for this is the presence of trans fatty acids (often called trans fats), which consist of unsaturated fats, the normal molecular shape of which has been altered by hydrogenation, the chemical process that makes oils solid at normal room temperatures, and they are 'transformed' fats.

Many studies have demonstrated that trans fats have the same effect on blood cholesterol levels as saturated fats; they raise the level of LDL-cholesterol – the bad cholesterol – and reduce the blood levels of good cholesterol – the HDL-cholesterol. Some trans fats do actually occur naturally in dairy products, but these do not have the same potentially harmful properties as the trans fats in hydrogenated oils, and are not as potentially damaging to your health.

It is still early days and more needs to be known about trans fats before we can draw final conclusions – but the message has been serious enough to cause several brands to reduce – or aim for a reduction in – the amount of trans fats in their products. Already the Flora range has reduced its trans fat content and Vitaquell and Whole Earth Super Spread have none.

The essential fatty acids

As we have seen, there are fats that are bad for us and fats that are good for us, but some fats are actually vital for the correct functioning of our metabolism. Recent reports from Boston University Medical Centre in America claims a diet very low in fat is not good for your heart. Such diets may lack essential fatty acids (EFAs). Research indicates that those with low levels of EFAs in their blood are also deficient in HDL-cholesterol, the 'good' cholesterol that protects against heart disease (see above).

The essential fatty acids are almost all to be found in vegetable oils like olive and sunflower oils, as well as the omega-3 oils in oily fish like salmon, mackerel and

GUIDELINES ON FAT INTAKE

UK Government advice issued by COMA, the Government's Committee on Medical Aspects of Food Policy, state that we should:

- Cut the total fat in our diet to protect us from heart disease.
- Eat less saturated (animal) fats.
- Use more oils high in monounsaturated fatty acids like olive oil.
- Eat more polyunsaturated fatty acids from oily fish.
- Try to cut down on trans fats.

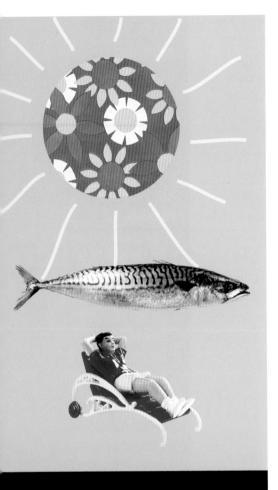

sardines. These are necessary for a healthy heart and a healthy body. Some of us today get most of the omega-6 we need from vegetable oils. However, we are nearly all deficient in omega-3, which is mainly found in oily fish and linseed (flax seed) oil.

A deficiency of omega-3 oils has been strongly implicated as a principal cause of things like heart disease, cancer, immune dysfunction and many other modern maladies. Conditions such as allergy, asthma, alcoholism, arthritis, dry skin, eczema, inflammatory conditions, learning difficulties, poor memory, schizophrenia and a great many others, all relate to fatty acid deficiencies or imbalances.

The huge change to our diet this century means that almost everyone has a deficiency of these essential nutrients or at least an unbalanced consumption of them, which can also cause chaos in our chemistry. Understanding how to correct these imbalances could be life-saving. It could also help to heal long-standing symptoms and delay the progress of degenerative disease. There is evidence that we are already lowering the collective IQ by feeding babies formulas deficient in essential fatty acids. Most breast-feeding mothers are deficient, too.

In 1992, in his book *Nutrition and Evolution*, Dr Michael Crawford, director of the Institute of Brain Chemistry at the University of North London, put forward the revolutionary theory that nutrition was the true driving force in evolution and that the development of the human brain was dependent on existence in locations with unlimited access to sea foods and fish, high in the omega fatty acids.

Dr Lesley Rhodes a consultant dermatologist at the Royal Liverpool University Hospital says: 'There is a big link between the effect of fish oil in preventing sunburn and what we suspect will prove to be its effect in helping prevent skin cancer, because the same wavelengths of light are responsible for both. What we also know is that the process which triggers sunburn and the process involved in the development of skin cancer over a period of time are the same.'

Dr Rhodes goes on to explain that sunburn is the result of tissue damage which is, in turn, part of the process that leads to skin cancer. Through trials, they discovered that tolerance to sunlight increased the more fish oils were consumed – in fact, the threshold for sunburn doubled!

FISH OILS AND SKIN CANCER

Fish oils may be as powerful a sun block as commonly used SPF creams and also may help prevent skin cancer. Eating a meal of fish rich in omega-3 fatty acids every day may boost your immunity to skin cancers and reduce the risk of sunburn through overexposure to the sun.

Everyone needs fat in their diet

Although most people may still eat too high a level of saturated fat from fatty meats, lard, etc., or too much trans fats – the kind found in most margarines and processed foods like biscuits, cakes and pastries (see page 41) – others are cutting out too much of the right kind of fats from their diet.

As well as being aware of the problems that high fat intake may produce, we must never forget that fat is essential to good health. Fat is:

- Our most important energy and heat source; the body burns off fat calories when active.
- Vital in providing a protective cushion around the vital organs and in insulating the body against heat loss. Obviously fat is even more vital in cold climates, and you need more in winter than in summer.
- A source of the fat-soluble vitamins A, D, E and K.
- Important in the diet of women to help them make the hormone oestrogen.
- A source of the essential fatty acids, linoleic acid (omega-6 oils) and alpha-linolenic acid (omega-3 oils), that are essential to your health and which help your body make other polyunsaturated fatty acids necessary to your well-being. They also help your body metabolize cholesterol.

The glycaemic index

The glycaemic index measures the effect of eating a particular food on your blood sugar levels against a pure glucose standard, which rates 100 on the index. Foods with a low glycaemic index (GI) rating are absorbed more slowly than foods with a higher rating, therefore affecting blood sugar levels less radically. You should try to include plenty of these foods in your diet because they provide long-term, sustained energy with fewer highs and lows. High-GI foods, on the other hand, provide quick-release, short-term bursts of energy, which is useful for people like athletes; for the rest of us, however, these foods should only be eaten in moderation.

The index rates only high-carbohydrate foods, because high-protein foods and fats do not have much of an effect on blood sugar. However, both types of food eaten in small amounts with a carbohydrate help to lower its GI rating, so it does help to have a little protein and fat with your carbohydrates (for instance, salad dressing or parmesan on pasta).

Some common foods and their glycaemic index:

Apple	39
Banana	62
Beans, kidney	29
Beans, lima	36
Beetroot	64
Brown rice	66
Carrot	92
Cherries	23
Chickpeas	36
Corn	59
Cornflakes	80
Glucose	100
Grapefruit	26
Grapes	45
Honey	87
Lentils	29
Milk, whole	34
Milk, skimmed	32
Orange	40
Peanuts	13
Pears	34
Peas	51
Plum	25
Porridge	49
Potato, baked	98
Potato chips	51
Raisins	64
Shredded wheat	67
Spaghetti	50
Sweet potato	51
Tomato	38
White bread	69
White rice	72
Whole-wheat bread	72
Yoghurt	36

liquid refreshment

LIQUID REFRESHMENT

Water

It is a fascinating fact that water makes up about 70–75 per cent of our body. Without this 'elixir of life' we would burn up or dry out; our very core temperature is regulated by drinking water and we couldn't survive without it. In fact, dehydration is a very serious – and potentially fatal – condition, which must be addressed immediately if it occurs.

Some people seem to function quite normally and unknowingly walk around in a state of semi-dehydration. The skin becoming dull and dry is one of the first symptoms of dehydration. Water not only helps us regulate our temperature but, just as importantly, is a powerful internal cleanser, dissolving waste material for elimination to prevent toxic build-up, and essential to the process of absorbing the nutrients we need to live.

For these reasons it is recommended that we drink at least 8 glasses of water daily. This may not be too easy for those brought up in a tea-, coffee-, juice-, cola-, beer- and alcohol-drinking culture like our own! People on high-fibre diets, especially, must drink at least the recommended minimum in order to avoid intestinal problems, particularly constipation.

As the recognition of water's vital role in our health has widened, there has been an enormous rise in concern over the level of pollutants in our water supply. This has unfortunately been matched by an increase in reports of contamination in the last decade. In the UK, this concern involves much more than the differences between hard and soft water. Chemicals have been added to our drinking water as a matter of course for various reasons, although some occur quite naturally.

Ammonia and chlorine are added to our water as disinfectants, but they can also cause skin problems. Some regional water companies also add fluoride to help prevent tooth decay, but this too is not good for your skin or bones. Pesticides get into the water system, too, via rain water in the fields moving into the rivers and streams. Some pesticides contain chemicals that mimic the action of the hormone oestrogen, and fertility researchers are linking the rise in male infertility to the increase in pesticide residues in our water. Latterly, it is also affecting female fertility by competing for oestrogen receptors.

The UK government has been taken to court several times in the last decade by environmental groups bringing attention to drinking water that doesn't measure up to European standards of quality. Government figures show that in 1990 there were occasions when over 16 million people were supplied with pesticide-contaminated water, and a further 5 million homes suffered from nitrates polluting their water.

Although millions have since been spent to clean up our tap water, and there are some real improvements, we still cannot assume our tap water is always perfectly pure and, in fact, its safety may be questionable. Is it any surprise that sales of water filters and bottled water has increased by 50 per cent every two years since the late 1980s?

Alcohol

The question of whether or not alcohol is good for you continues to spark a lot of debate in medical and non-medical circles alike. Most experts are agreed, however, that there is nothing harmful about drinking in moderation, but excessive drinking is very damaging to your health and well-being, and will dramatically affect you and your family.

Your alcohol tolerance is a very individual thing and can greatly vary depending on your age, sex and other physical and psychological considerations. Your own body and mind are your best guides as to how much you can drink. There are, though, measures you can take to prevent problems with your alcohol consumption, or more seriously, moving down the path to alcohol-related disease.

Moderate intake of red wine is reputed to be beneficial and may even protect the heart and lungs. In countries where moderate amounts of red wine are frequently drunk with meals, the incidence of heart attacks is much lower than it is in the UK, for example. One or two small glasses per day, with water to accompany the wine, would be considered a moderate amount.

Water filters generally work on the principle of passing the water through activated carbon and ion exchange resins to remove impurities such as lead, nitrates, pesticides and herbicides. Nowadays many types of water filter are available; the favourites in terms of effectivity, safety and taste appear to be the Brita Fill & Pour, Wayward Glass Cascade and Boots Aquacool Fridge Filters. Some people opt for filters that are installed directly in the plumbing of their home; these are much costlier but very convenient, and can be more effective if reverse osmosis filters are used.

Whichever filter system you may choose, be sure to follow all the manufacturer's instructions exactly or you could make the quality of your water much worse.

- Keep your filter reservoir and water container clean.
- Change the filter cartridge regularly, as per the manufacturer's instructions.
- It is safer to keep filtered water in the refrigerator, and the water will taste better. (A new design from Brita is shaped specifically to fit in fridge door shelves.)
- Continue to boil water for babies' food or drink.

If you can't find bottled water when travelling and are unsure of local water quality, always boil your water before drinking or cooking with it. Also don't assume all bottled water is clean and safe, because it may not be so. Water from a natural spring, free from pollutants and parasites, is best – but that too is not necessarily safer and certainly not subject to the same health regulations as tap water. Some spring water may contain dangerous levels of pesticides and nitrates, for instance; it depends very much on the terrain through which the water has travelled.

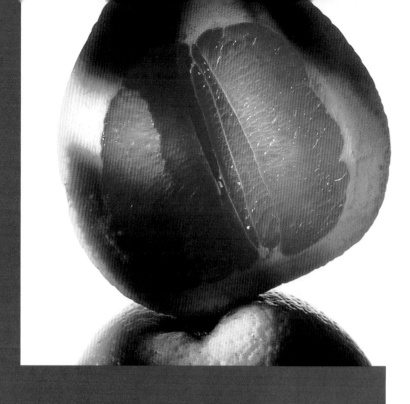

the medicine chest in your food

'Superfoods' is a recent term for some fairly everyday foods of all types that, as well as being highly nutritious, possess powerful properties for promoting well-being and helping to prevent or fight all kinds of illnesses. Most of the superfoods are common vegetables, fruits, seeds or herbs. It is the quality, quantity and regularity with which you eat the superfoods that count. A wide selection, eaten regularly, is a good way of getting all the nutritional and medicinal benefits they offer.

Almond

A very concentrated highly nutritious food, full of protein (a third more than eggs), almonds are rich in some B vitamins and minerals like potassium, zinc, calcium, magnesium and phosphorus. The body absorbs these nutrients best when eaten together with foods rich in vitamin C. Almond milk is an ancient natural remedy for respiratory and digestive problems. The soothing properties of almond oil have been widely recognized for centuries.

Apple

The power of the apple has been documented at least since biblical times. Modern-day nutritionists can only support what our great-grandmothers and the ancients already knew; an apple a day does keep the doctor away. As well as being full of antioxidant vitamin C, they are rich in pectin, which helps protect us from the ravages of pollution by binding to toxic heavy metals in the body like mercury and lead and carrying them out. This delicious, highly nutritious fruit is a natural aid to healthy digestion, and its tartaric and malic acid content helps the body cope with rich fatty foods or excessive protein. People with rheumatic pain often experience relief from their symptoms after adding apples to their daily diet.

Apricot

This small but powerful fruit is packed with beta-carotene and iron, which combat free radical activity and help fight respiratory and other infections. Some researchers claim they help in the prevention of cancer. Dried apricots are a good source of iron.

Avocado pear

This delicious and nutritious fruit is an amazing, almost complete food, rich in the antioxidant vitamins A, C and E, some B complex, potassium, a little protein, starch and monounsaturated fats. Make avocados a regular part of your diet to help lower LDL-cholesterol levels (see pages 40-41). Reputed to be good for your heart, digestion, skin and sex life; researchers have also found in avocado flesh a unique antibacterial and antifungal.

Banana

This sweet, soothing, easy-to-eat, easy-to-digest fruit has calming and restorative qualities, perhaps the reason it is one of the very earliest solid foods introduced to babies. They are a good source of potassium, which is so important to the healthy function of every cell in our body. Bananas are rich sources of many other nutrients, including vitamin B6, calcium, folate, iron and zinc, as well as being a source of the valuable fibre, pectin, which helps in the elimination of toxic wastes.

Barley

A soothing, strengthening, highly nutritious, easily digested tonic, people have been growing this grain for thousands of years – Roman gladiators ate it for strength. Relieving inflammation, constipation and diarrhoea, improving digestion, respiratory and liver function, it is reputed to help stress and fatigue and strengthen the nervous system. Rich in the B and E vitamins, calcium and potassium, barley is good for convalescents and improves brain function and mental alertness. Barley water helps to relieve a sore chest or throat and to soothe cystitis.

Basil

This very popular herb is reputed to be a natural tranquillizer, helping to calm the nervous system. Some people swear basil helps them sleep!

Beans

Beans of all types, fresh and dried as pulses, are high in fibre and protein, and low in fat. Rich in soluble fibre, they slow down the rate of digestion, reduce blood cholesterol, steady blood sugar and combat anaemia. High levels of iron and folate rival those of meat and fish, and they are rich in potassium.

Young green barley shoots and wheat grass juice are also among the new superfood stars and are used in many natural health centres for cures and fasts. They are rich in proteins, vitamins and minerals, and form the basis for many fasting programmes to cleanse and regenerate the body.

Berries

Berries, particularly blackberries and blueberries, are renowned for their high vitamin C content and antioxidant properties. Strawberries are also known as protectors against free radicals.

Beetroot

For many centuries this sweet vegetable has been known for its positive effect on the entire digestive system, but most particularly the liver. Eastern Europeans have particularly valued the healing and tonic qualities of this plant, the fresh raw juice being used there to cleanse and 'build' the blood, and to treat people recovering from serious illness by strengthening their immune system. Beetroot is best eaten raw for the full power of its healing properties.

Black cumin seed

The Prophet Mohammed said, 'Black cumin heals every disease – except death' and so it has become known as 'the medicine of the Prophet'. Containing nigellin, which stimulates digestion, it has many other qualities, including being a heart-protector and an antibacterial. Used externally, it can treat skin diseases and many allergies. It is a valuable source of the essential fatty acids.

Blackcurrant

Best known for their high vitamin C content, blackcurrants' dark-purple colour comes from flavonoids, which are known to strengthen the walls of the small blood vessels. Blackcurrants are also rich in vitamin E and carotenes, making them a valuable source of antioxidants. Also a very good source of potassium and a diuretic, their health-giving properties include helping to relieve inflammation and lowering risk of heart disease, stroke, cataracts and cancer. They are rich in anthocyanins, flavonoids which counter the common bacteria that can cause food poisoning and urinary tract infections, and their high pectin levels can help relieve diarrhoea. The seeds also contain the fatty acid, gamma-linolenic acid (GLA) used to treat the inflammation associated with rheumatism, skin conditions, eczema and psoriasis.

Brazil nut

This is one of the richest vegetable sources of the antioxidant mineral selenium, so important for fertility and hormone metabolism. It also helps the thyroid gland function.

Broccoli

Part of the crucifer family, which includes cauliflower, kale, Brussels sprouts, cabbage and radishes, this iron-rich vegetable is stocked with beta-carotene and vitamin C, antioxidants reputed to have the power to inhibit free radical activity, help prevent certain cancers and heart disease, and treat joint problems and fatigue. They are also the best source of anti-carcinogenic glucosinolates.

Brown rice

This complete food is high in fibre, which soothes, cleanses and protects the intestinal tract. It is also rich in the B vitamins which keep the nervous system healthy and in the antioxidant vitamin E. Brown rice is also a good source of methionine, needed to make enzymes that combat free radicals.

Brussels sprout

The Brussels sprout is another member of the nutritious crucifer family, rich in powerful free-radical-fighting carotenes. They also contain natural chemicals which help the liver break down the toxins that promote degenerative and age-related illnesses like Parkinson's and Alzheimer's. An excellent source of vitamin K, they are also very useful for preventing osteoporosis. Brussels sprouts are an excellent source of fibre, folate and vitamin C, and the second-best source of the anti-carcinogenic glucosinolates after broccoli.

Cabbage

A member of the brassica or crucifer family, cabbage has healing qualities that have been known for centuries. Cabbage is a tonic and disinfectant in respiratory infections, and its raw juice treats ulcers successfully. It is a notable cleanser, particularly of the liver, blood and skin. Anaemics would benefit greatly from eating lots of it as it is rich in both iron and chlorophyll, chemically very similar to human blood haemoglobin. Cabbage is also rich in vitamins A, B, C and E, as well as iron, sulphur, silica, magnesium and calcium. It boosts the immune system and helps protect against stress and in treating cancer. See also Sauerkraut, page 54.

Camomile

Camomile is renowned for its relaxing properties and has been widely used in Europe since at least the 17th century by those seeking restful sleep. Its uses are varied and it is valuable in treating stomach upsets, irritable bowel syndrome, period pain, headaches, migraines and muscle spasms. See more on page 107.

Cardamom

Cardamom is an excellent digestive tonic and is also used to treat some respiratory disorders. The seeds contain volatile oils, including borneol, camphor and pinene. Chewing them releases these to give a comforting, not-too-fiery warmth that eases indigestion, flatulence and colic.

Carrot

These sweet brightly coloured vegetables are rich in vitamins A, B and C, minerals like calcium, iron and potassium, and other antioxidants. They are good sources of beta-carotene; you can get your full RDA of vitamin A in just one carrot, hence the vegetable's reputed efficacy in eye and skin disorders, as well as respiratory infections. The mighty carrot is also high up on the list of foods that protect against cancer. Raw carrot juice is a wonderful tonic and often recommended for supporting the liver and for keeping wrinkles at bay, making it a popular anti-ageing food.

Cauliflower

Cauliflower is another member of the nutritious crucifer family (see more in Brussels sprout, opposite) and a good source of folate, antioxidant vitamin C and the cancer-fighting glucosinolates.

Celery

Celery is a good substitute for sea salt because it is higher in sodium than most vegetables. It is also a good source of potassium, which counterbalances sodium in the body to help prevent raised blood pressure, and contains a phytochemical which lowers blood pressure and blood cholesterol. Celery juice can help reduce acidity levels, which makes it an excellent preventative food for osteoarthritis. Celery, taken as a juice or eaten raw or used liberally in vegetable soups, is also an excellent natural diuretic. Celery is also known to act synergistically with cabbage, for example, in breaking down fat cells, so it is a useful food for those wishing to lose weight in a healthy way.

Cinnamon

Latest research indicates that cinnamon can inhibit growth of E. coli bacteria. This comes as little surprise to herbalists, who have known of its antibacterial, antifungal and antiviral effects for many years. It can treat stomach upsets and vomiting, and reduce cold and 'flu symptoms. A dash of ground cinnamon in a honey-and-lemon drink can soothe a sore throat. In the form of a tea, it is also an antispasmodic and eases menstrual cramps.

Chillies

Chilli peppers are, in fact, a fruit and they provide three times more vitamin C than oranges. Moderate amounts of any type of fresh or powdered chilli will induce sweating – a cooling mechanism that could explain the seemingly perverse popularity of chillies in hot climates. The unique chilli pepper heat comes from a component called capsaicin, concentrated in the internal pale rib membranes and seeds. Capsaicin can relieve nerve pain and is used in a medically prescribed cream to

DIET GUIDELINES FOR KAPHA TYPES (see pages 11–15)

Kapha types favour bitter, pungent and astringent tastes.

It is beneficial and restorative for them to eat hot dry food and spices, such as chillies, peppers, mustards – anything warming, particularly if red, gold or russet in colour. They should favour anything that moves the system and clears a sluggish liver.

Kaphas are better not eating large meals after 6pm. They will benefit from a monthly detox, drinking milk thistle and dandelion tea.

ease the pain of shingles. Herbalists advocate chilli to warm the body, improve the circulation and stimulate metabolism. However, chillies may be contraindicated in certain 'hot' conditions, such as acne rosacea, which causes abnormal facial flushing.

Cloves

Cloves are a well-known toothache remedy. Simply apply clove oil to the affected area or clamp a whole clove between your teeth. It is thought to act as a mild anaesthetic. Cloves also have strong antiseptic and germicidal qualities.

Cranberries

The juice is excellent for the treatment of cystitis and for preventing urinary tract infections, as it helps flush out the bacteria that are known to cause these conditions.

Fenugreek

High in ingredients that soothe and heal, freshly ground fenugreek seeds can be used in cooking or as an infusion to ease inflammatory conditions of the stomach and intestines. Alternatively, they can be sprouted, and the green parts eaten, together with the seeds. Fenugreek can be used in a soothing poultice for abscesses and boils. It should not be used medicinally in pregnancy.

Garlic

A member of the onion family, along with chives and shallots, this plant is now widely recognized as one of the most potent medicinal plants. It is a natural diuretic, increasing kidney function, and is traditionally used to clean and treat wounds and bites. It is a natural expectorant, helping the expulsion of mucus from the lungs and throat.

In ancient times a remedy for most pains and disease, it is now highly recognized for its natural antiseptic and antibiotic qualities. Recently published research claims that garlic powder can kill bacteria known to cause stomach ulcers. Another recent study showed that natural chemicals found in garlic can suppress tumours and that these may even help to prevent cancer.

Garlic is renowned for lowering the risk of heart disease and strokes, helping to reduce cholesterol and improving the circulation. It also has a powerful effect on blood clotting mechanisms by 'thinning' the blood and helping purify it.

The sulphur in garlic is responsible for its pungent aroma; garlic contains hundreds of components, with sulphur being involved in most of them. Allicin is the most notable of these and on crushing garlic, the allicin is released. Allicin is believed to be responsible in helping to reduce cancer risk. Recent research has shown that regular consumption of garlic reduced the risk of stomach cancer by 25–50 per cent.

A research team from Chelsea & Westminster Hospital in London have shown that taking garlic during pregnancy reduces the risk of pre-eclampsia (raised blood pressure and protein retained in the urine), which affects up to 1 in 10 women in the UK.

Everyone can benefit from regular consumption of raw and cooked garlic to fight common colds, 'flus, coughs and bronchitis, as well as other respiratory and digestive infections. Garlic is highly effective as a liver cleanser and can help reduce blood sugar.

Ginger

Ginger root is valued for its cleansing, warming and stimulating qualities. It aids digestion, helps remove gases from the stomach and intestines, is valued for its antiseptic qualities and helps loosen mucus. It is widely used to alleviate the symptoms of colds and 'flu. Ginger helps improve circulation and, with its warming qualities, can be useful in the treatment of rheumatism and arthritis.

Grape

This cleansing and strengthening fruit is best eaten fresh or as a juice and on its own, because it ferments in the gut so quickly. One of the most popular, effective cleansing fasts practised is a grape fast. Grapes seem to have the effect of stimulating the body's regenerative powers and are very effective for combating stress and fatigue, and are often included in the diet during convalescence.

Horseradish

Horseradish acts as a digestive aid and increases urinary flow. An infusion with some added crushed mustard seeds can help disperse excess fluid and reduce water retention.

Lemon balm

This plant, native to Southern Europe, can help to treat anxiety and tension or even mild depression.

Lentils

These are a very nutritious source of protein, cholesterol and blood-sugar-regulating fibre, as well as iron, magnesium, potassium and B vitamins. They are also rich in lignans, which fight hormone-dependent cancers.

Mango

Raw, this delicious tropical fruit is a useful source of vitamin E, iron and vitamin C. It is also a rich source of beta-carotene (100g/3½oz ripe flesh contains 300–3,000µg) and therefore has valuable antioxidant properties.

Melon

Cleansing and mildly stimulating to kidneys and bladder, melons are gently laxative – perfect for a summer fast.

Mushrooms

The Chinese have understood the usefulness of mushrooms in medicine for centuries, and the Japanese in a recent study showed that eating only 90g (3¼oz) of shiitake mushrooms every day caused blood cholesterol levels to plummet after only one week. Mushrooms contain vitamin B, potassium, iron and protein, as well as beneficial chemicals called polysaccharides, which are known

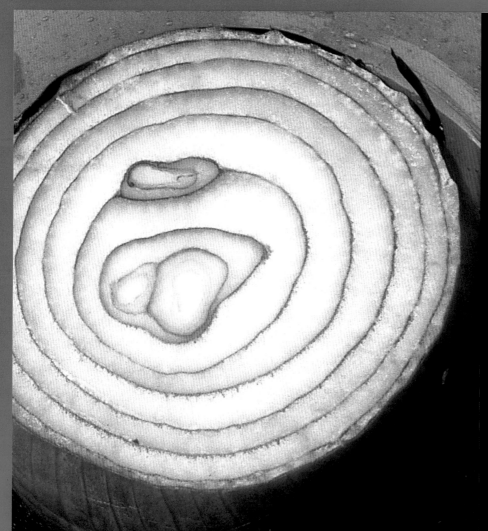

THE TOP 20 ANTIOXIDANT VEGETABLES

Aubergine
Bean, green
Beetroot
Broccoli
Brussels sprouts
Cabbage
Carrot
Cauliflower
Celery
Corn
Garlic
Kale
Lettuce, Iceberg
Lettuce, leaf
Onion
Pepper, red
Potato
Potato, sweet
Spinach
Squash, yellow

to stimulate the immune system because they are so similar to the bacteria cell walls.

Nutmeg

'Traditionally added to milky drinks given to convalescents, nutmeg contains myristin, a substance that, in small amounts, can cause drowsiness and a sense of well-being,' says diet consultant Joanna Hall. Just a pinch of the finely grated spice can also treat flatulence, nausea and vomiting. Grated nutmeg in a suitable carrier ointment is reputedly excellent for haemorrhoids. Too much nutmeg taken internally, however, is highly dangerous – as little as two whole nutmegs could be fatal.

Oats

This staple food is perhaps the most important grain after brown rice and should hold a regular position in our diet. Oats are highly stabilizing to blood sugar levels, making them excellent for people with diabetes. Oats have been shown to help lower blood cholesterol levels, one of the reasons people with heart or circulatory problems are advised to eat oats, particularly as porridge and some oat bran. Many digestive disorders, including constipation, respond to regular eating of oats and its demulcent quality soothes the stomach and intestines. Oats are traditionally known for their qualities as a sedative and nerve restorative, which is not surprising when you consider how nutritious they are, and rich in the B complex vitamins and vitamin E, calcium, magnesium, potassium and silicon.

Oily fish

Fish like herring, mackerel, salmon and sardines are rich in the important omega-3 fatty acids, which help lower blood cholesterol, protecting against heart disease, stroke, cognitive decline and skin conditions.

Olive oil

This delicious, healthy and popular oil is rich in cholesterol-neutralizing monounsaturated fats, and free-radical inhibitor, vitamin E. It encourages the digestive system and regular bowel movement, and is very good for easing rheumatic conditions.

Onion

High in the B vitamins and potassium, onions are considered to be in the food front line when helping to reduce heart disease, stroke and cancer risk. They also help us process fatty foods, preventing the blood-clotting rise in cholesterol after a fatty meal. People who eat raw onions regularly have more balanced, healthier cholesterol levels. Onions are a popular folk remedy for all kinds of conditions, including colds, arthritis, asthma, bronchitis, and gastric and urinary infections, early ageing, rheumatism and gout.

Orange

Renowned for their infection-fighting qualities, oranges help the body's defences, with their high content of vitamin C, beta-carotene and bioflavonoids. The latter aid the support of the immune system by strengthening

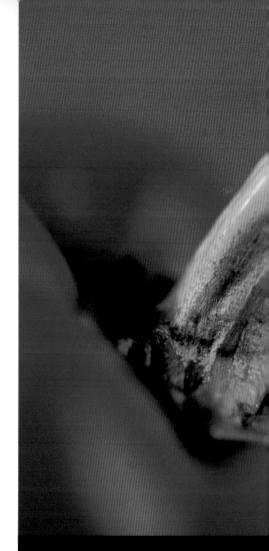

HOW TO GET ENOUGH!

The best sources of each of the major antioxidants should be:

VITAMIN C – red and green peppers, oranges and orange juice, blackcurrants, kiwi fruit, broccoli and green leafy veg.
VITAMIN E – nuts, seeds, vegetable oils, avocados and whole-grains.
SELENIUM – Brazil nuts, shellfish.
CAROTENOIDS – red peppers, cantaloupe melon, spinach, mangoes and oranges.

vitamin C's antioxidant powers, helping to enhance the strength of the blood capillary walls. Oranges eaten fresh provide pectin, which helps reduce blood cholesterol.

Parsley

This popular herb is so widely used raw in cooking, we do take it for granted and forget how much it can help improve our health as well as the taste of the dishes to which we add it. It is an excellent source of potassium and calcium, and is particularly rich in the antioxidants, carotenes and vitamin C. Recognized as quite a special herb at least since Roman times, parsley also has expectorant and diuretic powers. It is also considered an emmenagogue – with the power to stimulate the menstrual process. Pregnant women should not eat medicinal doses and take it only lightly and occasionally as a garnish, if at all.

Peppers

The capsicum, or sweet pepper, has very high levels of vitamin C, especially the riper yellow and red ones. They are also an excellent source of beta-carotene, iron and potassium. Red and yellow peppers rank high in the antioxidant army's war against cancer and heart disease. As with most plant foods, it is best to eat peppers raw and fresh to get the maximum nutritive value you can from them.

Peppermint

This plant is renowned for its usefulness in a wide range of digestive disorders. It apparently works by reducing the time

food spends in the stomach, by stimulating the gastric lining and also relaxing the stomach muscles. It is also a useful antispasmodic. See also page 108.

Pineapple

Hundreds of research studies have shown the positive action of the powerful bromelain enzyme found in the fresh raw juice or full fruit of pineapple. This enzyme can digest many times its own weight of protein in a few minutes. Pineapple is a delicious and juicy cure for all manner of digestive ailments and is also prized for its anti-inflammatory action and for speeding up the healing process.

Prune

These contain twice as much antioxidants as any other fruit or vegetable. They also have a high fibre content, which is why they are so popular as a natural laxative.

Pumpkin seed

In Eastern Europe, pumpkin seeds are said to protect the prostate gland and to be a good tonic for men generally. These tasty seeds are good for everyone and a valuable source of the B complex vitamins, calcium, iron, magnesium and zinc.

Radish

An important member of the crucifer family, radishes are hot and astringent in their action. They should be eaten fresh, regularly but not in excess. Their powerful juice stimulates the discharge of bile from the gallbladder, but too much

can irritate both the gallbladder and liver. A good source of calcium, potassium and sulphur, they have long been recognized for their detoxifying liver-toning qualities.

Raspberry leaves

For centuries, a tea made from raspberry leaves has been taken by women during late pregnancy. The leaves are now known to help relax the uterine muscles for labour and delivery. Raspberry tea also soothes throat irritations and mouth ulcers.

Rosemary

This astringent tonic herb has a deserved reputation for its toning and strengthening effect on everything from muscles to hair. It increases perspiration as well as having a calming action on the stomach, showing a nervine or sedative quality. It can help psychological tension, head colds, lethargy, giddiness and windiness, as well as relieve many varied symptoms like bad period cramps, excessive bleeding and circulation problems. It has natural antibacterial, antifungal, antiseptic and relaxant powers, and is a good brain and memory tonic. See more on page 108.

Sage

This pungent herb has traditionally been regarded as aiding the memory and fighting the symptoms of ageing, especially failing eyesight. It has strong antiseptic, antispasmodic and astringent properties, fighting infection and boosting the immune system. Sage tea and/or infusions are excellent for asthma, catarrh, colds, 'flu, sore throats, swollen

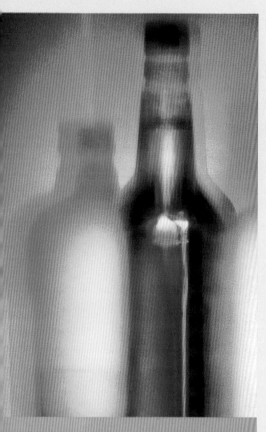

glands and respiratory infections. Sage is an excellent tonic if you are suffering from stress, anxiety or exhaustion, or convalescing. However, pregnant women and epileptics should avoid it.

Sauerkraut

This amazing medicinal food is the result of the fermentation of slices of raw cabbage layered with sea salt and a few juniper berries. The cabbage ferments in its own juices over the 3–4 weeks it takes to create this nutritious food, packed with important enzymes and high in calcium and vitamin C. It helps eliminate the toxins in the gut, arrests intestinal putrefaction and autointoxication, regulates digestion and helps cultivate intestinal flora. Some even say that, by promoting a healthy colon, it helps prolong youth.

Sesame seed

Rich in protein, important antioxidant vitamin E, iron, magnesium, calcium, zinc, essential fatty acids and important amino acids, these tasty little seeds are excellent for toning up the kidneys and liver, stimulating circulation and fertility, treating fatigue and enhancing your sex life and your sense of vitality. Try to have halvah (pounded sesame seeds and a little honey!) habitually...! You can mix the seeds with other foods, whole or ground up, or use tahini (sesame seed paste) instead of butter.

Soya bean

Soya beans and most soya products, like tofu and soy milk, are very nutritious foods rich in the B complex vitamins, calcium, iron and lecithin, and are known for their positive effect on the nervous system, especially when eaten in moderation and, as in the Japanese diet, fermented and combined with sea greens and rice. Recent research has shown that soya beans contain materials that, on digestion or fermentation, release genistein and daidzein, which help prevent breast and prostate cancer and form a natural hormone-replacement therapy for those in the menopause. They are referred to as 'plant oestrogens' and, in fact, are a type of flavonoid which is a good oestrogen balancer.

Spinach

To maximize the nutritious value of this dark green leafy antioxidant iron-rich food, it is best to eat it fresh and raw or very lightly cooked. Also very rich in potassium, this vegetable eaten raw a couple of times a week increases antioxidant protection and may help reduce the risk of cancer and eye degeneration in later years.

Sprouted seeds

Sprouted seeds are a storehouse of food energy and have a regenerative effect on your body. Generally eaten raw, they are packed with vitamins and minerals, as well as being rich in enzymes and complete proteins. A seed's nutrient value increases many times over when sprouted. The vitamin E content of wheat, for instance, increases 300 per cent after 4 days of sprouting. Sprouts are an excellent source of the B complex vitamins and the antioxidant vitamins A,

DIET GUIDELINES FOR VATA TYPES
(see pages 11–15)

Warm, well-cooked oily foods are best for vatas. They prefer sweet, salty and sour tastes.

The majority of their diet should be foods that are warming and grounding: brown rice, oats, couscous, lentils, root vegetables, all nuts and seeds, tofu, honey, live yoghurt, bananas, berries, cherries, grapes, pineapples, apricots, lemons and limes.

They should favour foods that are orange, red and yellow in colour, as well as warming spices.

C and E. They are one of the main foods of the Hunzas of the Western Himalayas, renowned for their longevity and vitality. Their rich enzyme concentration stimulates a heightened enzyme activity in the metabolism, leading to the regeneration of many of your body's processes, particularly those in the digestive and circulatory systems. For more detail on how to sprout your own seeds, see page 82.

Sunflower seed

Rich in the B vitamins and polyunsaturated fats, protein and minerals, these are a concentrated nourishing food that provides energy and helps to check irritability, fatigue and depression when eaten regularly.

Sweet potato

This delicious low-fat food is not related to the ordinary potato and possesses a much higher content of vitamins, minerals and antioxidants. It has a particularly high level of vitamin E, which can help lower the risk of many degenerative conditions, and is also a good source of iron and potassium.

Thyme

This herb has many medicinal uses, as it is a good astringent, anti-microbial and expectorant, that can be used for digestive and respiratory infections. It helps to ease the symptoms of asthma, bronchitis and whooping cough, can be used as a gargle to ease general irritable coughs and sore throats, and can help to reduce spasm. See more on page 108.

Tomato

People all over the world, but most especially in the Mediterranean countries, enjoy this juicy, sumptuous fruit regularly in their diet. As well as being the vegetable most commonly eaten raw, it is used in countless dishes and made into a wealth of different sauces, especially for pasta and other vegetables.

Long regarded as having the power to enhance your love-life, tomatoes are filled with nutrients, including the minerals iron and potassium and the antioxidant vitamins C and E, as well as beta-carotene. Lycopene, the main form of carotenes found in tomatoes and the reason for their vivid red colour, works in a unique way with vitamin C to make it an even more powerful protectant antioxidant.

People who eat large amounts of tomatoes are known to be less likely to suffer from heart disease and cancer, particularly of the prostate, lung and stomach. Worldwide studies recently carried out on women who consume high levels of tomatoes and tomato products showed that they are also less likely to suffer from breast, cervical and ovarian cancers.

The quantity of lycopene in a tomato depends more on the fruit's degree of ripeness than on type, and does not seem to be much affected by cooking, which means that sauces, soups, purées, concentrates and ketchups are as valuable in this respect as fresh tomatoes. Of course, some of these products contain high percentages of salt and sugar, so be careful of this. Children do usually love tomato ketchup on everything, so do let them eat this product. Try buying an organic brand with no additives.

Lycopene might also slow down the onset of age-related mascular degeneration (AMD), perhaps the commonest cause of poor vision and blindness in old age.

Turmeric

Turmeric contains liver-protectant compounds. Herbalists use extracts to treat conditions such as hepatitis, cirrhosis and jaundice. It is antiseptic and calms the digestive system as well as stimulating the gallbladder to release bile, improving the digestion of fats. Adding turmeric to pulses can help reduce wind and bloating. Curcumin, an active component, is thought to have anti-inflammatory and antitumour effects. A University of Miami School of Medicine study suggests that curcumin causes breast cancer cells to self-destruct.

Watercress

This is an excellent nutritious source of vitamins A and C, with some good amounts of B vitamins, together with iodine, calcium, iron, potassium and zinc. This reputed tonic food helps treat and prevent anaemia, infections of all kinds, eczema and countless other more serious degenerative diseases. Rich in antioxidants, especially when eaten raw, this leaf is purported to offer some protection against various cancers, particularly of the lungs and gut.

superfood recipes

Stuffed sardines Italian-style *serves 2*

6 small or 4 larger sardines, about
    400g (14oz), heads and backbones
    removed, gutted and rinsed
knob of butter
2 tablespoons lemon juice
a few sprigs of parsley, to garnish
lemon wedges, to serve

for the stuffing:
about 40 g (1½ oz) fresh breadcrumbs
40g (1½oz) Parmesan cheese, grated
1 tablespoon chopped parsley
1 teaspoon chopped basil
½ small beaten egg

Make a stuffing: mix the breadcrumbs, cheese, parsley and basil with the egg.

    Lay the sardines flat, skin side down, and spread the stuffing over them. Roll up each fish, starting from the neck end, and fix with half a cocktail stick.

    Heat the butter in a small shallow pan and arrange the stuffed sardines in the pan. Fry gently for a minute or two, turning once.

    Add 4 tablespoons of water and the lemon juice. Cover with a lid and cook for about 10 minutes, turning once again after 5 minutes.

    Arrange the stuffed sardines on small serving plates and pour over the juices from the pan. Garnish with a few sprigs of parsley and lemon wedges.

Rainbow vegetables *serves 2*

You can substitute peppers, broccoli or cauliflower florets for any of the vegetables.

6–8 cherry tomatoes, cut in half
2 celery stalks, sliced at an angle
5 cm (2 in) cucumber, thickly sliced
6–8 baby carrots,
a few sprigs of flat-leaf parsley

for the avocado dressing:
½ large avocado, peeled and stoned
½ small garlic clove, crushed
juice of ½ lemon
2 tablespoons low-fat live yoghurt
sea salt and freshly ground
    black pepper

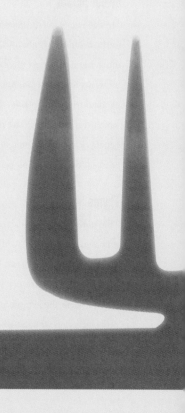

Make the dressing: place all the ingredients in a blender with 2 tablespoons of water and process until smooth. Add a little more water if the mixture is too thick. Arrange the vegetables in a colourful pattern on two serving plates. Spoon over the dressing and decorate with the sprigs of parsley. Serve at once.

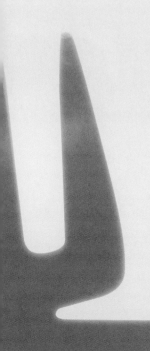

APPLE/CARROT/ CELERY JUICE

For a delicious and highly nutritious fresh raw juice, process together 1 apple, 3 carrots and 2 celery stalks. Season with freshly ground black pepper and/or lemon juice if you like.

Teriyaki salmon with tossed steam-fried vegetable noodles *serves 2*

2 fresh salmon fillets, each about
    150–175g (5½–6oz)
2 tablespoons grated root ginger
2 spring onions, finely chopped
2 tablespoons teriyaki or soy sauce
2 tablespoons sherry or white wine
parsley, chervil or dill, to garnish

for the noodles:
2 celery stalks
1 small red pepper, deseeded
16–20 mangetout peas
6–8 spring onions
1 teaspoon extra-virgin olive oil
100–150g (3½–5½oz) noodles

Prepare the noodles: bring a large pan of water to the boil. Cut the vegetables into thin sticks. Steam-fry in the oil and a little water for about 3 minutes until cooked to your taste. Meanwhile, add the noodles to the boiling water and cook for about 3 minutes or as directed on the pack. Drain and add to the vegetables.

Place the fillets, skin down, on 2 serving plates and spread with ginger. Sprinkle over the onions, teriyaki or soy sauce and sherry or wine. Fill 2 large pans with water and bring to the boil. Reduce the heat and place a plate on each pan. Cover the fish with another plate and steam for 7 minutes. Carefully turn the fillets over and steam for 5–7 minutes more, depending on their thickness, until cooked through. Try not to over-cook. Drain the juice into the noodles. Pile the noodles on to 2 serving plates. Very carefully arrange the salmon fillets on top. Garnish with herbs and serve.

Date and orange flan *serves 2*

75g (3oz) dried dates, pitted and chopped
50g (2oz) ground almonds
1 tablespoon honey
4 tablespoons Greek-style yoghurt
2 oranges, peeled and with zest removed and sliced separately

Chop the dates even further in a food processor, if possible. Mix in the almonds and honey and press the mixture into the base of a 15cm (6in) flan tin. Place in the fridge and chill for at least an hour or until required.

Remove the flan base from the tin. Mix the yoghurt with the grated zest of ½ an orange and spread over the base. Arrange the orange slices on the top and serve.

Recipes from *The Optimum Nutrition Cookbook*, Patrick Holford & Judy Ridgway (Piatkus)

the mediterranean diet

With the increased travel to the Continent over the last 30 years or so, many, many more of us are enjoying the benefits of a diet similar in content to that eaten by the people of the Mediterranean region. The Mediterranean diet is a rich blend of colourful and enticing foods, with a very high fruit and fresh raw vegetable content. The diet is also high in oily fish, now known to provide the essential fatty acids and omega-3 and -6 oils, as well as garlic and olive oil. In Italy, for example, the benefits of olive oil are widely acknowledged by doctors and it is revered as virtually an elixir of life.

Today foods produced in the area and enjoyed by most include complex carbohydrates such as pasta, pulses and rice; the region's abundance of vegetables, particularly those that are known to have protective properties, such as dark green leafy vegetables like broccoli; yellow, orange and other brightly coloured vegetables such as peppers of all kinds, carrots, pumpkins and salads and many of the orange-coloured fruits, such as melons, apricots, peaches, nectarines and oranges, which all help to boost the immune system and fend off infections.

Dairy products are kept to a minimum and they cook primarily with olive oil, which has many health-giving properties (see page 52). Protein is eaten in small amounts and is mainly in the form of oily fish, such as mullet, tuna, sardines and salmon, which contain essential and valuable quantities of omega-3 oils. They receive their fibre quotient from complex carbohydrates like pasta and rice, which are known to lower blood cholesterol and reduce the risk of some cancers.

The Mediterranean diet also includes plenty of garlic, which contains an active ingredient, allicin, now proved very effective in reducing blood pressure and preventing blood clots. It is also antibiotic, antiviral and antifungal, as well as being a general tonic for the body when eaten regularly in small amounts, preferably raw or lightly cooked, as a topping or in a salad dressing (for more on garlic, see page 50).

FOODS IN THE MEDITERRANEAN DIET WITH PROTECTIVE PROPERTIES

Complex carbohydrates

Pasta, rice and other grains; beans, lentils and other pulses, fruits and vegetables; nuts and seeds.
Protective constituent: fibre and a wide range of vitamins, minerals and phytochemicals.
Beneficial effect: lowers cholesterol; may protect against heart disease and some cancers.

Fruits and vegetables

Brightly coloured vegetables, such as peppers, carrots and tomatoes.
Protective constituent: as above, especially antioxidants and phytochemicals.
Beneficial effect: protects against the damaging effect of 'free radicals' (see page 26).

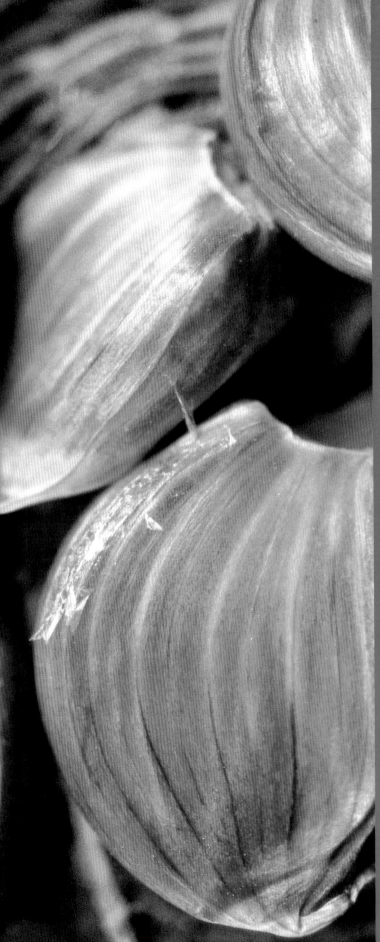

Dark green vegetables

Broccoli, peas and asparagus, salad leaves, spinach, watercress and cabbage.

Protective constituent: as for complex carbohydrates, especially antioxidant vitamins C and E, and beta-carotene which converts to antioxidant vitamin A.

Beneficial effect: combat damaging free radicals; reduce cancers of colon, breast and lung; delay and reduce effects of ageing.

Fats

Olive oil, oily fish such as tuna, sardines and anchovies.

Protective constituent: essential fatty acids, omega-3 oils.

Beneficial effect: reduce harmful LDL-cholesterol level and increase good HDL-cholesterol, stimulate pancreas to reduce risk of stomach ulcers.

Garlic

Protective constituent: allicin, sulphides, antioxidants.

Beneficial effect: antiseptic/antifungal and possibly antiviral, prevents blood clots, destroys free radicals, lowers blood pressure and blood cholesterol levels.

The variety of foods available from which to choose makes this a delicious, interesting and exciting way to enjoy food so vibrant in colour, flavour and texture.

the mediterranean way

The following is a week's eating plan that will whet your appetite and tempt you to try the Mediterranean way to health!

Every day

Breakfast Greek-style yoghurt with a little honey
Fresh fruit chosen from the following: apricots, cherries, grapefruit, grapes, melon, nectarines, peaches, plums, oranges, raspberries and strawberries

Day One

Lunch Taramasalata with pitta bread
Greek salad of tomato, red onion and feta cheese

Dinner Seafood risotto
Plate of assorted fruit sorbets

Day Two

Lunch Aubergine dip with a selection of crudités

Dinner Pasta with garlic and chillies
Grilled pepper salad with lemon dressing

Day Three

Lunch Grilled sardines with fresh tomato sauce
Fresh fruit salad

Dinner Braised lamb shanks with lemons
Mashed potatoes with olive oil and shredded basil
Baked figs

Day Four

Lunch   Salad niçoise with green beans, watercress and potatoes
Small baguette

Dinner   Tarragon roast chicken with grapes
Pears poached in red wine

Day Five

Lunch   Baked potatoes dressed with hummus and olive oil

Dinner   Spicy seafood tajine
Broccoli and cauliflower florets with pine nuts
Chilled melon balls and cherries

Day Six

Lunch   Grilled tomato, mozzarella and anchovy bruschetta

Dinner   Prawn and mushroom lasagne
Rocket salad
Fruity panettone pudding

Day Seven

Lunch   Frittata
Tomato and red onion salad

Dinner   Griddled lemon-marinated chicken breasts
Spinach and walnut salad
Mixed fruit compote with gingered fromage frais

DIET GUIDELINES FOR PITTA TYPES
(see pages 11–15)

Pittas favour bitter, sweet and astringent tastes. It is good for them to start and end meals with sweet-tasting foods. They should avoid very hot or spicy foods, like chillies and peppers. Pittas do better with cooling foods, such as salads and sea foods.

They should favour lots of green vegetables, melons, grapes and other fruits with a high water content, sweet fruit juices, mint, peppermint and alfalfa teas, and plain cool water.

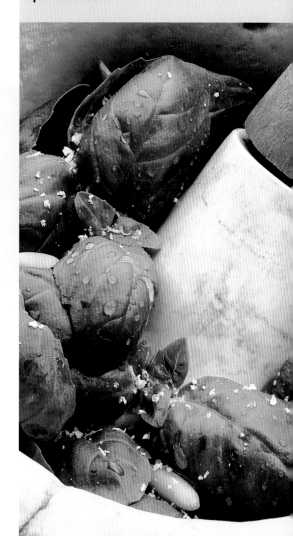

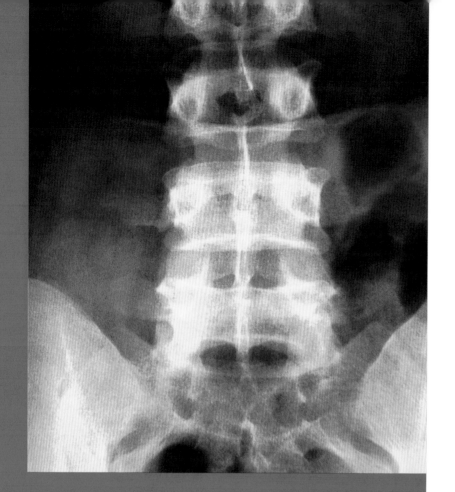

diets for your needs

Obviously what constitutes a good balanced diet does also vary considerably according to all sorts of factors, such as age, gender, activity level, time of year, climate, stress levels, even your genetic make-up. In this section we look at some of these in detail and try to make some suggestions as to how you can adjust your eating habits to best suit your own personal needs. This is an opportunity to make your life fit your mind/body and reap untold benefits in terms of health and well-being.

Recent research reported in *Higher Nature News* has revealed that your blood type can determine the conditions to which you may be prone. Eating foods and taking supplements that support your genetic make-up might be the key to optimum health. Dr Peter D'Adamo with Catherine Whitney, in their book *The Eat Right Diet* (Century), have made this link between food and disease and blood types. There has been much literature in the area, but D'Adamo amd Whitney are the first to research it in great depth. The blood group links have historical and anthropological origins. For example, originally there was only one group among the peoples of Europe, type 'O', and this is still the most common there. Whereas type 'B' began among the Mongols.

TYPE 'O'

Type 'O's were the hunter-gatherers who lived on meat, fish, vegetables and fruit. As this was pre-agriculture, going back over 200,000 years, farmed grains and dairy products just weren't available. 'O' types cannot effectively digest these foodstuffs even today.

Health problems 'O's may experience: low thyroid activity, leading to fatigue and weight-gain; ulcers because of high stomach acids (for digesting animal protein); allergies, arthritis, blood clotting problems.

Sensitivities: 'new' foods, i.e. farmed foods such as wheat and milk, can lead to arthritis and allergies.

Positive attributes: strong defences against infection; hardy digestive system; with sufficient exercise and the right diet, they metabolize food well and stay lean and strong.

Type 'O' Diet

Eat freely: fish, meat, vegetables, fruit (except oranges).

Restrict intake of: oranges, dairy products, corn, wheat.

Ideal supplements: iodine (kelp), vitamin B, vitamin K, calcium.

Ideal exercise (energetic): aerobics, running, martial arts.

TYPE 'A'

Descended from the first farmers, these were the earliest vegetarians, going back a mere 10,000 years. They thrive on vegetable proteins, grains and beans, and were the first to cultivate wheat, but should restrict their intake as their muscles may develop acidity. They are not genetically disposed towards dairy foods, as these can cause them blood sugar problems.

Health problems 'A's may experience: cancer, anaemia, liver/gallbladder problems, diabetes (type 1), heart disease.

Positive attributes: these are not as specific as for 'O's, say, as this group did not have as many demands made on them. They make good followers and community members.

THE GREAT MILK DEBATE

After suffering 5 bouts of breast cancer, geochemist Professor Jane Plant decided to treat herself by diet. Her researches, outlined in her book, *Your Life In Your Hands*, showed that incidence of breast and prostate cancer is much less in China and Japan than in the West. She put this down to our 'unnatural' reliance on dairy foods and eliminated them from her diet. Her tumour shrank and she is convinced that her diet saved her life. She also eliminated or reduced levels of harmful chemical additives in her food by eating organic whole food and cutting out refined, preserved and over-cooked foods, at the same time including as many foods known to combat cancer as she could.

Type 'A' Diet:

Eat freely: tofu, grains (except wheat), beans and other legumes/pulses (except kidney and lima beans), fruit, soya foods, seafood.

Restrict intake of: dairy products, kidney and lima beans, wheat, meat.

Ideal supplements: folic acid, vitamin B12, vitamin C, vitamin E.

Ideal exercise (calming): yoga, t'ai chi.

TYPE 'B'

'B's evolved after 'A's, and originated in the Himalayan highlands, as Caucasian and Mongolian tribes mingled. Mongols then brought the type B blood group to Europe. Many Jewish people from Eastern Europe are type 'B'. They are sturdy and can often resist most killer diseases, like cancer and heart disease.

Health problems 'B's may experience: immune disorders; multiple sclerosis; lupus; chronic fatigue syndrome, diabetes (type 1).

Positive attributes: with correct diet they can live long and healthy lives. Type 'B's can eat the widest variety of foods, including dairy products, lamb and venison.

Type 'B' Diet:

Eat freely: dairy products, beans and other legumes/pulses (except lentils), vegetables, fruit, meat (but not poultry).

Restrict: poultry, lentils, peanuts, sesame, buckwheat, wheat, corn.

Ideal supplements: magnesium.

Ideal exercise (moderate): hiking, cycling, tennis, swimming.

TYPE 'AB'

This, the rarest of all major groups, is found in less than 5 per cent of the population and is only 1,000 years old. It is a blend of type 'A' Caucasians with type 'B' Mongolians.

Health problems 'AB's may experience: certain cancers, anaemia, heart disease.

Positive attributes: they combine the best of all worlds and are resistant to allergies, arthritis and other auto-immune diseases.

Type 'AB' Diet:

Eat freely: seafood, dairy products, tofu, beans and other pulses (except kidney and lima beans), fruit, grains (except buckwheat), meat, vegetables (except corn).

Restrict: kidney and lima beans, corn, seeds, red meat, buckwheat.

Ideal supplements: vitamin C.

Ideal exercise (calming/moderate): hiking, cycling, tennis, yoga, t'ai chi.

the circadian diet

A book very recently published in the USA, *The Circadian Prescription*, by Dr Sidney MacDonald Baker and Karen Baar (to be published in the UK under the title *The Body Clock Diet*, Vermillion Books) assures us that the smooth functioning of the body is reliant on the types of food we give it at specific times of the day. Getting your eating habits in tune with your body clock is a powerful disease deterrent.

Our body clock, or circadian rhythm, goes through many stages in a 24-hour period. We cannot affect the natural pace at which our personal body clock progresses, but we can make the processes it goes through more effective; for example, by eating the right foods at the right times of day for us. It is obvious that our bodies utilize less energy at night, when we are resting and sleeping, than they do during the day, when energy is expended to enable us to function at work and play. Why is it then that so many of us eat huge meals at the end of the day, when we don't actually NEED the energy that the food provides? What goes into those meals is also important.

Often, in the mornings and during the day we load up on carbohydrates in the form of sandwiches, chips, croissants, muffins, cereal, even fruit juice – all high in carbohydrates – and dinner can often be high in protein, such as chicken, fish or red meat. In fact, it is during the 'day shift' that protein is actually needed. At this time it creates the correct chemical reactions in the body that enable us to stay mentally alert and physically active. If we are low on protein during the day, we suffer from poor attention span, confusion and low energy – even apathy. The 'night shift' is the time for carbohydrates, which are essential then as they enable the body to perform crucial repair work to damaged cells and produce new ones, detoxifying our systems and ensuring we get adequate rest and healthy beneficial sleep.

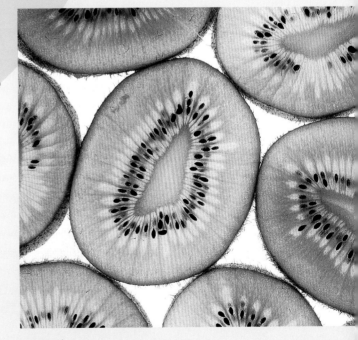

Following such a regime is quite a tall order for people whose normal habits will literally need to be turned head over heels. However, the general indication is simply that benefit can be achieved if the majority of protein is eaten in the morning and at lunchtime, and the majority of carbohydrate in the evening. It is believed that adopting this eating pattern could be instrumental in alleviating or even curing a variety of recurring health problems.

Our cultural habit is to eat too much carbohydrate, in the form of starchy and sugary food, too frequently. This is a fairly recent occurrence, historically, and we just have not evolved as quickly as our eating habits have changed. Problems with processing carbohydrates in the body and, specifically, a disorder called insulin resistance or carbohydrate poisoning are responsible for many conditions blamed on high cholesterol, such as weight gain, and some cardiovascular disease. Generally too much carbohydrate causes overly high insulin levels, which can lead to insulin resistance, which in turn can contribute to heart disease, diabetes and chronic inflammatory problems. The circadian diet, therefore, addresses this common problem by tending to reduce to one the number of times per day that carbohydrates are eaten, as would have been the common practice of our ancestors.

Conditions that are known to respond to the circadian diet include asthma, arthritis, pre-menstrual problems, infertility, and menopause and prostate problems, to name but a few.

CIRCADIAN MEALS

10 POWER BREAKFASTS:
Sliced fruit, cottage cheese
Herb omelette
Ham omelette
Crème fraîche over slices of melon and strawberries
Peanut butter thickly spread on a thin slice of toast
Nut protein bar
2 eggs and ham fried in olive oil
Grilled tomatoes with kippers
Chopped bacon and scrambled eggs
Honey and nuts in Greek-style yoghurt

10 PROTEIN LUNCHES:
Green salad, lamb and onion kebab
Salad with egg mayonnaise
Salad with clam chowder/fish soup
Green salad with cauliflower cheese
Green vegetables with grilled pork chops and apple sauce
Smoked salmon salad
Beef stew
Salad Niçoise
Chicken casserole
Coronation chicken

10 CARBOHYDRATE DINNERS:
Green salad with vegetable crumble
Wholemeal roll and pasta salad with peppers
Salad and vegetable burger in seeded bun
Thick vegetable soup, green salad and warm bread
Potato and mushroom pie
Dolmades (vine leaves with rice) with hummus and pitta bread
Tomato macaroni, onion and herb sauce and green salad
Warm focaccia bread, large potato, onion and chive salad, carrot and sultana salad and watercress salad
Vegetable casserole with dumplings
Vegetable lasagne

seasonal diet

Seasonal eating

Your dietary needs, and even your lifestyle habits, naturally change with the season. The changes seem obvious when we look at them, but how often do you really think about the way you eat, for instance in the summer as opposed to the winter? Or your different sleeping patterns in winter and summer? We respond quite instinctively to the natural cycles, the seasonal patterns within which we live. For example, in winter you need more than extra layers of clothing; you also feel the need for extra inner padding and therefore hunger for more warming soups, stews and hot food in general. Whereas, in summer you hanker after more fruits, salads and cold drinks.

Here we look at some of the simple healthy foods you can eat to help avoid the winter blues.

Warming food and drink for the winter blues

Brown Rice: an excellent winter food. Filling and warming, it is a very healthy, balanced grain which makes a good replacement starch for potatoes or pasta in your weekly menu plans.

Garlic: eating raw garlic may not be the easiest thing to do, but you do get the most benefit from its potent healing and antiseptic qualities. There are other ways you can ingest garlic – you can take garlic capsules or cook it lightly in your food; but in its natural state it is reputed to be a food that gives you strength. What could be better? That's just the thing you need in winter: when you are feeling low, without energy, fighting off yet another invading germ, garlic can help pick you up and fight off infection.

Ginger: to reap its full warming benefit, this root is best ingested in the form of a tea. It helps fight colds and 'flu, aids digestive problems, improves a sluggish circulation and is excellent for aches and pains, particularly those brought on by damp.

Oats: on top of all its health-giving, cholesterol-lowering qualities, oatmeal is essentially one of the best comfort foods there is. Warming and filling, it meets the most important criteria for a winter food.

Mustard: this is a very warming food and great for sustaining warmth as well. Good for preventing or treating muscular pain, you can eat it and bathe in it to treat potential or existing rheumatic or arthritic conditions.

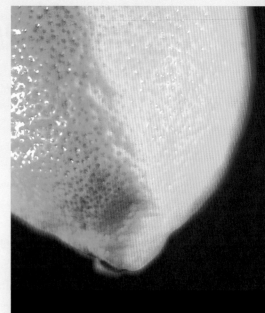

SOME SURPRISING WARMING FOODS:

APPLES: this healthy fruit helps with rheumatic pain, so can be quite useful in your winter diet. Apples also have a calming and relaxing effect on the digestive system.

LEMONS: an excellent food for inner cleansing, they are really effective for cleansing the liver and kidneys, and are also very good for treating colds, 'flus and circulation problems.

ONIONS: these can help prevent or ease rheumatic pain, respiratory problems and ear disorders. This vegetable is also good for your sex drive.

SPINACH: an excellent leafy vegetable to eat in plenty. Longer nights in winter means we need brighter eyes! Spinach helps prevent night-blindness because it is so rich in the 'eye' vitamin, A.

eating through the ages

We all also need to eat well at every stage of life. To live life to the full and keep illness and degenerative conditions at bay, a diet rich in fresh foods, fruit, salads and vegetables will aid this at every stage. Bring in plenty of physical activity according to your needs during the different stages of life, and you can be assured of continued good health into old age. Eating well and exercising regularly will also help in preventing stress and providing adequate satisfying and nourishing sleep, the third and equally important component of ensuring a healthy individual.

There are general rules of thumb which traverse time and age.

- Fruit and vegetables must play a significant role in everyone's diet.
- Limiting your fat intake and opting for essential fats (see The Fat Crisis, page 40) in correct quantities will help prevent conditions associated with high-fat and wrong-fat intake.
- Protein is also an integral part of everyone's diet, but not in the high proportions to which so many of us are nowadays accustomed.
- Complex carbohydrates, found in vegetables, some seeds and grains, are essential for energy and for a well balanced diet.

There are many schools of thought regarding order of intake, quantities and how often. 'Little and often' is a good guide and philosophy to adopt. Do not overeat and strain the digestive system... especially if you are inactive. It is a good idea to try whatever appeals to you and find the 'diet' that works for you and best fits in with your lifestyle.

Parents can play an important role in their children's lives by 'training' them into healthy eating habits from the beginning! So many of us are unlearning the bad habits passed on to us: those habits formed such an important part of our early years they are often hard to shake off, even if we know them to be bad for us. Children learn quickly and well, and seeing you eating healthy food will encourage them to do the same.

As it is important for children to eat well, so it is for us all. The middle years are perhaps the most significant in terms of our health in the later 'golden years'. This is the time when the metabolism is beginning to slow down, we no longer have the unlimited energy supplies we had in our youth and we are now realizing that we really do need to take care of ourselves at this stage to ensure good health and fitness in later life.

The foregoing are guidelines that we should adhere to throughout life, making

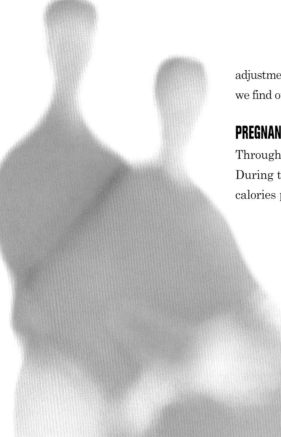

adjustments as detailed later according to the different phases in which we find ourselves.

PREGNANT WOMEN

Throughout life, women have a daily requirement of 2,000 calories. During the last three months of pregnancy this increases by 200 calories per day and while breast feeding by 400-600 calories. It is important that the diet remains healthy during both pregnancy and breast feeding to ensure good health for both mother and baby.

Tips for a healthy pregnancy for mother and baby

- Green vegetables and fruit are musts during pregnancy, to provide sufficient intake of vitamins, folic acid, iron and fibre. Always buy the best quality available, preferably organic.
- The need for dairy products increases, because of their high calcium content. For those who eat dairy-free diets, calcium-enriched soya milk is a good alternative. For those eating dairy products, try semi-skimmed milk, low-fat cheeses and yoghurts, and organic products.
- Eat small amounts regularly to ensure your energy levels remain constant.
- Protein needs are high. Fish provides high amounts, together with essential fatty acids. Avocados are a useful alternative for vegetarians, vegans or allergy sufferers. Eggs are full of protein.

Avoid

- Refined or processed foods, junk and fast foods.
- Excess salt and sugar in foods, and added to them.
- Tobacco.
- Alcohol should be excluded, or at least limited.
- Vitamin A can be harmful in very high quantities, so liver and any products that contain liver (which is very high in Vitamin A) should be avoided.

Trying to conceive?

- Try to take folic acid supplements for three months before aiming to become pregnant and during the first three months of pregnancy to prevent neural tube defects, such as spina bifida.
- Limit or exclude alcohol.

PRE-ADOLESCENCE (UP TO 14)

Pre-adolescent children are growing rapidly. They need plenty of starchy carbohydrates, like rice and pasta, and calcium-rich foods to ensure healthy bones. At this stage children need saturated fats, so avoid low-fat versions; instead, buy organic milk and cheeses, for instance. Introduce nuts and seeds into the diet, as they are an excellent source of calcium and essential fats.

Although many children would love to live on junk food alone, they can be encouraged to eat a diet full of fresh fruits and vegetables, essential to ensure good health. Growing uses a lot of energy and you may marvel at the amount of food a child can get through in a day! They usually know instinctively just how much they need. Encourage them to use their instincts and to enjoy food!

These instincts are good; they will carry them into later life and should be encouraged. It may not be appropriate to sit at table with a huge plate of food to be tackled, with constant probings from parents or carers. In other cultures, for example, a small bowl is proffered to each at the table and appropriate quantities of each food item taken from a large serving dish and placed in the bowl. This way what is needed and desired will be eaten, not what is forced into one's mouth.

This habit comes, perhaps, from historical times of hunger, particularly in Western culture. Feeding children well was a status symbol, and it was important for families to show they could! Now, we have more money and choice where food is concerned. Listen to your child's needs and let them decide, while encouraging them in healthy habits.

Tips for diet in childhood

- Limit sweet eating. Try introducing a 'sweet day' (or days) – special days when children are allowed to eat sweets – to avoid them becoming a daily necessity.
- Satisfy their need for sugar with fresh or dried fruits. For example, children often love white grapes, as they are soft, sweet and very juicy.
- Encourage them to drink plenty of water (without anything added!). This is a wonderful habit to get them into in their early years and will help to reduce the risk of sugar addiction that sweet and carbonated drinks can help create. Furthermore, their teeth will rot into the bargain (remember, even fruit juices may have sugars added to make them more appealing to children)!

- Salty, fatty snacks, like crisps and chips, should be limited to indulgent treats like sweets, not part of their daily diet.
- Helping them to understand food (getting involved in its preparation, for example) can be fun for them and will help to increase their awareness about good and bad foods.
- If their schools provide meals, make yourself aware of the weekly menu. If they have to have school meals, ensure that whatever is missing gets provided in the evening meal or at breakfast, where appropriate. If possible, give them packed lunches.

ADOLESCENCE (15–18)

Calcium still plays a vital role in the diet during this period, as adolescents' bones are still growing. A healthy balance of foods, with as much variety as possible, is highly recommended at this time. The calorie requirement at this time in life is higher than at any other time, due to the amount of energy expended just living an adolescent life! Males need 2,755 calories and females 2,100 per day. They will amaze you with the quantity of food they can get through and the extent of their appetites! They need it because they are still growing, going through puberty, studying hard and playing hard, and going through the often troublesome process of transition from child to young adult.

Emotions can often run high and will need sensitive and intelligent nurturing. Emotional energy can burn up a lot of calories. Ensure adolescents continue eating well, especially when they have the blues, are preparing for exams and generally going through the ups and downs of puberty. They are still instinctive at this age and, as much as they use energy, they require sleep – and lie-ins into midday and beyond are not unusual.

During this time it is important to encourage them to eat foods that supply energy without causing damage. Continue with the vegetable and fruit theme, ensuring that adequate quantities of all food types are eaten.

Tips for diet in adolescence

- Your own habits in this area will come into play now as adolescents often start experimenting with alcohol at this time. If you are a moderate drinker, your children will probably follow your lead to an extent. Peer-group pressure – and just the desire for FUN – will potentially increase the desire for alcohol and experimentation. Talk to them about this and advise them of the possible side-effects and safe limits.
- With their hunger levels being at an all-time high, encourage them to eat foods that include plenty of starchy carbohydrates, to provide energy, and limit or cut out junk foods.

ADULTHOOD

All the general recommendations of healthy eating apply throughout adulthood, and healthy patterns established in early adulthood will prove their worth in middle-age and later life. Throughout adult life, men have a consistent calorie requirement of 2,550. A man who exercises frequently, or has a very physically active lifestyle, should increase his intake under guidance. Women, however, tend to need fewer calories from around the age of 50, although the same recommendation applies to women as men regarding exercise and physical activity. Pregnant or breast-feeding women require higher calorie levels (see page 69). All the general rules of healthy eating apply throughout adulthood.

Tips for diet in adulthood

- During this period, taking care of your health will help to avert problems in later life. Exercising regularly and eating well will help you maintain good, consistent and appropriate energy levels.
- Get your energy requirements met by eating starchy carbohydrates found in fruit, vegetables and grains.
- Limit the amount of fat in your diet.

Establishing healthy patterns for prevention of disease

- Bowel problems such as colon cancer can be minimized by eating plenty of fibre-rich complex starchy carbohydrates.
- The benefits of moderate drinking (no more than two glasses of red wine per day) are now common knowledge. It is advised, of course, not to go over this amount and certainly not to binge-drink, as this can be more harmful than regular drinking. The reputed benefits, to men in particular, include reduced blood cholesterol and lowered risk of heart disease.
- To encourage a healthy heart, salt levels should be greatly restricted. Even better, don't add ANY salt to food in cooking or when raw. This will help to prevent high blood pressure and other heart-related problems.
- Keep to your calorie levels between ages 40 and 50. This is the time of middle-aged spread, often caused by lack of activity and more indulgence in food. Of course, food can – and should still be – a source of pleasure and socialization. With potentially increased earnings, you can also afford to take the time out to indulge yourself in luxury foods that are good for your health. It is important to continue to keep physically active to keep your flexibility and mobility at a healthy level. If you have not been an avid enthusiast at the gym, start now! You will enjoy it and appreciate it now and definitely in the future.

THE GOLDEN YEARS (50+)

As men and women mature, their calorie requirement changes – earlier for women than men. From around the age of 50, women need about 1,900 calories per day up to age 75 and 1,810 from then on. Men on the other hand have a consistent need up to about age 60, with a gradual decline to 2,100 per day by the age of 75.

Tips for diet in old age

- As you become less and less active, you need less energy from food. Reduce your intake, sensibly maintaining a healthy balance and exercising to retain flexibility, mobility and good health, and avoid weight-gain and any degenerative diseases that seem to be the modern-day plague in the Western culture – and need not be!
- Everyone should eat a cooked meal every day – but especially after retirement and beyond. Always eat a varied and well-balanced diet, rich in fruit and vegetables.

Anti-ageing foods

As the population continues to grow worldwide, with more people living longer than 85, and with one-fifth of the world population destined to be over 65 by the year 2020, the issue of defying age-related conditions becomes ever more relevant to us all. We want to live longer and stay healthy at the same time. Age-related disease is not inevitable.

Research consistently bears out the theory that eating right not only promotes longevity but defies age-related diseases that we may have come to accept as almost inevitable. The theories behind why we age seem to rest in two main courts: one, thinks that cells are lost due to oxidative stress, when our cells are attacked by free radicals; and two, is that of 'glucation', a process by which damage is caused to our tissues by excess sugar in the blood.

ten foods that can help you to live longer

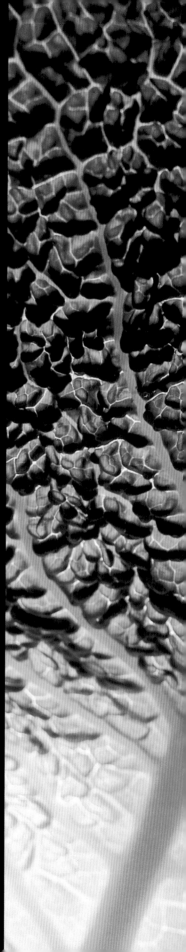

1   DARK FRUITS:

Red or purple fruits, black grapes, blueberries, black cherries, blackberries and bilberries contain much vitamin C and flavonoids.

2   WHOLE-GRAINS:

They include brown rice, wholemeal bread and porridge, all keeping bowels regular and efficient to prevent toxins, that have been processed by the liver and sent to the intestines, from re-entering the blood. Whole-grains are also rich in vitamins E and B, which keep your nervous system healthy. Brown rice contains methionine, which forms enzymes that fight free radicals.

3   CABBAGE FAMILY:

All members of the cabbage family, especially broccoli, Brussels sprouts and spring and winter greens are rich in chemicals that help the liver break down cancer-causing toxins and pollutants. They are also rich in carotenes, more agents against free radicals. The cabbage family helps prevent osteoporosis, as it is an excellent source of vitamin K, needed for bone formation and repair.

4   OILY FISH:

The omega-3 oils found in oily fish, particularly mackerel, herrings and sardines, may help prevent red blood cells from clumping and blocking blood vessels. Oily fish are also rich in zinc, which helps prevent prostate problems in older men.

5   SOYA BEANS:

Recent research has shown that soya beans contain materials that can be converted by digestion and fermentation to genistein and daidzein, which help prevent breast cancer and prostate cancer and also form a natural hormone-replacement therapy for those in the menopause. Referred to as 'plant oestrogens', they are, in fact, a type of flavonoid which is a good oestrogen balancer. To receive all the benefits soya has to offer, eat tofu, soya yoghurt, soya flour and soya milk, but more especially fermented soya products such as miso and tempeh.

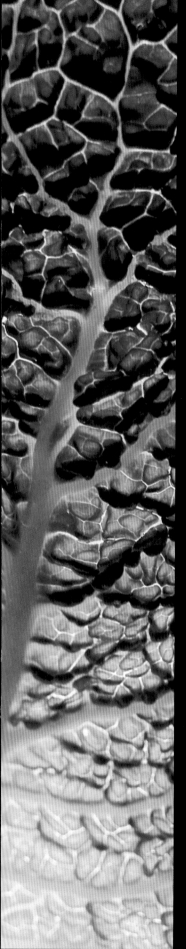

6 BRAZIL NUTS:

Selenium is found in Brazil nuts, which are actually one of the very few good sources of this mineral, needed in the body to make the antioxidant enzyme called glutathione peroxidase, which helps prevent free-radical damage to your cells. Studies continue to show that people who eat selenium-rich food greatly reduce their risk of developing cancer and heart disease. Research also indicates that selenium helps the kidneys to clean toxins from the body more efficiently. Other sources include whole-grain cereals, seafood and seaweed.

7 CELERY JUICE:

Meat eating can cause over-acidity which, can lead to illnesses such as osteoarthritis. Celery juice, made with an extractor or juicer, will help reduce acidity. It is credited with being one of the best treatments for the prevention of osteoarthritis. Drink 1–2 glasses daily, even more if it seems to be helping.

8 SESAME SEEDS:

Although bones obviously need calcium to remain strong and healthy in later life, they also need the osteoporosis-fighting nutrients magnesium and zinc. Sesame seeds are rich in both and contain high levels of calcium. Mix them with other foods or use tahini (sesame seed paste) instead of butter.

9 ORGANIC LIVER:

Liver is rich in vitamin A and zinc, which are both high in the anti-ageing nutrient list and help to prevent hormone deficiencies. Liver also contains folic acid and other B vitamins, which could help prevent heart attacks and Alzheimer's. Furthermore, it contains chromium, which helps keep blood sugar levels down. Not everyone likes to eat liver; those who prefer not to but who are happy to eat meat can buy desiccated liver tablets, though they are quite difficult to find in organic form. Vegetarians need to eat a varied diet and take vitamin A (up to 10,000 i.u.), or safer beta-carotene which is converted to vitamin A (but not readily in diabetics), and mineral supplements. It is not advisable for pregnant women to eat non-organic liver as it has a high retinol content.

10 WATER:

Dehydration affects about 60 per cent of the UK population. Stimulants, such as tea, coffee and alcohol, increase our need for water as they cause dehydration and thus increase the potential of kidney problems and damage. The average adult must drink at least 8 glasses of water daily to flush out toxins, maintain good health and adequate hydration. People who exercise a lot must drink more.

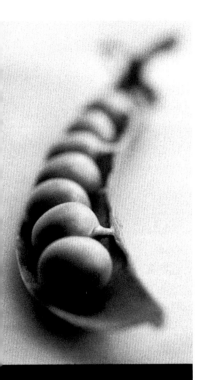

the de-stress diet

Your body/mind needs the appropriate and best-quality fuel to run at optimum performance levels. A poor diet destroys more than our physical health – our mental health and well-being may be totally undermined. The symptoms of deficiency of most nutrients usually show up first in the brain and central nervous system. Your moods, memory, ability to concentrate and make decisions, are all affected by what you eat and drink.

You can also help control and cope with the symptoms of stress by eating regularly a varied, balanced and nourishing diet. In fact, this can do more than de-stress; it can improve your memory and overall mental performance, enhancing your mental well-being, improving your behaviour and moods.

When you are under prolonged stress, your immune system can become depressed along with your mood. You are more prone to digestive problems because the autonomic nervous system, which governs stomach action, is stimulated by anxiety. This triggers the secretion of excess stomach acid juices which can eat away at the stomach's coating, and over time can lead to inflammation and ulcers.

Stress also doubles your risk of catching a cold and other viral infections, as well as triggering all sorts of other health problems, from asthma and eczema to high blood pressure, heart disease and even possibly cancer. You can counteract many of the unhealthy effects of excessive stress by choosing healthy meals and snacks to calm your nerves and increase your vitality.

It's not only what you eat, but how you eat that matters when looking at your diet and how to reduce stress levels through developing balanced and nutritious eating habits. It is well known that it is better to eat little and often than to eat large meals that may overtax an already stressed system, with large spaces between meals, when your blood sugar levels can fall dramatically.

A nutritious diet is the best defence against the destructive effects of stress in a healthy body. Although it is generally considered good advice to avoid eating when you are very angry or rushing around in a stressed state, it is obviously not practical or healthy to diet or eat irregularly when you are under prolonged stress or pressure. During these times, it is especially important to stop what you are doing and allow yourself to relax before eating. Eating wholesome foods that are easy on the digestive system will help you cope with stressful situations while maintaining your health.

Foods rich in the B vitamins, vital to the brain and nervous system's well-being:

Milk and other
   dairy foods
Eggs
Chicken
Beef
Liver
Brewer's yeast
Wheatgerm
Whole-grains
Dark green leafy
   vegetables
Peas
Hazelnuts
White fish

Here are some guidelines for stress-free eating habits:

- Give yourself time off to eat. Acknowledge the importance of nurturing your body and mind by allowing enough time to enjoy each meal.
- Take time to eat, and put some thought into what you eat and the environment in which you eat.
- Don't eat if you are very anxious or angry; wait for the moment to pass.
- Don't bolt your food or eat on the run.
- Eat breakfast. During stressful times it is important to keep your blood sugar level steady to sustain your mental as well as physical energy. Breakfast is an essential high-carbohydrate meal that will set you up for the day and at least keep you going for hours. If you starve yourself in the morning it can play havoc with your blood sugar levels.
- Chew food slowly and well. The mouth is where digestion begins. Good chewing and saliva production help break down and process the food you eat.
- Choose fresh food, preferably home-cooked.
- Eat plenty of whole unprocessed foods, like oats, barley, rice, whole-grain breads and cereals, fresh fruit and vegetables, nuts, seeds, sprouts, dried beans and peas.
- Eat fresh fruit and vegetables every day. Some experts recommend at least five servings a day.
- Don't eat too many high-sugar or fatty manufactured snacks. They have practically no nutritional value and can alter your moods and clog your system.
- Don't add salt to your food. It can stimulate a state of high blood pressure.
- Replace unhealthy salty or sugary snacks, like crisps and sweets, candy, biscuits and cakes, with healthy snacks like sunflower and pumpkin seeds. Mixed seeds provide concentrated nourishment, packed with B-complex vitamins, calcium, iron, zinc and protein. Mixed seeds are ideal for countering irritability, depression and lack of energy. This healthy snack contains important nutrients to help maintain you under pressure. Bananas are another brilliant snack. Whole and nourishing, they are packed with minerals, and are delicious and filling.

The following are considered excellent for protecting you against the ravages of stress:

Apples
Apricots
Asparagus
Avocado
Bananas
Barley
Beetroot
Broccoli
Cabbage
Carrots
Celery
Figs
Grapes
Kiwi fruit
Lettuce
Oats
Oranges
Peaches
Peppers
Raspberries
Spinach
Strawberries
Watercress

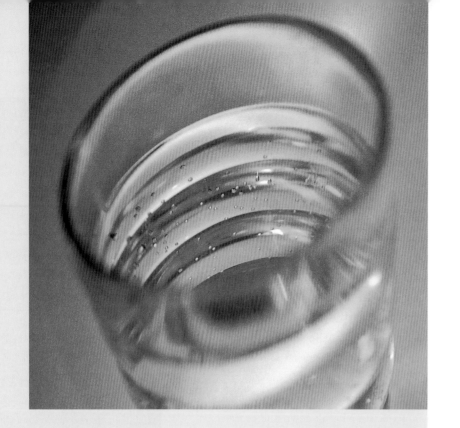

is a good diet enough?

It's not just what you eat that matters for health, but how you eat it. Grabbing snacks at work in a standing position, or sitting in front of the TV, or even on the move can all lead to a build-up of toxins in the body and malabsorption in the digestive system. You may well be eating the healthiest diet possible but your body may just not be assimilating correctly. Poor assimilation of food could be the root of many minor and more serious illnesses from headaches, lethargy, tiredness and weight-gain to irritable bowel syndrome. Sitting down to eat a meal – even if you are alone – and making sure you chew slowly, aids correct absorption.

it's not just what you eat

Good health can be attained by reducing toxicity and maintained by keeping the body free of impurities. Clear systems can have a profound effect on the mind, emotions and spirit – you will lose weight, have glowing skin, more energy, be calmer and more able to concentrate. The following 10 simple steps will encourage you to eat properly and will aid digestion:

1.   Don't eat too much at any one sitting. Eat regularly to avoid getting over-hungry and being tempted to indulge.

2.   Chew food well. Saliva contains predigestive juices – these start the breaking down of starchy food before it even reaches the stomach. Gulping food means it fails to break up properly, is harder to digest and will not be absorbed well.

3.   Drink plenty of water (not with meals, as it dilutes the digestive juices). About 8 glasses per day or 1½ litres (3 pints) is recommended. Fruit juices and herbal teas are also advised, to dilute toxins and expel them through the kidneys more easily.

4.   Eat at least three times as much vegetables as starch or protein.

5.   Never eat in a rush, when angry or upset. Eat calmly.

6.   Avoid processed or convenience foods at all costs.

7.   If you are taking antibiotics, ensure you also take acidophilus tablets at the same time. Antibiotics kill off the benevolent stomach bacteria which aid digestion. Alternatively eat plenty of live bio yoghurt, which will also maintain a level of healthy bacteria.

8.   Try to listen to your body. Keeping your blood sugar level on an even keel throughout the day will ensure that your energy levels are consistent. Are you very tired after eating lunch? You may have a plummeting blood sugar level in this case. Many people find that eating as many as five small meals throughout the day maintains a consistent energy level without causing the familiar after-Sunday-lunch siesta!

9.   Breakfast is a very important meal. The old adage, 'Breakfast like a king, lunch like a prince, dine like a pauper,' is very appropriate! You utilize the energy gained from food throughout the day, so it makes good sense to eat more at breakfast than in the evening, especially if you expect to expend little or no energy after eating. Eating breakfast will kick-start the metabolism into action, otherwise your body will react and go into 'starvation emergency mode' and start to store food rather than process it, encouraging weight-gain.

10. Make food exciting with herbs and spices instead of salt and heavy sauces.

TEN GOOD REASONS TO BUY ORGANIC (FROM THE SOIL ASSOCIATION)

1 Benefit from nutritious and flavoursome foods.
2 No chemicals in your foods.
3 Saving energy and reducing global warming.
4 Helping restore biodiversity.
5 Ensuring water quality.
6 Protecting future generations.
7 Preventing soil erosion.
8 Have an independent guarantee.
9 Helping small farmers.
10 Paying real money for real food.

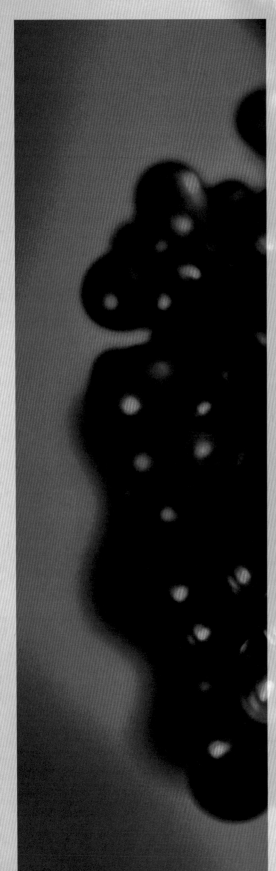

Fasting and cleansing

Fasting is one of the most natural and effective methods of stimulating and regenerating your body's own dynamic healing power. It can help you fight many minor and major ailments and has been employed as a therapeutic treatment for over 2,000 years. Some natural therapy practitioners recommend one 24-hour fast once a month, or every other month, as well as at least one longer fast every year. Only liquids, preferably pure water or freshly pressed vegetable or fruit juice, or a gentle cleansing herb tea, should be ingested in the monthly fast.

If your diet is rich in meat and processed/packaged food you should seriously consider a regular fasting programme. Short-term fasting allows the body to concentrate on cleansing and detoxifying. It can help with obesity, high blood pressure, arthritis, rheumatism, food allergies, eczema and even psychiatric problems like schizophrenia and depression. Short-term fasting is perfectly safe if properly undertaken, but longer-term fasting should be done under professional supervision and at the most appropriate times of the year (not high summer or deep winter).

Cooked foods and protein foods, especially flesh foods, produce more waste matter than raw food and tend to cause a build-up of waste material in the digestive system, particularly the bowel. This can inhibit intestinal absorption of nutrients. If you regularly eat meat, you might consider a longer fast annually or even biannually.

A water fast is not for everyone. If you are suffering from any debilitating illness, then a more nourishing fast would be more appropriate. Seek professional advice.

A popular 3–5-day fast is the white grape fast. Just replace your normal three meals a day with a filling portion of grapes and only drink water. For best results (and least discomfort during the fast), this fast should be preceded and followed by a 1–2-week cleansing diet.

A cleansing diet is made up predominantly of fresh raw foods and juices – vegetables, fruit, salads, seeds and some cooked vegetables – cutting out all fats, meats, sugar and starches. This annual 'spring clean' is actually best done in summer, when we might expect to need less food to keep warm and there's plenty of fresh local food, and we are more relaxed and likely to be outdoors taking the air and sun, as well as gentle exercise like walking.

It is always a good idea to prepare for fasting by eating organically grown vegetables, fruits, seeds, sprouts and pulses for two or more weeks before; and to do the same after you fast, to minimize the discomfort and maximize the healing effect of the fast. Some people experience headaches, nausea, irritability, fatigue and aching muscles while fasting. You may feel cold and lethargic, and alternate from a state of euphoria to exhaustion. Certainly, towards the end of your fast you will experience light-headedness. This is because the body starts quickly to release and eliminate stored toxins that have accumulated over time, which irritate muscles, tissues and nerves.

These reactions should pass after a few hours and it is generally a good idea to rest and drink some water whilst symptoms persist. Be sure to rest a lot when you are fasting, taking only mild regular exercise. Never time a fast during a busy or demanding period.

Some experts recommend starting a fast by taking a heaped teaspoon of Epsom salts in 300ml (1/2pint) of hot water and then drinking a hot cup of herbal tea. This helps purge the bowels and can be repeated at the start of the second day of your fast, together with a 600ml (1 pint) warm-water enema at bedtime. Carbon is strongly attracted to Epsom salts (magnesium sulphate). When taken this way, the salts saturate the lining of the digestive tract and, by osmosis, attract and remove the carbonaceous wastes out of the bloodstream and into the digestive tract – eventually reaching the intestines and being eliminated by the body. If the space around the cells is clogged, then nutrients and oxygen cannot reach the cells and they starve and die. This is why the accumulations of waste matter and impurities is so detrimental to health.

A 'mono-fast', similar to the grape diet outlined on page 80, is also possible – eating just one food type throughout the fasting period. You may choose to eat nothing but apples, which should be peeled, grated and left to turn brown (once oxidized the apple loses its acidity and won't harm the stomach) before eating.

Ideally, all fruit and juices should be organic and water should be pure spring or low in minerals, especially sodium, like Evian, Volvic and Malvern. Alkaline waters, like Vichy, are the most beneficial if they are available. You can increase the effectiveness of your elimination functions during the cleansing period by taking daily doses of 1g of vitamin C and Cynara and extract of globe artichoke. These stimulate the liver and enhance the process.

GUIDELINES FOR FASTING

- Do not fast if you are under a lot of stress.
- Do not fast if you are pregnant.
- Do not fast during a physically demanding or active patch.
- Do not fast if you are ill, unless advised to do so by your doctor and your naturopath.
- Do not fast if you are menstruating or if you are breast-feeding.
- Children should not fast, but a wholesome cleansing diet, rich in organic fruits and vegetables, will always be a good thing to replace all the junk food they love to eat!
- Do not do a water fast if you eat mostly flesh foods and packaged and refined foods. Try a preliminary 2–3 day fast, ingesting only organic fresh-fruit juices and raw vegetable juices, together with your choice of mineral water and cups of herb tea, to which you can add lemon juice and a little honey.
- Do fast only when you have the time and freedom to rest whenever you feel like it.

raw food diets

Sprouts and seeds

These comparatively unrecognized superfoods are wonderfully easy to grow and can help immeasurably on the road to optimum health and well-being. They can be grown in any climate and take only 3-5 days to reach maturity. As they do not require either soil or sunshine, they can be grown indoors by anyone, in any environment. There is no correct growing 'season', as sprouts may be grown any time of the year. Their nutritional value is extraordinary, as they compare favourably to meat and have as much vitamin C as tomatoes for example. As they are a live, raw food that is ingested in its purest state and uncooked, they provide very high levels of nutrients.

Raw sprouts have a regenerative effect on your body and are one of the essential foods in the diet of the Hunzas, Himalayan tribesmen who are renowned for their longevity and vitality. The sprouting seed is a storehouse of food energy, its rich enzyme concentration stimulates a heightened enzyme activity in your metabolism, leading to regeneration of many of your body's processes, particularly your digestive and circulatory systems.

According to nutrition expert, Dr Francis Pottenger Jr from the USA, sprouted legumes and grains contain a complete protein and they are easily and completely

HOW TO SPROUT SEEDS

You can buy sprouting jars and kits or you can make your own using large, tough glass jars or unpainted flowerpots, making a lid with a stainless-steel screen or cheesecloth mesh. Wash the seeds well and soak them overnight in a container of tepid untreated water, preferably distilled or well water.

For the best nutritional value use organically grown seed. Use two parts water to one of seed. Small seeds, like alfalfa, need only to soak for 3-6 hours, while the larger seeds, like chickpea and mung, may be soaked for 15-20 hours. Drain off the water and wash the seed; then drain off the water again. Place your seed container in a warm dark place, preferably between 15-20°C (60-70°F) in temperature.

While your seeds are sprouting, rinse them twice a day in tepid water and drain off, placing the container back in its warm, dark place. Remove the seed hulls that come away from your seeds; they will usually float to the surface of the water for easy removal while you are rinsing your seeds.

assimilated into the body. A seed's vitamin content increases tremendously when sprouted; they are a very good source of the antioxidant vitamins, A, C and E, plus the B vitamins. Sprouted wheat, for instance, is less mucus-forming and more easily digested than wheat prepared in any other way, plus the vitamin E content of the wheat increases 300 per cent after four days of sprouting.

The best seeds for sprouting for good health are: oat, buckwheat, soybean, alfalfa, mung bean, aduki, wheat grass, fenugreek.

The principles of a raw food diet

Avoid meat and fish and any other animal products such as dairy. Advocates of raw food diets vary from athletes to those afflicted with cancer to the overweight. All argue that raw food has put them on the right track to gain strength, stamina and improve recovery rates, or help to cure cancer or lose excess weight. Eating 50 to 100 per cent raw food helps with everything from general day-to-day aches and pains to curing long-standing and chronic conditions.

Olivia Silverwood-Cope, co-director of The Raw Food Centre in Brighton says, 'I've been on a 100 per cent raw food diet for some time and I feel light and energized, lucid and as if my senses are alive. I used to suffer from frequent minor illness, such as cystitis and colds. Now they've disappeared.'

Raw food possesses live vital energy and it is this that our bodies crave. We are used to eating 'dead' foods, foods that are so refined, or cooked until all the natural goodness has been drawn out of them, that we have forgotten what food is supposed to be like and do for us!

Our body's cells must be supplied with food that also possesses live, vital energy. Of course we can survive on cooked and refined foods, but our health will continue to deteriorate, and various degenerative processes will occur, with loss of energy and vitality. It needn't be this way. 'Eating raw foods ensures that you get optimal levels of vitamins, minerals and fibre, easily assimilated proteins and top-quality essential fatty acids,' writes Leslie Kenton in *The Raw Energy Bible*.

She further advises, 'Most of the health-boosting plant ingredients exist in perfect form in raw plants, not in cooked ones. Raw foods also contain a virtually unlimited variety of health-enhancing factors in pristine conditions. These range from the carotenoids (which enhance immune functions) to the powerfully detoxifying isothiocyanates to flavones (which inhibit the spread of cancer and guard against premature ageing).'

Many professional athletes claim their strength and endurance are enormously improved by greatly reducing the presence of cooked foods and greatly increasing the amount of raw food in their diets.

Many are put off the raw food diet by believing they will have to survive on masses of tasteless green leaves, fruit and the odd tomato here and there. This is

FOOD COMBINING

Early this century, William Hay, an American doctor, devised food combining as a means of self-cure. In principle, it means not eating starches and sugars at the same time as proteins and acid fruits, in order to allow the body's own natural curative processes to get to work unhindered. Because it also stresses eating less proteins, starches and fats and much more whole food, especially vegetables and fruits, it is basically a very healthy regime that helps people lose weight and return to good health.

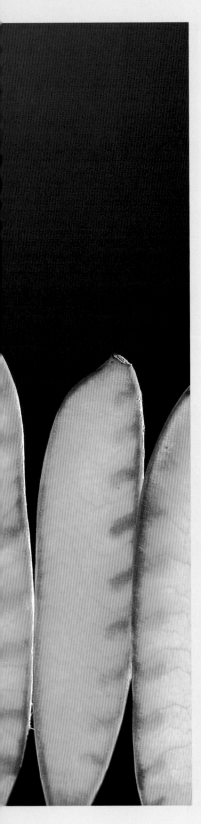

not necessarily the case and, of course, would be unbalanced and detrimental to the body in the long run. Arming yourself with some knowledge of the components of food often helps to awaken you to the potential of raw food dieting. For example, green leafy vegetables contain as much calcium as cheese; fruits provide carbohydrates; fatty plant foods provide calories; nuts and seeds contain essential fats and protein.

Raw food diets used for fasting, for example, can be wonderfully beneficial in clearing out toxins from the body and increasing the efficiency of the body's organs. However, long-term 100 per cent raw food diets, according to Catherine Reynolds of the Institute of Food Research in Norwich, are '… not healthy, nor balanced. You need to get food from a variety of sources and eating this way stops you doing so.' Reynolds believes a raw diet would turn into an unhealthy obsession rather than a normal part of life.

Tom Billings, ex-raw fooder and US editor of the web site 'Beyond Vegetarianism' says, 'I lived for a while on fresh foods of superior quality, but I experienced serious health problems.' He goes on to say 100 per cent raw food diets seem to boost energy and make you feel good in the short term, but have a dismal record of failure in the long run. He accuses many raw-food gurus of making 'simplistic and over-idealistic claims' about its powers.

Generally it is accepted that increasing your intake of raw food to about 50–70 per cent daily intake is wonderfully beneficial. It is all a matter of personal choice, and learning what suits your body best is imperative. It is widely accepted that those of us living in the colder climates of the Northern hemisphere cannot live on raw food alone. We need hot, cooked foods to provide energy and warmth in the cold winter months. In the hotter months of summer, plenty of cooling foods such as salads and green vegetables are a wonderful tonic for the body and for your health generally.

Eating plenty of citrus fruit for some is the be-all-and-end-all of cleansing and an integral part of their daily diet, but for others citrus means internal discomfort and eliminations. It really is all about what suits you best according to the climate you live in and your body type.

At the end of a long winter, eating lots of meat and heavy meals, and getting less exercise than usual, your body can feel run down and sluggish. You may be suffering from constipation, other bowel conditions, skin problems like rashes, spots or more serious conditions like eczema or acne, or just have a dull lifeless complexion needing some nourishment and a breath of fresh air!

There are any number of persistent small symptoms like bad breath, cellulite and smelly feet that suggest we have an overload of toxins in our body. It is unfortunately all too easy to pollute ourselves, creating a toxic inner environment that we are not even aware of until the damage manifests itself.

detox - a spring clean for the body

Many experts believe that excessive toxicity of the body creates all manner of serious illnesses, from osteoarthritis (where toxins settle in the joints), to heart disease, cancer and diabetes. To prevent such illness you need to be in tune with your body, aware of its condition and its needs, and be committed to giving yourself a good, thorough internal spring-clean at least once a year. At that time, also, implement the good eating and exercise habits that will help prevent the build-up of a toxic state again. A spring-clean for the body is an essential part of any preventative system of health care.

Spring is a time of rebirth and renewal – what better time to put into action a detoxifying programme to revitalize and strengthen your body. Give your energy levels the boost only a clean, toxin-free body can achieve. To restore the balance it is essential to flush out the toxic substances that have built up in the main organs responsible for cleansing the body – the intestines, liver, kidneys, gallbladder, spleen and skin.

The ideal way to start a detox programme is to begin with a 24-hour fast, if you feel up to it and are not on any medication. Seek your doctor's or nutritionist's advice if you are unsure. Choose a day when it is not necessary to be very active – preferably a day when you are not physically challenged. You also need to drink lots of fluid during a fast, as dehydration must never be allowed, but drink only water or hot water and fresh lemon juice. To aid inner cleansing, a very good health habit is to both begin and end the day with a drink of hot water and fresh lemon juice. This has a cleansing effect on the liver and kidneys, as well as the rest of the digestive system.

After the first stage in your detox programme, your 24-hour fast, the idea is to eat as much raw food as possible for the rest of the week. Raw fruit and vegetables are not only the easiest food for our body to digest, and the means of getting the most nutrition from food, but they also have a brilliant cleansing effect on the body. Cooked food is more complicated for the digestive system; uncooked food enhances the metabolism and strengthens the immune system. Instead of a slow sluggish constitution, the body finds its best level for peak performance.

Eucalyptus is a fantastic herb and folk remedy to use as an antiseptic and decongestant, and has excellent detoxifying properties. Eucalyptus stimulates the circulatory system and is diaphoretic (causing you to sweat), which greatly aids your body in getting rid of toxins. Tea made from eucalyptus leaves can benefit your health by increasing blood-flow to the skin, encouraging sweating and a detoxifying action.

The high fibre content of fruits and vegetables is excellent for flushing toxic residues out of the body. If you try this approach, you will see an improvement in your overall health, with many minor niggling symptoms disappearing altogether. Whether you suffer from skin rashes, headaches or heart disease, you owe it to yourself to build your body with the right materials.

Try to buy produce that is as fresh as you can get it and buy organic fruit and veg where possible, as they obviously have fewer toxins. A good greengrocer will usually have much fresher fruits and vegetables than the large supermarket chains. The fresher the food, the higher the nutritional value. Fresh herbs are also full of healthful properties, so use them liberally. The ideal, of course, is to grow your own herbs and vegetables, but this is not possible for most of us.

We are lucky to have such a wide range of available food from all over the world. However, the mainstay of your diet should be fresh food from close to home and in season. At least, this is the purist's view. Do remember, though, that rules are made to be broken. For example, many exotic tropical fruits contain enzymes that have an excellent effect on the digestive system.

When you do cook your vegetables, remember that many vitamins and minerals are destroyed by the heat in cooking. When we boil vegetables, the nutrients are leached out into the water and poured away down the drain! So, whenever possible, gently steam or stir-fry vegetables for just a few minutes instead, until they are tender – but only just – to preserve their nutritious goodness. Also aim to eat a good variety of fruits, salad and other vegetables every day.

detox action plan

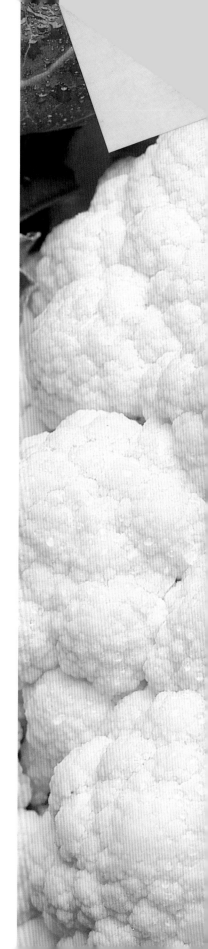

- Begin your detox at the weekend or during a time when you don't have too much going on.
- Walk for at least 15 minutes every day.
- Drink at least 2 litres (3½ pints) of water a day – purified, distilled, filtered or bottled. You can also drink dandelion coffee or herb teas.
- Have ⅓ litre (½ pint) of fruit or vegetable juice – either carrot and apple juice (you can buy these two separately and combine with one-third water) with grated ginger, or fresh watermelon juice – a day. The flesh of the watermelon is high in beta-carotene and vitamin C. The seeds are high in vitamin E, as well as the antioxidant minerals zinc and selenium. You can make a great antioxidant cocktail by blending fresh fruit and seeds in a blender into a great-tasting drink.
- **Eat in abundance:** Fruit – the most beneficial fruits with the highest detox potential include fresh apricots, all berries, cantaloupe melons, citrus fruits, kiwis, papayas, peaches, mangoes, melons, red grapes. Vegetables – especially good are artichokes, peppers, beetroot, Brussels sprouts, broccoli, red cabbage, carrots, cauliflower, cucumber, kale, pumpkin, spinach, sweet potato, tomatoes, watercress and beansprouts.
- **Eat in moderation:** Grains – brown rice, corn, millet, quinoa – not more than twice a day.
  Fish – salmon, mackerel, sardines, tuna – not more than once a day.
  Oils – use extra-virgin olive oil for cooking and in place of butter, and cold-pressed seed oils for dressings.
  Nuts and seeds – a handful a day of raw, unsalted nuts and seeds should be included. Choose from almonds, Brazil nuts, hazelnuts, pecans, pumpkin seeds, sunflower seeds, sesame seeds and flax seeds (linseeds).
- **Avoid:** All wheat products, all meat and dairy produce (including eggs), salt and any food containing it, hydrogenated (trans) fats (most margarines and spreads), artificial sweeteners, food additives and preservatives, fried foods, spices, dried fruit. Limit potatoes to one portion every other day and bananas to one every other day.
- Don't be surprised if you feel worse for a couple of days before you start to feel better. This is especially likely if you are eliminating foods to which you are allergic or on which you are dependent.
- Take a double dose daily of quality multivitamin/mineral supplements, plus two 1,000 mg vitamin C capsules and antioxidant complex.

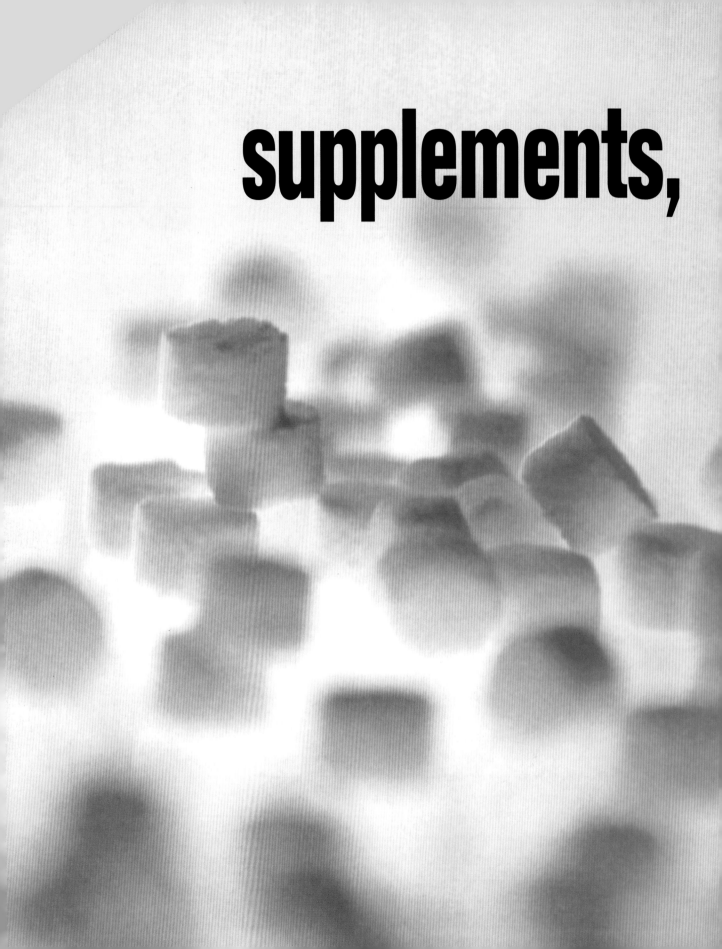

supplements,

herbs & tonics

Although healthy eating is essential to our well-being, there are often times when it is just not enough and we do have to boost our intake of nutrients from non-food sources. We should be able to get all we need from a balanced diet, rich in whole grains, fruit and vegetables, but many leading nutritionists believe that, as modern life is so demanding and stressful and our food and environment so polluted, nutritional supplementation is an essential part of healthy living. Also in many vitamins, herbs and natural tonics we have an amazing treasury of totally natural preventative medicines that we can use to fend off everything from colds and 'flu to heart disease and cancer, as well as help us boost our immune system, deal with stress and generally improve our frame of mind.

In this section, we take a detailed look at each of the vitamins and minerals, as well as the more important herbal tisanes, Chinese herbs and tonics, and the many other tonics and elixirs available, both those that have been around for centuries and some more recent discoveries.

supplements
vitamins
minerals
herbs
herbal tisanes
borage
camomile
dandelion
elderflower
fennel
lemon balm
lemon verbena
marjoram
parsley
peppermint
rosemary
sage
thyme
chinese herbs
tonics and elixirs
acidophilus
agnus castus
alfalfa
aloe vera juice
black cohosh
cat's claw
catuaba
chlorella
cider vinegar
citricidal
clary sage
cod liver oil

vitamins

supplements

What role do vitamins and minerals play in our lives? How and why are they so important that our total well-being is dependent on a sufficient daily intake of these nutrients? How do we achieve a way of eating that ensures our intake of vitamins and minerals meets the RDA or Recommended Daily Amount?

In order to prevent nutritional deficiency diseases like scurvy, governments set levels of RDAs that can vary widely from country to country. RDAs are not designed to create optimum health – they are designed to impart information for the prevention of nutrient deficiency and the many diseases that result.

It is much more difficult than we realize to eat a diet that meets the RDA levels. Even when we are very conscientious about eating a well-balanced diet, we can fall well short of the mark. One survey (The Bateman Report, 1985) found that more than 85 per cent of people who believed their diet was well-balanced failed to meet RDA levels.

Some nutritionists are concerned with the low RDA levels, believing they would not be high enough even if they were doubled. In the last decade, RDAs were mostly replaced by DRVs (Dietary Reference Values) in the UK. The practical part of DRVs are the Reference Nutrient Intakes (RNIs). These are the amounts that should be enough for 95 per cent of the population according to experts in the field. To complicate matters further, European government laws increasingly require labels on products to display EC RDAs.

Founder of The Institute for Optimum Nutrition in London, Patrick Holford, a leading nutrition expert and educator in the UK, does not believe it is possible to meet individual needs if we use RDAs and RNIs as guidelines. He is in agreement with the view held by medical researcher Dr Stephen Davies, who tested thousands of people to measure levels of vitamin B in their blood. He

WHEN TO TAKE SUPPLEMENTS

The best time to take most supplements is with the first meal of the day or just after it. If you have difficulty sleeping, don't take B vitamins late at night. However, taking some minerals, particularly calcium and magnesium, in the evening can aid sleep.

SUGGESTED OPTIMAL VITAMIN ALLOWANCES COMPARED TO EC RDAS

	EC RDA Male/Female	SUGGESTED OPTIMAL INTAKE age 25–50	51+
Vitamin A (retinol)	800 µg (micrograms)	2,000 µg	2,000 µg
Vitamin C	60 mg (milligrams)	400 mg	800/1,000 mg
Vitamin E	10 mg	400 mg	800 mg
Vitamin B1 (thiamine)	1.4 mg	7.5/7.1 mg	9.2/9.0 mg
Vitamin B2 (riboflavin)	1.6 mg	2.5/2 mg	2.5/2 mg
Vitamin B3 (niacin)	18 mg	30/25 mg	30/25 mg
Vitamin B6 (pyridoxine)	2 mg	10 mg	25/20 mg
Vitamin B12	1 µg	2 µg	3/2 µg
Folic acid	200 mg	800 µg	1,000 µg
Biotin	150 µg	150–500 µg	150–500 µg

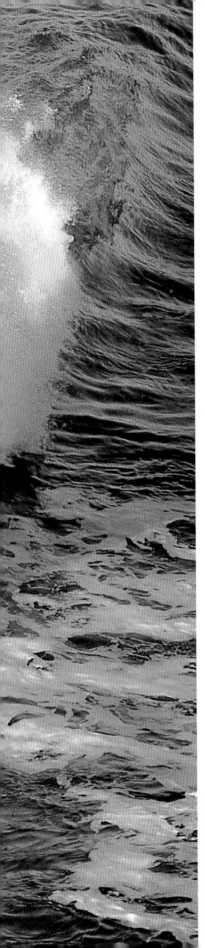

found more than seven in every ten to be deficient. If you drink alcohol, smoke heavily, live in the centre of a polluted city or are pregnant, pre-menstrual, on the pill or menopausal, or just simply in a particularly stressful patch, your nutritional needs can easily double.

During the spring of '95, The Institute of Optimum Nutrition hosted a debate on 'What is Optimum?' One of the guests was Dr Emanuel Cheraskin from the University of Alabama, USA, which was part of an international think tank on the subject.

Over a 15-year period, he and his researchers carried out in-depth studies of the health of 13,500 people living in six different parts of America. They found the intake of nutrients associated with optimum health was many times higher than RDA levels. The people who were the healthiest were eating a nutritionally rich diet and taking vitamin and mineral supplements that far exceeded the RDAs.

Dr Cheraskin and his colleagues have so much evidence to date that they have established new guidelines, called SONAs (Suggested Optimal Nutrient Allowances), to promote the idea of achieving and maintaining optimal health, rather than intake levels that suggest we will not get a deficiency disease but that not much else will be achieved either.

Recent research confirms the view that vitamins and minerals play a very important role in making and keeping us healthy. There are, however, two quite contradictory schools of thought concerning the intake of nutrients. What is the best way to ensure we meet our individual vitamin and mineral requirements? One school believes that if we eat a balanced nutritious diet we don't need to take supplements, and in some cases too much of a good thing is bad and even dangerous.

Synthetic vitamins and minerals are considered useless – or worse, toxic – by some nutritional therapists, who advise that natural organic supplements are the only ones to consider. Of course, the purists believe even these are quite worthless and harmful, that fresh raw fruits and vegetables contain most of all our nutritional requirements in their most healthy, accessible state. (Remember, boiling and soaking food considerably reduces the mineral and vitamin content.)

Mother nature, of course, did not intend to nourish our bodies with man-made supplements alone, but largely with delicious fruits and vegetables that are full of natural water, cleansing the insides at the same time. Foods with a high content of water can catalyse this 'inner bath' so necessary to our well-being. Our bodies are made up of at least 70 per cent water and obviously we need to replenish our supplies regularly.

Water, food and air are absolutely vital for our survival and our optimum well-being.

Moreover, in just the last few years, research has started to catalogue a whole new level of 'micronutrients' present in fruit and vegetables, that have a wide range of powers to combat disease. Among these phytochemicals are the organosulphides present in such high quantities in the onion and garlic family and the glucosinolates found in broccoli and other greens, which stimulate the immune system and help fight cancer and heart disease. It is the rich content of such chemicals that has led to some produce being termed 'superfoods'. Most of the benefits offered by such 'micronutrients' will not, of course, be obtained by supplementation.

The other school of thought believes that because so many people live at a very fast pace, with a lot of stress and little access to fresh fruit and vegetables and also perhaps drink alcohol or smoke etc., our nutrient needs double. Environmental pollution, sick buildings, whether we are male or female, young or old, all these factors and more influence our individual vitamin and mineral requirements.

There is a consensus of belief in one area only – the only one where all the experts agree – eating more fresh, raw and organic (pesticide-free) fruits and vegetables is a great booster to better health and a real sense of well-being.

TOP 10 SUPERFOODS

Almonds
Apples
Apricots
Avocado Pears
Bananas
Beetroot
Berries
Broccoli
Cabbage
Carrots

OTHERS TO EAT REGULARLY

Grapes
Melons
Oats
Oily fish, like sardines, herring, mackerel, salmon
Olive oil
Pineapples
Soya beans
Watercress

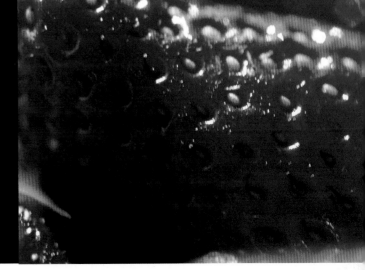

Vitamin A

Vitamin A is very important for good vision, skin and hair. It helps maintain healthy tissues throughout the body, including the skin and retina, and is important in the formation of strong teeth and bones. Because vitamin A is fat soluble, excesses are stored in the liver, where it can build to toxic levels. Therefore, it is important not to take too much of this vitamin.

Safe daily regular intakes should not exceed 7,500 µg for women (25,000i.u.) and 9,000 µg for men (30,000i.u.). Pregnant women should not exceed 3,000 µg (10,000i.u.) and consult their doctor before taking supplements or dramatically changing their diet. Recommended daily intake for infants and children is 350 µg (1,167i.u.) to 900 µg (3,000 i.u.), depending on age and state of health.

Deficiency signs: mouth ulcers, poor night vision, acne, frequent infections, dry flaky skin, dandruff, thrush/cystitis, diarrhoea.

Food sources: animal livers, dairy products, vegetables – spinach, broccoli, lettuce, asparagus, squash, pumpkin, tomatoes, carrots, peppers and sweet potatoes – fish oils, eggs, melons and mangoes.

Beta-carotene

This is an important nutrient with antioxidant properties that inhibit the activity of 'free radicals' in the body. It is also thought to help reduce the risk of cancer and heart disease, and is easily converted by the body into vitamin A (see above).

Food sources: fruit – particularly yellow- and orange-fleshed varieties – and dark green vegetables.

Vitamin B1 (Thiamine)

B1 is crucial in the digestion and metabolism of fat and carbohydrates in food, and helps to maintain the healthy function of the nervous system. Because it is needed to burn calories, the amount you need depends on the amount of carbohydrates you eat.

Deficiency signs: this is the vitamin that prevents beriberi. Thiamine deficiency can be very serious and is linked to depression, sleep disturbances, irritability, chronic fatigue, confusion and poor memory, eye pains, stomach pains and constipation, anaemia, impaired immune system, water retention, tender muscles and even heart failure and lung damage. A principal cause of deficiency is alcoholism, as Vitamin B1 is destroyed by alcohol. It also is most readily attacked by environmental conditions.

Food sources: wheatgerm, soya beans, nuts, brown rice, whole-grains, wholemeal pasta, bran, pumpernickel bread, lean pork, liver, brewer's yeast, potatoes, milk, eggs, orange and grapefruit juice.

Vitamin B2 (Riboflavin)

One of riboflavin's most important contributions is to enzyme activity controlling chemical reactions within the body, including digestion, energy release and the synthesis of fatty and amino acids. Riboflavin forms the essential co-enzymes for converting nutrients into energy and helps cell growth. It factors into the maintenance of healthy eyes, mouth and skin, and can be an effective treatment for migraine. The action of the adrenal glands is influenced by riboflavin levels. It is not easy to overdose on riboflavin, but excess will turn urine bright yellow.

Deficiency signs: may manifest in or around the mouth, in sore tongue or cracked lips, sometimes lesions of the skin, mouth and genitals. Burning, itchy eyes, blurred vision, sensitivity to bright light, even cataracts, have been associated with deficiency, as have dull or oily hair, eczema, dermatitis or split nails.

Food sources: mostly meat, dairy products, bread and cereals, breakfast cereals, cheese, eggs, liver, kidneys, almonds, green vegetables and avocados.

GUIDELINES FOR VATA TYPES (see pages 11-15)

Vatas have a need for all antioxidants, especially vitamin C and beta-carotene. They also benefit from nervous system regulators, like vitamins B5 and B6, and the minerals calcium and magnesium, which are all excellent for stress.

Vitamin B3 (Niacin)

Together with thiamine and riboflavin, niacin is a pivotal factor in the release of energy from carbohydrates.

Too much of this vitamin can cause liver damage. Niacin has been successfully used to improve blood cholesterol status by raising 'good' cholesterol, HDL (see pages 40–41). However, the doses required are 'mega doses' and you need to be under the supervision of a doctor or nutritionist to use this supplement in this way.

Deficiency signs: long-standing deficiency can lead to pellagra, a very serious and ultimately fatal illness, the symptoms of which are all sorts of mental conditions, from depression, anxiety, confusion, hallucination and memory loss to dementia, along with serious dermatitis, diarrhoea and vomiting leading to emaciation. More minor deficiencies show symptoms of depression, exhaustion and a dulled memory, as well as insomnia, headaches, bleeding or tender gums, acne, eczema and dermatitis. Those who drink too much alcohol are commonly deficient in niacin as well as other vital B vitamins.

Food sources: poultry (chicken and turkey), fish (particularly salmon, tuna and halibut), oysters, lean red meat, liver, eggs, nuts, seeds, wholemeal bread.

Vitamin B5 (Pantothenic acid)

It is virtually impossible to be deficient in vitamin B5 because it is found in such a wide variety of foods and is essential to so many vital bodily processes. It is converted into the co-enzyme A, which plays a major part in the metabolism of nutrients in food and, therefore, in the release of energy. It also affects the functioning of the adrenal glands and helps in the formation of antibodies.

Large quantities are required to repair tissue damage. As a supplement, B5 is often called calcium pantothenate.

Deficiency signs: symptoms of fatigue, muscle tremors and weakness, apathy, poor concentration, propensity to get headaches, dizzy spells and an upset digestive system. Burning feet or tender heels, nausea or vomiting and teeth grinding may also be exhibited.

Food sources: brewer's yeast, eggs, poultry and meat (particularly liver), lobster, peanuts, wheat bran and wheatgerm.

Supplement: 3–7 mg daily is sufficient, but perhaps more if you eat lots of protein.

Vitamin B6 (Pyridoxine)

B6 is readily converted into co-enzymes that are crucial to a variety of metabolic processes. It aids the action of the many neurotransmitters that directly affect the brain, assists in the absorption of several minerals, helps to break down proteins and fats in food and affects hormone production. This versatile vitamin also helps to manufacture red blood cells. Research is being done into this vitamin's value in treating asthma, cancer and heart disease. Many women are successfully treated for PMS (pre-menstrual syndrome) with this or the entire B complex. Diabetes and food intolerance may respond well to pyridoxine therapy.

Exceedingly high doses of B6, above 500 mg, may result in nerve damage, so it is safer to seek a doctor's advice when considering B6 therapy. The general rule is not to take more than 100 mg per day. The amount of B6 you need daily is

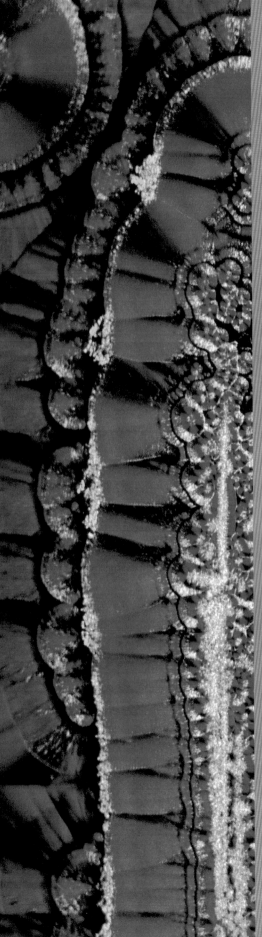

relative to your protein intake.

Deficiency signs: water retention, tingling hands, depression or nervousness, irritability, muscle tremors or cramps, lack of energy, flaky skin.

Food sources: nuts, cereals, grains, pulses, white meat/fish, beef, bananas, broccoli, peas, beans, cauliflower and wheatgerm.

Vitamin B12

This vitamin plays a key role in cell production and protection, particularly red blood cells, and in maintaining a healthy nervous system. Most water-soluble vitamins are not stored in the body, but B12 – also known as cobalamin because it contains cobalt – is stored in body tissues, so a deficiency may take a long time to show up. When it does, it can result in anaemia. It helps to synthesize DNA, to metabolize fatty acids and works with folic acid to control an amino acid that, in excess, can create the conditions for heart disease. We cannot manufacture it, so we must have it in our diet.

Deficiency signs: symptoms are pernicious anaemia and menstrual problems. A vitamin B12 deficiency can be difficult to detect and care should be taken not to let it go on for too long, to ensure your neurological health. Signs include poor hair condition, eczema or dermatitis, mouth over-sensitive to heat or cold, irritability, anxiety or tension, lack of energy, constipation, sore or tender muscles, pale skin. Vegans and those who drink a lot of alcohol are at risk.

Food sources: lean red meat, particularly liver and kidneys, fish and shellfish, brewer's yeast, eggs and cheese.

Folic acid

Essential for blood-cell formation and cell division, this B complex vitamin helps to maintain a healthy nervous system. It is an important growth nutrient and is thought to be particularly crucial in the pre-conception and early pregnancy stages to help prevent spina bifida and birth defects. It also helps the body manufacture the iron-carrying component in blood and to synthesize nucleic acid. Alcoholics benefit from a folic acid supplement (or B complex with folic acid) as they tend to have depleted levels. 200 μg a day is recommended for men and women, 400 for pregnancy and during breast-feeding.

Food sources: beans, wheatgerm, yeast, green leafy vegetables like spinach, citrus fruit, watercress, cereals, wholemeal and wholewheat bread, poultry.

PABA (Para-aminobenzoic acid)

PABA is a component of folic acid, rather than a vitamin in its own right. It has antioxidant and skin protection properties, and helps to produce red blood cells and to metabolize amino acids. High doses, under professional care, are used to treat some serious skin disorders like vitiligo, a condition where there is skin depigmentation, lupus and scleroderma, in which the skin thins. Because of its ability to protect the skin, PABA is a common ingredient in sunscreen. It is best to take PABA in a B-complex supplement, rather than on its own.

Food sources: wheatgerm, whole-grains and bran, molasses, eggs, kidney and liver.

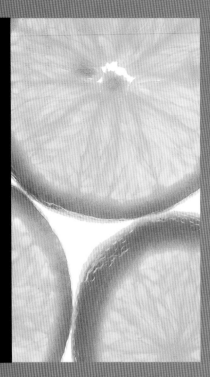

- Aspirin increases the need for vitamin C.
- Paracetamol increases the need for antioxidants, like vitamins C and E and selenium.
- Antibiotics increase the need for B vitamins and beneficial bacteria.
- HRT and birth control pills increase the need for vitamins B6, B12, folic acid and zinc.

Biotin

Biotin is the last in the B complex group and is an essential acid for growth and general well-being. It aids in several important bodily processes, including the metabolism of carbohydrates and the formation of fat, as well as helping the body use carbon dioxide. Biotin is thought to help prevent *Candida albicans* from developing into its fungal form, which then becomes much harder to treat.

Deficiency signs: can lead to a scaly dermatitis, other skin conditions and premature greying or hair loss, particularly in babies. Extreme deficiencies are very rare, but may manifest in depression, hallucination, anorexia and nausea.

Food sources: egg yolk, kidney, liver, bran, chicken, brewer's yeast, wheatgerm.

Vitamin C (Ascorbic acid)

This vitamin is a carbohydrate-like substance that aids various metabolic processes around the body, such as the release of hormones from the adrenal gland, the maintenance of cell-structure strength and the metabolism of several amino acids, including folic acid. It is perhaps best known for its role in maintaining an efficient immune system, as it is a powerful antioxidant; many people take vitamin C supplements to protect against, and reduce the severity of, colds and 'flus and to fight the effects of free radicals, which attack healthy cells and are thought to be a contributing factor in many serious degenerative conditions, including heart disease and cancer. Breast cancer research shows that women with diets rich in vitamin C are least at risk.

Vitamin C helps maintain the skin as it is important in the formation of collagen (cellular glue), and for tissue repair, growth and for the healing of wounds. It helps your body absorb iron and aids energy release, and even helps your breathing and heartbeat.

As this is a water-soluble vitamin and the body cannot manufacture or store it, it needs to be taken daily, preferably as citrus fruits, green leafy vegetables, tomatoes and peppers. It is also very unstable and easily destroyed by water, heat and air and cooking. Smokers need more vitamin C, too, as one cigarette can use up about 25 mg!

It is accepted that, as well as smoking, alcohol, stress and antibiotics also deplete the body's vitamin C and that, as explained, during times of illness your levels are considerably reduced. There is good evidence that large doses of vitamin C, 1,000 mg and above, help prevent the common cold.

Deficiency signs: include frequent colds or infections, scurvy, slow wound healing, red pimples, bleeding, inflamed gums, loose teeth, bruising and nose bleeds, general weakness, irritability, chronic fatigue and muscle and joint ache.

Food sources: fruit, particularly citrus, strawberries, nectarines, mangoes and blackcurrants, and raw vegetables, especially peppers, broccoli and greens.

Vitamin D (Calciferol)

This vitamin is converted in the body into a hormone that controls calcium and phosphorus metabolism, particularly important for the teeth and bones. Vitamin D is formed in the skin when exposed to sunlight and it is particularly important for children, who need more for proper growth.

Deficiency signs: hair loss, tooth decay, skeletal deformity, painful bones/joints and muscle cramps and weakness, tenderness in the pelvis, spine, shoulders and ribs. Those at risk are usually house-bound or vegan.

Food sources: dairy products, eggs and fish and fish oils (especially cod liver oil).

Vitamin E (Tocopherol)

The fat-soluble vitamin E is a powerful antioxidant and is believed to slow down the ageing process in cells. It helps repair the skin, as well as promote growth and formation of new blood cells. Vitamin E also works to prevent nerve and muscle degeneration, promotes healing and combats atherosclerosis and thrombosis. Other conditions it is said to help prevent include: cancer, cataracts, circulatory problems, fibrocystic breast disease, heart disease, Parkinson's disease and PMS (with evening primrose oil).

Deficiency signs: lack of sex drive, easy bruising, slow wound healing, varicose veins, loss of muscle tone, infertility.

Food sources: corn oils, sunflower seeds, peanuts and peanut butter, almonds, wheatgerm, whole-grain cereals, leafy vegetables, asparagus.

Vitamin K

Vitamin K helps to manufacture the coagulant proteins the body needs for proper clotting of the blood. It is also required for the proper laying down of bone. Digestive bacteria synthesize around half the needed amount.

Deficiency signs: may manifest in nosebleeds or excessive bleeding.

Food sources: some green, leafy vegetables: sprouts, cabbage and spinach, liver.

Bioflavonoids (Vitamin P)

These are a large group of antioxidants that help the body assimilate vitamin C, strengthen capillaries and speed up the healing of wounds, sprains and muscle injuries. Some flavonoids are now credited with strong properties against cancer and heart disease. The body is robbed of these 'semi-essential' nutrients by free radicals, and the best supplements for it are rosehip extract, citrus bioflavonoids and berry extracts.

Deficiency signs: bruising easily, frequent muscle pain/sprain, varicose veins.

Food sources: berries, cherries and citrus.

Inositol

The brain and spinal cord need this 'semi-essential' nutrient. It is needed for cell growth and for the formation of nerve sheaths, and helps to reduce cholesterol and maintain healthy hair. Lecithin and brewer's yeast are the best sources.

Food sources: eggs, fish, liver, pulses, nuts, wheatgerm, melons and citrus fruits.

Choline

This component of lecithin helps break down fat in the liver, aids movement of fat into cells and the synthesis of cell membranes in the nervous system, and also helps protect the lungs.

Food sources: eggs, fish, lecithin, liver, nuts, pulses, whole-grains, soya beans, peanuts, wheatgerm and citrus fruits.

minerals

Minute but mighty, the tiny elusive mineral plays a big part in good health. A natural substance, minerals are inorganic. Many are actually elements, the basic building blocks of all matter. The amount of minerals you need may be small, but their influence on your well-being is huge – about 1 per cent of our total nutritional needs is for minerals – but without them we wouldn't last long!

Minerals not only help the body to perform some crucial functions, but also contribute to general well-being and help prevent the onset of disease. Recent research suggests the role of minerals in your continued well-being is crucial and often underestimated. Minerals come to us from the earth's crust and it is its erosion over time that results in minerals seeping into the sea, soil and groundwater, which is how they are absorbed into the fruits, vegetables and grains that we eat. Your body needs minerals to efficiently absorb and utilize vitamins, enzymes and amino acids, as well as to build healthy new cells.

Many experts believe that mineral deficiencies that cause cell breakdown, resulting in weak and vulnerable cells, may cause degenerative disease. Every day we lose millions of cells and to stay healthy we must replace them. Your body can only do that efficiently if it contains the right mineral balance. Minerals play a major part in every internal function and are found in every part of your body, from blood to bones to brain, and are crucial to your ability to keep well and prevent illness.

There are more than 50 minerals commonly in the body, but only 22 are considered essential. Of these, seven (calcium, chlorine as chloride, magnesium, phosphorus, potassium, sodium and sulphur) are major minerals of which you need a substantial amount on a daily level to maintain healthy body functioning. The other 15 'trace minerals', or 'trace elements', so named because you need only tiny amounts or traces of them, are also extremely important on a daily level and are crucial for the absorption of the major minerals, as well as the vitamins, amino acids and enzymes.

In an ideal world it should be possible to get all your mineral requirements by eating a diet rich in vegetables, fruits and grains, meat and fish. Unfortunately, the soil that produces much of the produce we eat is undernourished and over-farmed and therefore not as mineral-rich as it probably was in the past. So, depending on your circumstances, even if you eat a brilliant diet, if it is from a poor or polluted soil area you may still need a mineral supplement. (Also, remember, boiling and soaking food considerably reduces the mineral and vitamin content.) It should be OK to take a multi-mineral supplement made by a reputable manufacturer, but ask your doctor or nutritionist for help if you feel you need some advice, particularly if you have special health needs or are taking medication.

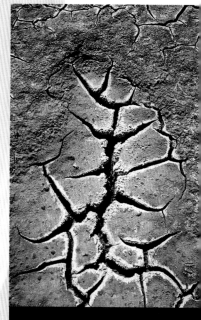

SOME SYMPTOMS OF MINERAL DEFICIENCY

- dull, dry and lifeless hair and skin
- weak teeth prone to cavities
- brittle and easily broken finger nails
- very pale (not pink) tongue
- slow-to-heal bruises and cuts
- chronic fatigue
- muscle cramps
- premature ageing and menopause
- depressed immune system
- PMS
- painful and exhausting periods

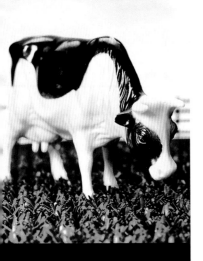

SUPPLEMENTS AGAINST OSTEOPOROSIS

Calcium and magnesium are vital in maintaining bone density.

Other bone-building nutrients include vitamin D, vitamin C, vitamin K, boron, phosphorous, silica and zinc.

Natural progesterone cream has proved four times more effective than synthetic oestrogen HRT in restoring bone density.

Calcium

Calcium is both the most abundant mineral in the body and the mineral most likely to be deficient. Calcium is crucial for building strength and density in the bones and teeth – 99 per cent of the body's calcium is held there. The rest of the calcium supply circulates in the blood and plays a role in some important bodily processes, including blood clotting, nerve impulse transmission and heartbeat regulation. Malabsorption of calcium resulting from a vitamin D deficiency can lead to rickets – softening of growing bone. Long-term calcium deficiency can also place women at risk of osteoporosis (loss of bone density, making bones easy to break and fracture). Although calcium-rich foods are abundant, supplements are often recommended. Calcium helps the metabolism of iron and, in combination with magnesium, aids muscle movement.

This essential mineral is also known to protect the body from the effects of pollution and the presence of damaging heavy metals such as lead and cadmium. When combined with potassium and magnesium, it helps to lower blood pressure and cholesterol levels and protects against intestinal cancer.

Depleted calcium levels are a characteristic of several very serious conditions, osteoporosis in particular, which causes a loss of bone density, making bones weak and prone to fracture. Over 2 million people – mainly women – in the UK alone suffer from osteoporosis, resulting in 40 premature deaths a day. The UK National Osteoporosis Society recommends an intake of 1,500 mg calcium each day for women over 45 years old.

Deficiency signs: calcium deficiency may manifest in PMS, severe period cramps, depression, irritability, insomnia, nervousness, muscle ache, cramps or tremors, arthritis, stiff joints, high blood pressure, bloating, fluid retention, bowel sensitivity and irregularity; in extreme deficiency, rickets and malformed bones.

Food sources: dairy products – milk (and powdered milk), cheese and yoghurt; leafy green vegetables, like broccoli, spinach and cabbage; root vegetables, e.g. pumpkin; seeds, including sesame, sunflower and pumpkin; salmon and sardines (with bones); tofu.

Supplement dose: 500 mg calcium; 250 mg magnesium.

Chlorine as chloride

Chloride works with potassium to normalize water and sodium levels in the cells, and is a factor in breathing and digestion. It also helps form healthy hair and teeth.

Deficiency signs: difficult digestion, hair and teeth in poor condition.

Food sources: salt, kelp, olives and yoghurt. Because it is abundant in most foods there is normally no need to supplement.

Chromium

Chromium plays a crucial role in the prevention of diabetes, by enhancing the effect of insulin on the metabolism of glucose and blood sugar levels. It helps growth, reduces blood cholesterol levels and helps to prevent high blood pressure and arteriosclerosis. It is difficult to difficult to absorb this vital mineral in excess because it is often lost during food processing.

Deficiency signs: excessive or cold sweats, cold hands, dizziness or irritability after six hours without food, diabetes, excessive thirst, addiction to sweet foods, chronic fatigue, mood swings, hardening of the arteries (arteriosclerosis).

Food sources: liver, kidney, wheatgerm, whole-grains, broccoli, brewer's yeast, mushrooms, legumes, nuts and shellfish.

Supplement dose: 100 µg a day.

Cobalt

This helps the body synthesize insulin and other enzymes essential to the process of breaking down carbohydrates and fats. It also helps protect against anaemia. Cobalt occurs as part of Vitamin B12, see page 96.

Food sources: milk, meat, liver, oysters, clams.

Copper

Copper is important in the formation of haemoglobin, the oxygen-carrying component of our blood cells, and helps the body absorb iron and vitamin C. It also affects the action of many enzymes and contributes to skin pigmentation. Too much copper can be toxic, while a copper-deficient diet may cause anaemia.

Food sources: prawns, liver, peas, pulses, mushrooms, prunes, whole-grains.

Deficiency signs: anaemia and oedema (too much fluid in the tissues), hardening of the arteries, cirrhosis of the liver, hepatitis, osteoporosis.

Supplement dose: take as part of a balanced vitamin and mineral supplement, not on its own. There is normally no need to supplement.

Symptoms of too much copper: anaemia, eczema, rheumatoid arthritis, hyperactivity, manic depression, high blood pressure, insomnia. Supplement with zinc and manganese to bring copper levels down.

Fluorine

In its natural state in your food, this mineral can help strengthen your teeth, bones and tissues. The synthetic version can be toxic and should not be taken.

Deficiency signs: tooth decay.

Food sources: seafood, egg whites, cabbage, radishes, beets, lettuce, garlic, whole wheat and gelatine.

Iodine

This mineral burns off excess fat, aiding a balanced metabolism, efficient energy release and stimulating growth. An iodine deficiency may impair the functioning of the thyroid gland, resulting in dry skin, fatigue, weight gain and apathy.

Deficiency signs: underactive thyroid, lack of energy, unusual and excessive weight gain and hair loss.

Food sources: seafood, kelp, iodized salt, vegetables grown in rich soil, and onions.

Supplement dose: kelp, and seek advice.

Iron

As with copper, iron is a key factor in the production of haemoglobin, the oxygen-carrying component of blood. It also helps to produce the enzymes that regulate the metabolism and aids muscle activity. Iron is essential for the proper absorption of B vitamins.

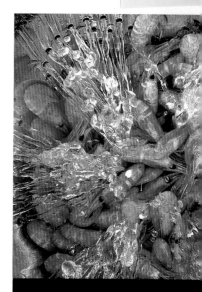

CAN YOU OVERDOSE ON MINERALS?

At exceedingly high doses all minerals are toxic to some extent. It is more advisable to take high-quality balanced formula multi-mineral supplements. Excessive copper is to be avoided. A strong antagonist of zinc, copper also depletes manganese. Do not take supplements containing copper unless they contain at least 10–15 times as much zinc, as this will help prevent copper accumulation.

Iron deficiencies are common because iron is often hard to absorb and is easily lost. Tannic acid in coffee and tea inhibits iron absorption. Iron deficiencies are usually easy to treat.

Deficiency signs: anaemia and haemorrhage, pallor, inflammations, listlessness, loss of appetite, nausea, sensitivity to cold.

Food sources: red meat and liver, green leafy vegetables, whole-grain bread, eggs, nuts, seeds, cereals, beans, and molasses.

Supplement dose: females, puberty to menopause, take 15 mg a day with vitamin C after or with heavy periods; all others take 8–10 mg a day.

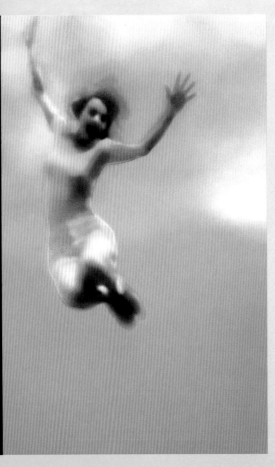

IRON DEFICIENCY IS ON THE INCREASE

A recent American survey found that 90 per cent of children between 1 and 2 are getting less than the RDA of iron. They also found 50 per cent of 3–5-year-olds and 95 per cent of women aged 20–45 do not get the RDA. Eating a diet rich in whole-grains and vegetables, and limiting cups of coffee and tea, should help avoid iron deficiency.

Magnesium

A large proportion of magnesium in the body is associated with calcium and each needs the other in order to function properly. These interdependent minerals control muscle activity – magnesium forms charged particles that stimulate nerves and muscles. It is known as the 'nerve mineral' because it is so important in keeping the nervous system in balance. Magnesium plays a part in countless processes around the body, from DNA function to the release of energy, where it aids in cell nutrient breakdown. A steady balanced intake of magnesium and calcium can help prevent and treat stress, insomnia, depression, PMT and cramps and sugar cravings. Magnesium is sometimes called the 'anti-stress' nutrient because it has tranquillizing properties, but stress affects the body's use of magnesium dramatically. In times of pressure, take a supplement that also includes calcium.

Deficiency signs: sleeping problems, anxiety and irritability, nervous energy, hyperactivity, fits and convulsions, depression, insomnia, confusion, poor memory, PMT, high blood pressure, irregular heartbeat, headaches, muscle spasms, tics, constipation, kidney and gall stones. Heavy and regular tea/coffee/alcohol drinking can cause deficiency, and it is much easier to be deficient than we might think.

Food sources: cereals and whole-grain bread, green vegetables (particularly dark leafy ones like spinach), tropical fruit as well as apples, figs, grapefruit and lemons, some nuts, seeds and pulses, seafood, and dairy products.

Supplement dose: 250–400 mg a day, with at least an equal amount of calcium.

Manganese

This mineral promotes normal and efficient cell functioning. Manganese aids the transmission of nerve impulses, as well as calming the nerves and reducing irritability when necessary. As with many other minerals, manganese is involved in many processes around the body, including the synthesis of cholesterol, the metabolism of blood sugar and fats, the release of thyroid hormones and the formation of bone and tissue. It also helps blood clotting and can substitute for magnesium in the release of energy. Manganese may help to reduce fatigue and poor digestion.

Food sources: green leafy vegetables, egg yolk, avocados, seeds and nuts, whole-grain cereals, some tropical fruit and green teas.

Deficiency signs: not enough of this little-known mineral can lead to that 'tired all the time' feeling and to excessive irritability, dizziness, chronic fatigue, poor digestion and sluggishness, muscle twitches, fits and convulsions, childhood growing pains, sore knees and joint pain, poor memory, infertility and diabetes.

Supplement dose: 2–4.5 mg a day, best taken with B and C vitamins to redress the body's balance and build strength.

Phosphorus

Phosphorus is the second most abundant mineral in the body (after calcium, with which it works closely) and is essential for growth, maintenance and repair processes around the body. This crucial mineral helps to synthesize proteins, to produce energy in cells and to transfer nerve impulses, and plays a major role in the maintenance and repair of cells and tissues. Phosphorus is the 'mood mineral'. It helps the formation of strong, healthy teeth and bones (where most of

the body's phosphorus is stored), and also aids heart regularity.

Research shows that adequate phosphorus intake plays a major role in the prevention of stress disorders, stiffness in the joints (including arthritis) and even cancer. However, it is important to balance phosphorus and calcium intake, because excess phosphorus can reduce the performance of calcium and lead to depleted stores in the body that, over time, can create the right environment for osteoporosis.

Deficiency signs: gum disease, osteoporosis, rickets, a general feeling of weakness and over-sensitivity, loss of appetite, arthritis, aching and stiff joints, stress disorders.

Food sources: dairy products (the most balanced ratio of phosphorus to calcium) and eggs, tofu and soy, fish, poultry and meat, pulses, nuts, seeds and grains.

Supplement dose: generally, there is no need to supplement as there is an abundance in most diets. For those with any of the signs above, however, 500 mg each phosphorus and calcium, and 225 mg magnesium a day. Those suffering from arthritis and/or osteoporosis may need double or even triple the supplement, but always seek advice from a doctor or nutritionist.

Potassium

Potassium helps regulate the delicate equilibrium of the cells by maintaining the balance of water and sodium inside and outside the cells. This process is crucial for nerve and muscle efficiency, ensuring the healthy functioning of your nervous system. Potassium is the 'brain mineral' because it helps send oxygen to

the brain. It also helps convert blood sugar into a form that can be stored in the liver and, because of its role in balancing the body's water levels, it also plays a vital role in eliminating waste products and reducing blood pressure.

It can be useful in treating allergies and relieving bloating due to water retention. Hypertension or fluid retention sufferers may need to supplement their potassium intake, as may those with high blood pressure or at risk of stroke. Because potassium and sodium are intricately linked in cells, it is important to maintain a balanced intake – research shows that high-sodium-low-potassium diets may create the right conditions for cancer and heart disease. Processed, packaged, refined and fast foods contribute to high salt (sodium chloride, see page 105) intake, so extra potassium is needed to counteract this. Also,

---

FOODS AND HABITS THAT STRIP THE BODY OF NUTRIENTS

Smoking and drinking alcohol depletes the quantity of vitamin C in the body. Around 25 mg of vitamin C is lost per cigarette you smoke.

A cup of coffee can cut your iron absorption to one-third of normal.

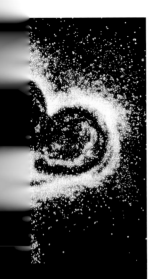

SUPPLEMENTS FOR A HEALTHY HEART

The renowned biochemist, Linus Pauling, found that vitamin C, together with the amino acid lycine, helped reverse cardiovascular disease. Vitamin C protects against the oxidation of the arteries. Vitamin E is important for healthy heart muscle. A Cambridge University study showed a minimum of 400 i.u. a day reduced heart attacks in patients who already had heart disease by 77 per cent!

potassium is very easily lost in cooking and in the body's excretion processes. Doctors may prescribe potassium supplements for patients on diuretics, as these promote potassium excretion.

Deficiency signs: rapid irregular heartbeat, easily upset, irritability and over-sensitivity, depression, fatigue and confusion, apathy, muscle weakness, 'pins and needles', slow reflexes, bloating, cellulite, nausea, diarrhoea, hypoglycaemia and malfunctioning neuromuscular system. If you drink a lot of alcohol, coffee and tea, you may lack potassium, as these neutralize this important mineral.

Food sources: bananas, potatoes, garlic, onions and green leafy vegetables, citrus fruits, pulses, nuts, dried fruit, fish, tomatoes, barley, whole-grains and dandelion and mint leaves.

Supplement dose: again, there is generally no need to supplement this mineral as it is so abundant in most diets. In fact, it is not normally included in a multivitamin/mineral supplement. Those exhibiting any deficiency signs should eat more fruit and vegetables.

Selenium

This mineral is a key antioxidant that works with vitamin E to protect the cells from free radicals and improve immunity. As well as its antioxidant properties, it contributes to the efficiency of the immune system by aiding white blood cell production. Selenium also protects the skin: it guards against UV radiation to minimize sun damage and prevents

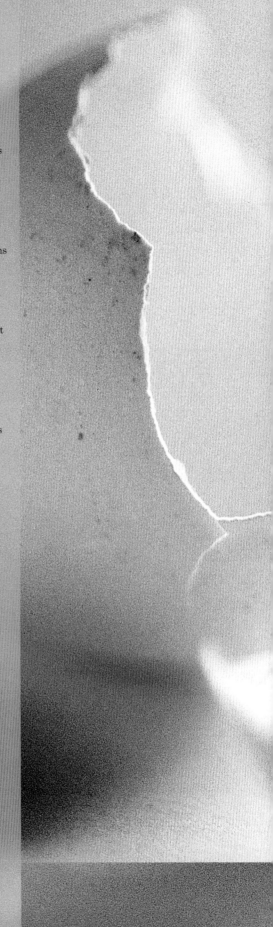

premature ageing, drying skin and scalp conditions like dandruff.

Selenium also helps maintain good eyesight, has an anti-inflammatory effect that relieves the symptoms of rheumatoid arthritis and is important to the functioning of the male reproductive organs. It is thought to alleviate some menopausal symptoms.

Research has linked selenium deficiency with some cancers.

Deficiency signs: diabetes, cataracts, premature ageing, male infertility, sluggish immune system and energy level, high blood pressure, frequent infections, dandruff, lowered liver function.

Food sources: Brazil nuts, fish (especially tuna), eggs, garlic, onions, wheatgerm, bran, whole-grains, seeds, liver.

Supplement dose: 60–70 µg a day.

THE 10 MOST COMMON SOURCES OF HIDDEN SALT

Potato crisps
Biscuits
All packaged processed foods
Pre-cooked convenience meals
Breakfast cereals
Mass-produced sauces and soups
Most tinned foods
Smoked fish
Yeast extracts

Sodium

Sodium, in combination with potassium, helps regulate water and pH levels in the body and aids efficient nerve and muscle function. Sodium deficiency is very unlikely because it is found in almost all foods, and only excessive perspiration can seriously deplete sodium levels. The link between sodium and the hypertension epidemic in the Western world is well-documented. High sodium intake may also contribute to calcium depletion. The general recommendation is to reduce intake of salt (40 per cent of which is sodium – see box, bottom left).

Food sources: kelp, salt, meat, fish, salted, cured and smoked foods, shellfish.

Deficiency signs: headache, dizziness, heat exhaustion, low blood pressure, rapid heartbeat/pulse, apathy, loss of appetite, nausea, indigestion and heartburn, muscle cramps.

Sulphur

Sulphur helps keep skin, hair and nails healthy and disease-free. It is essential for the maintenance of the 'elasticity' of proteins. Sulphur is a 'purifying' mineral that helps to detoxify the liver and fight bacteria to prevent infection. It also helps the brain to function properly.

Food sources: dried beans, fish, eggs, onions, garlic.

Deficiency signs: jaundice, liver ailments, yellow skin, headaches, boils, psoriasis, acne.

Zinc

Zinc is one of the body's most important trace minerals and plays a role in more body functions than any other mineral.

It is an important component of many enzymes in the digestive and reproductive systems and is found in the brain, eyes, heart, lungs, spleen, skin, hair, teeth, etc. It is essential for the maintenance of your body tissues and your immune system, for the functioning of the reproductive system, and for proper growth and development. Zinc, like iron, is easiest to absorb when ingested in animal foods, within which it is bound to proteins that aid its absorption. This 'healing mineral' speeds up the healing process, and helps to reduce cholesterol levels and to synthesize insulin.

Zinc is often used to treat depression and loss of sex drive and is important to the health of the reproductive organs – it may prevent prostate problems.

Food sources: shellfish, lean red meat, poultry, egg yolk, milk, yeast, wheatgerm, bran, pecans, seeds, maple syrup, mustard, chilli and cocoa.

Deficiency signs: poor sense of taste and/or smell, loss of appetite, pallor, skin diseases like acne and boils, stretch marks, dandruff, arteriosclerosis, enlarged prostate, wounds slow to heal, depression, poor concentration, learning disabilities, anorexia nervosa, lack of sexual function, infertility.

Supplement dose: 15 mg a day; seek professional advice for larger doses.

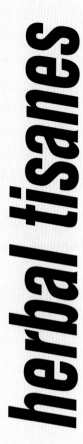

herbs

Ancient physicians and shamans used herbs to cure the sick – recorded use of this natural form of medicine can be found as early as 2,500 BC. Today we still appreciate refreshing, healthy and therapeutic herbal teas or tisanes. Herbs can even provide the stimulating pick-up we all need from time to time, in an easy and safe form. You can only enhance your health if you explore the delicious nutritional and medicinal plants that are the original inspiration for most modern orthodox synthetic drugs.

*'The Lord created medicines out of the earth
and a wise man will not abhor them'*
ECCLESIASTES

Apart from the medicinal value of herbs when they are administered as extracted medicines mixed by a professional herbalist (see Herbalism, page 269), there are many very different herbal teas you can choose to drink safely on a regular basis. It is important to vary them, as they all also have medicinal properties. Herbal tisanes are delicious healthy drinks that are easy to prepare. Just boil some water and, when the boil has gone off, pour the hot water over 1–2 teaspoons per cup of dried or ground herbs and allow to infuse for 5–10 minutes. Many herbal drinks now come in tea bags and can be found in your local supermarket as well as health food stores. Herbal tisanes are usually made from the leaves, flowers and, sometimes, the root; herbal medicines tend to use the seeds, stems, fruit, resin and bark.

You can drink herbal tisanes hot or cold. If you follow the instructions, they are harmless and healthful. There are many herbs from which to choose, but the following are the more common garden herbs in everyday use. If you need to treat any major or persistent symptoms, seek the advice of your GP and/or a professional medical herbalist, who can prepare a complex combination of herbs into a remedy individually suited to your needs, symptoms and body type. Professional herbalists train for four or more years and it would be unwise to believe you can treat yourself herbally other than using the popular herbs, which are harmless and healthy when used in your cooking or taken as a tasty tisane to quench your thirst as well as boost your health.

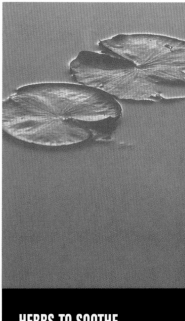

HERBS TO SOOTHE AND RELAX

**Camomile
Lemon balm
Lime blossom
Mistletoe
Peppermint
Skullcap
Valerian**

Borage

This cooling herb stimulates adrenaline production, so can help raise the spirits and allow you to fend off depression or cope with grief. A borage tisane is good for treating colds with accompanying fever and bad coughs. Breast-feeding mothers sometimes take borage in combination with fennel to increase their milk flow.

Camomile

This relaxing herb is also very good for the digestion, helping nausea, morning sickness and a poor appetite, as well as those who have overeaten. A cup at night is good for insomnia, and is reputed to ward off nightmares. Camomile tea is very useful externally to lighten hair and to relieve conjunctivitis as well as skin puffiness and inflammation.

Dandelion

This is one of nature's strongest diuretics and is very useful when you want to cleanse your system. It gently stimulates the digestive system, liver and kidneys, and is useful for treating many conditions, like skin impurities, where there is a build-up of toxins.

Elderflower

This cooling, sweet astringent tisane is reputed to be excellent for the prevention and treatment of colds and 'flus, along with any excessive catarrh and upper-respiratory inflammation, like that caused by hayfever and sinus infections. The cold tea makes a good eyewash and is reputed to be effective in preventing and treating conjunctivitis. The bark of the same plant, used in infusions, helps eliminate uric acid and relieves gout.

Fennel

This pungent, warming, sweet herb is known to aid digestion, to stimulate the circulation and to act as a diuretic and as an expectorant. Its essential oil quickly relieves asthma attacks. Eat fennel root in salad; use the seeds in a tea for period pains.

Lemon balm (Melissa)

For centuries the reputed soothing effect of this delicious herb has brought it to the forefront of the natural medicine chest. It makes a refreshing tea that helps sooth muscular cramp; a good reason to use it for period pains. It helps encourage sweating, making it very useful when treating fever or 'flu symptoms. It is also excellent for its calming effect on nervous stomachs and the entire digestive system.

Lemon verbena

With a strong scent of lemon, this is mainly used for stomach problems, but doesn't have the other properties associated with Melissa (lemon balm) above, although they are quite often confused.

Marjoram

A lightly bitter herb, warming as well as astringent, this has the reputation of being helpful in the treatment and prevention of menstrual cramp, along with soothing indigestion, coughs and asthma attacks.

Parsley

One of our most popular herbs in cooking, parsley also has many medicinal properties. Applied directly on a contusion, it reduces inflammation and can also reduce an abscess. Its diuretic and detoxifying properties are well documented; parsley seeds are useful in the treatment of hypertension.

Peppermint

This popular refreshing herb is widely used to help the digestive process, particularly indigestion, as well as to treat nausea (particularly the kind brought on during travelling) and bad breath, and to promote cooling when treating fever. It can help to soothe migraine headaches when combined with lavender.

Rosemary

Used to treat and prevent a wide range of conditions, including indigestion, headaches, fatigue, cold, 'flu, rheumatic symptoms and depression, this warming, pungent and bitter herb is a very good natural antiseptic.

Sage

With strongly antibacterial properties, sage was traditionally used as a mouthwash, and fresh sage leaves were simply used to clean teeth. Sage infusions are excellent for colds and 'flus, digestive problems and asthma. A handful of fresh sage leaves thrown in the bath has a tonic effect on the body and a calming effect on the nervous system.

Thyme

Its strongly antiseptic properties make an infusion of thyme an excellent gargle for sore throats, or a very effective mouthwash for bad breath, gingivitis etc.

Yarrow

Astringent, cool and bittersweet, this herb is brilliant for treating PMT and unpleasant menstrual symptoms. It is also good for the prevention and treatment of catarrh, and is even reputed to help alleviate high blood pressure.

Chinese herbal medicine is a vital part of one of the oldest medicinal systems in the world, traditional Chinese medicine or TCM. One of the early holistic systems, TCM has the aim of restoring and maintaining equilibrium and harmony within the whole person. Chinese doctors believe that, like everything in the universe, humans too are governed by the laws of yin and yang – the 'Great Principle'. There are two complementary forms of *chi* or energy: '*yin*' reflects the feminine, receptive, dark, cool, soft and moist; and '*Yang*' the masculine, creative, bright, warm, hard and dry. We need a healthy balance of *yin* and *yang* energy to maintain general good health and well-being.

Traditional Chinese medicine practitioners believe that clearing and stimulating the channels of energy within the body helps restore balance, thereby restoring health. They consider illness to be the result of the loss of balance between *yin* and *yang*, or that the circulation of *chi* through the body is blocked.

Chinese herbs have been used for their medicinal value and tonic properties for many millennia. Mixtures of herbs are created that can cleanse, cool or warm the blood, strengthen the immune system, and balance and regulate all the systems of the body to enhance mental – as well as physical – well-being. In their herbal formulas, the Chinese include the roots, seeds, stems, twigs and sap along with the berries, flowers and leaves.

Please note that traditional Chinese medicine experts take the ingestion of herbs and tonics very seriously and advise you seek the advice of a qualified practitioner and have a formula created for your unique needs and requirements. Even ginseng and ginger may be too much of a stimulant for a certain type and could be dangerous for people with high blood pressure.

Astragalus (Huang Chi)

This traditional Chinese herb is derived from the root of the perennial *Astragalus membranaceus*. In China astragalus is used in traditional medicine to strengthen the Wei Chi or 'defensive energy' of the immune system. Antibacterial, with ginseng it is helpful for young adults for energy production and endurance; its warming energy is helpful for hypoglycaemia, and it is used for 'outer energy' as ginseng is used for 'inner energy'.

Among the most popular herbs used in the Orient, it is a tonic, specifically for toning the lungs and spleen. One of the most powerful blood tonics in the Chinese pharmacopoeia consists of an infusion of Dang Gui (overleaf) and Huang Chi; the quantity may vary, but the proportion is always 5 to 6 times the amount of Huang Chi for Dang Gui. This simple formula is recommended for those suffering from anaemia, or recovering from a long illness or cancer treatment.

Scientists have isolated a number of active ingredients contained in astragalus, including bioflavonoids, choline, and a polysaccharide called astragalan B. Animal studies have shown that astragalan B is effective at controlling bacterial infections, stimulating the immune system and protecting against a number of toxins. A great immune-enhancer, astragalus boosts production of white and red blood cells, interferon, immunoglobulins and the adrenal cortex function. In the USA it is being investigated for use with cancer and AIDS.

Chinese angelica root (Dang Gui or Dong Quai)

Growing profusely throughout Asia and called the 'female ginseng', Dang Gui or Dong Quai is an all-purpose herb for a wide range of female gynaecological complaints. For centuries, Chinese women have used this herb to regulate the menstrual cycle and quell painful menstrual cramps caused by uterine contractions. Modern herbalists use Dang Gui to eliminate the discomfort of pre-menstrual syndrome, PMS, and to help women resume normal menstruation after going off 'the pill'. Rich in vitamins and minerals, including A, B complex and E, it also helps prevent anaemia. Dang Gui has been used to treat insomnia and high blood pressure for both sexes. Both men and women use it as a blood tonic.

Researchers have identified in Dang Gui several coumarin derivatives that are known to act as antispasmodics and vasodilators. Caution: don't use Dang Gui during pregnancy or menstruation (when you typically experience a heavy flow).

Chinese liquorice root (Gan Cao)

This remarkable root can detoxify the ill-effects of drugs, balance blood sugar levels and relieve digestive pain and spasms. Liquorice also stimulates the action of other herbs.

Codonopsis pilosulae or Pilose asiabell root (Dang Shen)

As famous as ginseng in China, this herb helps strengthen the lungs, spleen and stomach. A twining and climbing herbaceous perennial native to China, codonopsis is sometimes known as 'Poor Man's Ginseng' or 'Bastard Ginseng', as it builds vital force and tones the blood. It is also nutritious, sweet and warming, containing high levels of immune-enhancing polysaccharides. Dang Shen roots are used for energy deficiency, strengthening the immune system, lowering blood pressure, helping lack of appetite and invigorating the spleen.

Cordyceps fungus (Dong Chong Xia Tiao)

Also known as Caterpillar or Deer Fungus, this is a very effective herb for treating circulatory, respiratory, immune and sexual dysfunction. It is popular as a general health tonic because of its capability to improve energy, stamina, appetite, endurance and sleeping patterns. In traditional Chinese medicine, cordyceps is used for the kidney and lung meridians. Chinese athletes who used cordyceps in their athletic training programme surprised everyone when they broke the 10,000-metre World Track Record in 1993.

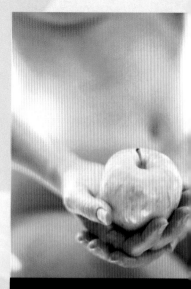

CHINESE HERBS FOR FEMALE REPRODUCTIVE HEALTH

Astragalus, Chinese angelica root, codonopsis, lycium. (Remember always to consult a qualified professional practitioner of traditional Chinese medicine.)

Western herbal formula for the menopause: 1 part each black cohosh, goldenseal, life root, oats, St John's wort; 2 parts each agnus castus and Mexican yam.

Fleeceflower root (He Shu Wu)

He Shu Wu is said to possess almost magical rejuvenating properties and is especially popular with the elderly who believe it can help maintain hair colour, preserve youthfulness and restore fertility.

It replenishes the vital essence and nourishes the blood; it is also a powerful liver and kidney tonic, clearing away toxins. It is used to relieve constipation, usually with Dang Gui (page 110) and hemp seed (page 120). He Shu Wu is also employed as a remedy for insomnia, diabetes and skin problems.

He Shu Wu contains a number of glycosides that account for the herb's use as a remedy for stomach disorders. In Chinese *materia medica*, it has been used effectively for neurasthenia, insomnia, excessive sweating, dizziness, elevated serum cholesterol, coronary disease, weakness, pain, backache, and tuberculous adenopathy.

Ginger (Sheng Jiang)

Because of its ability to help prevent blood clotting, ginger offers substantial protection from stroke and heart attack. For centuries, traditional Chinese medicine has valued ginger as a digestive tonic. It is still commonly used for indigestion today, because ginger absorbs and neutralizes toxins in the stomach. As the ginger eases the transport of various substances through the digestive tract, it decreases irritation to the intestinal walls. Ginger also improves the production and secretion of bile from the gallbladder. Bile aids in the digestion of fats, which helps to lower cholesterol levels.

In traditional Chinese medicine, ginger is used to reduce the toxicity of some herbs. Ginger relieves motion sickness, morning sickness and nausea. Ginger is also used for: colds and coughs, colon and stomach spasms, constipation, indigestion, gas or flatulence, headaches, sinus congestion.

Ginkgo biloba (Bai Guo, Xin Xing)

The ginkgo is one of the oldest living tree species, dating back over 300 million years, and individual trees can live for over 1,000 years. In China, extracts of the fruit and leaves of the ginkgo tree have been used for over 5,000 years to treat lung ailments, such as asthma and bronchitis, and as a remedy for cardiovascular diseases.

Recently, Western researchers have been studying Ginkgo biloba as a treatment for senility, hardening of the arteries and oxygen deprivation. Its ability to improve blood flow has been demonstrated in numerous studies with the elderly, leading researchers to study ginkgo as a treatment for atherosclerotic peripheral vascular disease. More than 34 human studies on ginkgo have been published since 1975, showing, among other things, that it can increase the body's production of the molecule adenosine triphosphate, commonly known as ATP. This activity has been shown to boost the brain's energy metabolism of glucose and increase electrical activity.

Ginkgo flavonoids act specifically to dilate the smallest segment of the circulatory system, the micro-capillaries, which has a widespread effect on the organs, especially the brain. Researchers have also reported that ginkgo extracts effectively increase blood circulation and increase oxygen levels in brain tissues. Ginkgo is a powerful antioxidant that prevents platelet aggregation inside arterial walls, keeping them flexible and decreasing arteriosclerotic plaque.

Ginseng (Ren Shen)

The ancient Chinese believed that the root of the ginseng plant was the crystallization of the essence of the earth in the shape of a man and that ginseng had rejuvenating, recuperative, revitalizing and curative action. The first Chinese *materia medica*, written by Shen-nong, stated that ginseng was used for its tonic and tranquillizing effects; that ginseng increased alertness, brilliance and concentration, and improved memory; and that prolonged use brought about longevity.

Ginseng's other claimed benefits include: increased physical stamina, enhanced blood flow, slowing of cell degeneration, reduced stress, calming of nerves, increased metabolism, strengthening of immune system.

There are two major ginseng species: Asian ginseng (*Panax ginseng*, Ren Hen) and American ginseng (*Panax quinquefolium*, Xi Yang Shen). The name 'panax' is derived from the Greek, meaning 'cure-all'. Ginseng, meaning 'wonder of the world', has been known and respected by the Chinese for centuries. The action of ginseng is neither local nor specific; i.e. it increases

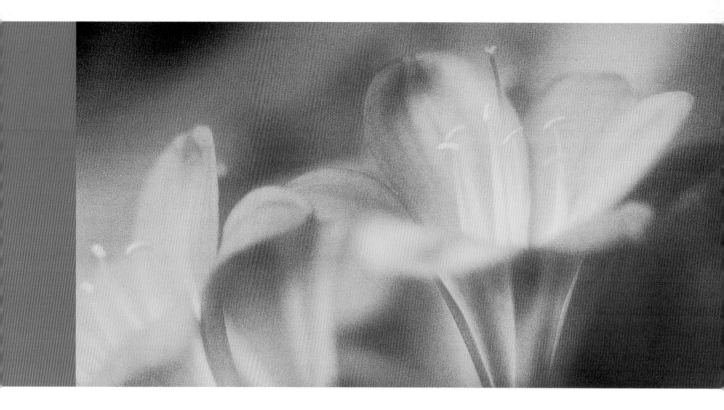

the body's strength and capacity for resistance to adverse stress or damage (by chemical, physical or biological agents). Ginseng stimulates both physical and mental activity and greatly protects the human body from severe or prolonged physical or mental stress. It stimulates the function of the endocrine glands and has been used in traditional Asian medicine for a long time as a general tonic and cardiotonic agent.

American ginseng has 'cooling' properties, while Asian is 'warming'. Those with 'warm' energy should therefore take only American ginseng, but those with 'cool' energy only Asian. American ginseng is often used to reduce stress and fatigue, but Asian has a stimulating effect. The former is effective against high blood pressure and cardiovascular diseases.

Lycium (Gouqizi)

Lycium's botanical name is *Lycium Barbarum L. Lycium* and it also has the common name Wolfberry fruit. For thousands of years, Asians have used lycium fruit and liquorice to help maintain good health. Lycium helps improve vision and prevent headaches and dizziness caused by liver and kidney deficiencies. It has been shown effective in mild forms of diabetes. It contains vitamins, minerals and phytonutrients, beta-carotene, polysaccharides and amino acids.

Rehmannia root (Shudihuang)

Used to treat anaemia and fatigue, and to promote the healing of injured bones, rehmannia is also a demulcent and laxative. It stops bleeding, provides energy and helps strengthen the immune system. Rehmannia also helps strengthen blood, bones, and tendons.

The rehmannia roots are prepared with wine, Amomum fruit (Sha Ren) and tangerine peel (Chenpi). The roots are steamed and dried in the sun several times until they become black, soft and sticky; then they are cut into slices.

Rehmannia nourishes blood and replenishes *yin*. The raw or dried root is a cooling herb often used in skin formulae. Rehmannia is a strong blood tonic, often combined with Dang Gui (page 110) for women's conditions.

Reishi mushroom (Ling-Zhi)

Shown in recent studies to be helpful for treating high blood cholesterol levels, normalizing blood pressure, regulating the circulatory system and helping cure allergies, reishi mushroom contains a high amount of polysaccharides which are essential for proper functioning of the immune system. It is used as a tonic and a sedative, and is useful in Chronic Fatigue Syndrome, diabetes, liver disorders, hypertension, arthritis and nervous exhaustion. Reishi has a strong antihistamine action that can help control allergies. Reishi mushroom extracts have been shown to exert many beneficial effects, which endorses their historical use as an 'adaptogen' – a substance that increases resistance to stress and generally improves the tone of the body and mind. In addition to Reishi's anti-cancer and immune-enhancing properties, it has been used to treat: insomnia, altitude sickness, high cholesterol and chronic hepatitis.

In pharmacognosy, reishi mushroom is actually the powder inside the spores of the fungus Ling-Zhi which are formed as Ling-Zhi matures. The powder collected from these spores, the essence of reishi, consists of 18.5 per cent high-quality protein, with all 18 essential amino acids, plus a combination of vitamins and critical trace elements essential for the proper functioning of the immune system, the remainder being polysaccharides.

Schizandra (Wu Wei Zi, Five-taste seed)

Highly prized by the Chinese as a youth tonic, schizandra is also reputed to increase sexual stamina among men. Until recently coveted by the wealthy and a favourite among the Chinese

emperors, schizandra is also considered an adaptogen and, like ginseng, is believed to increase stamina and fight fatigue; it also improves night vision.

Schizandra (*Schizandra Chinensis*) of the family Schizandraceae is a creeping vine with small red berries, native to Northern China. The dried berries are used as an astringent for the treatment of dry cough, asthma, night sweats, nocturnal seminal emissions, chronic diarrhoea, and as a tonic for the treatment of chronic fatigue.

During the early 1980s Chinese doctors began researching schizandra as a treatment for hepatitis, based on its potential for liver-protective effects. Schizandra is now a recognized 'adaptogen', capable of increasing the body's resistance to disease, stress and other debilitating processes. Eastern herbalists commonly recommend schizandra for the lungs, liver and kidneys, and to help with depression due to adrenergic exhaustion. Schizandra is also used to treat eye fatigue and increase acuity. CAUTION: Schizandra should not be used during pregnancy, except under medical supervision to promote uterine contractions during labour. Schizandra should be avoided by those with peptic ulcers, epilepsy and hypertension.

White peony (Bai Shao Yao)

In traditional Chinese medicine, white peony root is used for heavy bleeding, menstrual pain and premenstrual syndrome. White peony root is the single herb that will help with menstrual pain.

GUIDELINES FOR KAPHA TYPES (see pages 11-15)

B complex is very good for kaphas, as are the antioxidants, particularly vitamin E. Ginseng and ginger are also excellent for them, as they stimulate more sluggish digestive systems.

It is also relied upon to cure 'falling evil', epilepsy. It nourishes the blood, helps with hot flushes and night sweats, is antispasmodic and alleviates cramps.

Ziziphus seed, Wild jujube (Suan Zao Ren)

The seed of the Chinese red date nourishes the heart and the liver. Its natural tranquillizing properties are used to treat mental tiredness. It helps reduce sweating, especially anxiety sweating, and can be used effectively for insomnia and palpitations.

tonics & elixirs

Throughout history, all cultures have used various herbs and plants to purify the body and mind, to restore energy to a tired, over-stressed physique and to prevent illness in the future by building up the body's strength in the present. The modern-day person is no exception and the hunt for the ultimate and most effective stress- and age-buster continues globally. Today, tonics and elixirs are rapidly gaining in popularity – both with the general public and with health researchers worldwide.

The demands of modern living, the long winters in some parts of the world, etc., make us all feel a little below par at times and in need of a pick-me-up. Nature has conveniently created a very interesting and wide range of natural tonics.

If over a prolonged period you feel tired all the time, consult your GP to determine if there is any apparent physical cause for your 'chronic fatigue'. Otherwise you might want to try some of the popular tonics so widely available through health-food stores and chemists. The following are the most popular and widely available. Here and there are suggestions for the form in which to take them and the dosage. However, remember that, unless taking the preparation in question under the supervision of a doctor or other qualified practitioner, you should ALWAYS follow the manufacturer's instructions and heed any warnings they give.

Acidophilus

This is a probiotic, meaning that it is rich in beneficial bacteria. It can help reinstate healthy bacteria in the gut lost after an infection or course of antibiotics.

Agnus castus

Women have long used this herb, also known as Vitex, for combating menopausal symptoms. Containing oestrogen-mimicking substances, it has a balancing effect on hormone production and tends to normalize hormone levels. It can, therefore, function like a natural hormone replacement therapy. The active part lies in the berries, which are dried and ground in a tincture dosage of 1–2 ml three times a day (3–6 g). It also had a reputation for reducing the sex drive, earning it the names Chaste and Monk's Berry.

Alfalfa

Chinese and Indian physicians have long used alfalfa sprouts to treat digestive disorders, and in North America Native American Indians made use of its blood-clotting qualities. Alfalfa contains ALL the major vitamins and minerals, and is rich in chlorophyll and enzymes. It assists in detoxification of the body and, as it is rich in vitamin K, it is an excellent supplement for pregnant women, helping to promote blood clotting during birth.

Aloe vera juice

The rubbery leaves of the aloe vera plant, native to the tropical Americas, are filled with a gel-like substance that is reputed to heal wounds both internal and external. Held to be one of nature's most potent healers, it is particularly good for the digestive system and an effective preventative or treatment for irritable bowel syndrome and related disorders. All kinds of conditions respond to aloe taken internally: acne, arthritis, colds, candida, chronic fatigue, inflammations, ulcers, viral infections and IBS to name but a few. It is available in fresh juice and capsule form, but make sure that you buy the full-strength varieties rather than the adulterated versions; Aloe Gold is an excellent international brand.

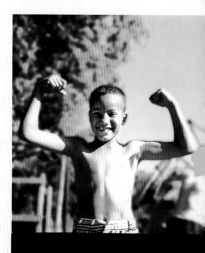

BEST IMMUNE BOOSTERS

Alfalfa
Aloe vera juice
Cat's claw
Co-enzyme Q10
Echinacea
Ginseng
Glutamine
Kombucha
Propolis
Reishi mushroom
Royal jelly
Sambucol
Selenium
Zinc

**BEST
SUPPLEMENTS
FOR HEALING**

Aloe vera
Cat's claw
Chlorella
Co-enzyme Q10
Echinacea
Floradix
Sambucol

Barley grass, see Grasses

Black cohosh

Traditionally used for many problems
associated with the menstrual cycle, this
root originated in North America, where
native Americans called it Squawroot or
Black Snakeroot, as it was also used to
treat snake bites. It is a normalizer of the
female reproductive system that helps
regulate the cycle and reduce spotting
and heavy bleeding. Because it contains
plant oestrogens, it is good for balancing
female sex hormones, and as part of a
tonic formula for treating premenstrual
tension. It is also used in the treatment
of rheumatic conditions, muscular pain
and arthritis, anxiety and mental stress.

Cat's claw

This new herb from the Peruvian rain
forest may turn out to be one of the most
important herbal discoveries yet made.

Cat's claw is a large creeping vine of the
Peruvian rain forest. It bears strong
thorns shaped like a cat's claw, hence its
name. The local Indians have used it for
thousands of years, but only in the last
few decades have Western researchers
taken serious notice of this amazing
plant. It seems that cat's claw works at so
many levels in the body that it can
potentially help everything from cancer
and candida to allergies, intestinal
disorders, depression and HIV. Studies
around the world are now revealing that
cat's claw is highly antioxidant, anti-viral,
anti-tumour, and anti-inflammatory, that
it has a pronounced healing effect on the
digestive system and seems to be able to
relieve chronic fatigue.

The first Western knowledge came
when a German researcher, Dr Klaus
Keplinger, brought specimens back to
Germany in the 1970s. He has since
obtained patents isolating six alkaloids

from the root. The most active,
Isopteredin, is a powerful immune
stimulator. Four others markedly enhance
the ability of white cells to digest bacteria,
viruses, cancer cells and other toxins.

The shamans of Peru recognize cat's
claw as a premier herb for cancer,
arthritis, rheumatism and digestion, with
the power to combat infections and
inflammation of all kinds. So far the
Western catalogue of clinical reports add
a beneficial effect on all forms of herpes,
Epstein-Barr, ME, asthma, acne,
circulatory and all intestinal problems,
toxin poisoning, lupus and diabetes.

Only the potent red inner bark
should be used for tea. The dried bark is
sold, but increasingly it is available in tea
bags and also in capsule form, sometimes
mixed with aloe vera to great effect.

Catuaba

The bark of this Amazon shrub or tree is
used to brew a tea, with a peculiar bitter
taste, that stimulates the central nervous
system and the desire for sex. This is one
of the ingredients of the tonic 'Love Bomb',
which also contains Korean and Siberian
ginseng, guarana and muirapuama, and
has gained some renown as an effective
tonic and aphrodisiac in recent years.

Chlorella

A green algae, chlorella comes from
Japan, where today it is one of the most
popular supplements. It has a very high
protein content and is also rich in beta-
carotene, B complex vitamins, zinc and
iron. Chlorella is high in RNA and DNA
nucleic acids – responsible for the growth

and repair of tissue. As it also contains chlorophyll, it helps to prohibit germs from spreading and assists in the speedy healing of wounds. It is also an excellent immune system booster and tonic.

Cider vinegar

Made from fermented apple juice, apple cider vinegar has been used for centuries to aid digestion. It is useful for those who lack stomach acids, such as the elderly. It is rich in potassium and other trace minerals and may be used in shampoos to make hair glossier.

Citricidal

This extract of grapefruit seeds may turn out to be the most potent, and benign, antimicrobial yet discovered. As well as bacteria, it has been shown to inactivate viruses, yeasts, parasites and worms.

Clary sage

The essential oil of clary sage contains sclariol, which mimics oestrogen and thus provides excellent natural HRT. It is very powerful in its effects and must not be taken during pregnancy or internally, but rather as one or two drops placed on the inner arm at the elbow joint to allow it to be absorbed through the skin.

Cod liver oil

Cod liver oil is a traditional supplement taken for its rich source of vitamins A and D. Vitamin A is good for the skin, eyes, bones and mucous membranes while D helps the body to absorb calcium and so helps to strengthen the bones. It also reduces arthritic pain and inflammation.

Research is being done in Strasbourg into the effectiveness of cod liver oil in reducing fatty tissue around the abdomen.

Co-enzyme Q10

Co-Q10, a viral component of every cell and found in the mitochondria, is involved in cellular energy production. Co-Q10 has potent antioxidant properties, which is how it earned its reputation for being an anti-ageing and immune boosting supplement. Clinical application includes against ME, diabetes, cardio-vascular disease, angina, congestive heart failure, high blood pressure, immune deficiency and breast cancer.

Damiana

This potent energy and sex tonic was originally used by the Aztec and Mayan Indians as a cure for impotence or as an aphrodisiac. It gets its reputation as a reproductive organ rejuvenator because it increases blood flow to the capillaries. This is a herb that is stimulating to the reproductive organs and may be used to enhance sexual performance. Damiana may be helpful for men in the treatment of impotence and combined with saw palmetto would be a useful tonic to ensure the health of the prostate gland.

Damiana is also known to be useful in treating depression and reducing anxiety and as a rejuvenator. Damiana is available in capsule form or as a dried loose herb for making into a tea.

Echinacea

Echinacea increases the production of white blood cells, making it a valuable herb in fighting viruses, bacteria and

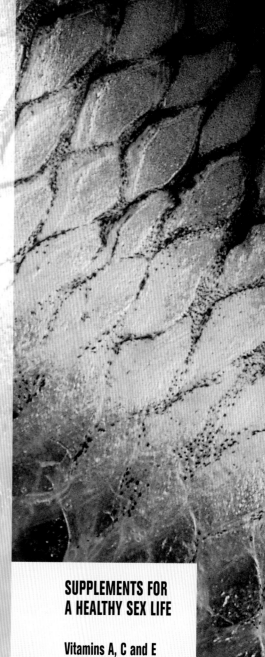

SUPPLEMENTS FOR A HEALTHY SEX LIFE

Vitamins A, C and E
  and B complex
  vitamins with biotin
Magnesium
Zinc
Damiana
Ginseng
Evening primrose oil
Linseed (flax seed) oil
Olive oil
Saw palmetto

infection. Echinacea is a popular tonic and is frequently used as an immune system booster during the winter months, either as a prevention against colds and 'flu or in their treatment, as well as helping to treat herpes and other infectious diseases. The exception, however, is the HIV virus, which attaches to immune cells – therefore, echinacea may stimulate replication of the virus too. As a tea it improves circulation and may help bronchitis. Cancer patients undergoing chemotherapy may find that supervised echinacea supplementation helps restore their immune system.

Evening primrose oil

We now know that certain types of fats are actually essential for health. The omega-6 essential fatty acids are important for healthy hair, skin and nails, brain function, immunity, hormone production and most importantly for the production of anti-inflammatory mediators. Evening primrose oil is an important source of these fatty acids, as well as of the hormone-like substances prostaglandins, which combat pain and inflammation, reduce blood pressure, prevent platelet clotting (keep blood thin), reduce cholesterol levels and prevent water retention. Although an important source of the essential fatty acid GLA (gamma linolenic acid), you have to look further to avoid deficiency of the essential omega-3 fatty acid.

Generations of women have successfully used this supplement to alleviate menopausal symptoms like hot flushes and pre-menstrual symptoms such as breast tenderness. Conditions that evening primrose may help to treat include arthritis, acne, eczema, psoriasis, MS, depression, allergies, hyperactivity, alcoholism and diabetes.

Eyebright

Used internally, this plant extract is a powerful anti-catarrhal, and can be used to treat sinusitis and other congestive disorders. As its name suggests, however, it is best known for its ability to treat eye conditions, particularly acute or chronic inflammations, stinging or weeping eyes, and over-sensitivity to light.

Feverfew

This plant extract is known to help relieve a number of conditions, including dizziness, tinnitus, period pains, sluggish menstrual flow, migraine headaches (in conjunction with hot compresses to the head) and arthritis in the inflammatory stage.

Fennel

This is excellent for toning up a sluggish system and for stimulating the appetite. An infusion of fennel on its own, or mixed with camomile and hops, helps constipation. Mix 10–20 drops of extract with one teaspoon of honey in warm water.

Flax/Linseed

The Cherokee Indians believed the flax was sacred and vital to the life processes of the body, and that its seed captured energies from the sun. They used the linseed to nourish pregnant women, for treating malnutrition, arthritis, skin diseases and fertility and virility problems.

Flaxseed is one of the best sources of the essential alpha linolenic acid, an important member of the omega-3 group of fatty acids, so vital to our health and well-being. Omega-3 is recognized as an essential nutrient – it is as vital to the body as a vitamin, but we cannot produce it in our bodies ourselves. In recent times we have lost many sources of fatty acids from our diet and some experts believe many of our chronic modern physical and

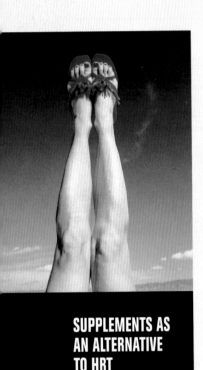

SUPPLEMENTS AS AN ALTERNATIVE TO HRT

Agnus castus
Black cohosh
Wild yam
Soyagen
Dang Gui
Natural progesterone
  cream
Clary sage

mental woes may be attributed to a deficiency of these fatty acids. Today it is widely recognised that the omega-3 fatty acids are important in the prevention of arteriosclerosis, cancer, heart disease, depression, mental illness, immune disorders and allergies. As well as the vital omega-3 acids, flax seed oil contains omega-6 (linoleic acid) and omega-9 (oleic acid) in the right balance, which is so important to our health.

You should take flax/linseeds that are organic and fresh on a regular basis. The ready-pressed oil from the seeds is now available from health-food stores, usually in the chill cabinet, as it has a short shelf-life. You cannot cook with it, but it makes an excellent salad dressing, as well as a simple way of taking flax as a supplement.

Floradix

This internationally renowned vegetarian food supplement, rich in an easily absorbable iron compound, combines selected herbs plus vitamins, minerals and fruit concentrates to create a tonic drink that is widely used for convalescing patients, and for people recovering from any long-term debilitating illness. This tonic is also useful in late autumn/early winter to build up your immune system so that you can fight off seasonal colds and 'flus.

Ginger

This is the herb the Chinese use for treating morning sickness, travel sickness, indigestion and nausea. Peel and grate the root to make an infusion of ginger tea for treating these digestive complaints or take one capsule up to three times daily. An infusion of ginger is also helpful in treating most forms of arthritis, as well as cheering those suffering depression. Tablets may also be used for treating period pains: take one up to three times a day. Ginger is said to stimulate lung function and a practitioner may prescribe a tincture for treating bronchitis. An infusion of ginger and spring onion is a traditional remedy for colds and 'flu.

Ginkgo Biloba

Ginkgo acts as a cerebral vasodilator, boosting circulation to the brain and enhancing the brain's ability to function under conditions of deprived oxygen and glucose supply. Ginkgo promotes healthy artery walls, prevents platelet aggregation (reducing the 'stickiness' of blood) and acts as a general tonic for the circulatory system, boosting peripheral circulation.

Ginkgo exerts an anti-inflammatory effect, inhibiting the production of a substance called platelet activating factor (PAG), which triggers asthma and allergies. Ginkgo also contains flavoglycosides, powerful antioxidants which offer protection from free radical damage.

This valuable supplement can be used to help treat tinnitus, vertigo, memory loss, senility, Alzheimer's, poor concentration, depression, angina, stroke, ischeamic attacks, brain injury, asthma and a range of allergies. Take up to three 40 mg capsules or tablets a day.

SUPPLEMENTS TO FEND OFF COLDS AND 'FLUS

Vitamins A, C and E, and beta-carotene
Selenium, zinc
Aloe vera
Cat's claw
Echinacea
Sambucol
Garlic
Ginger
Goldenseal
Mushrooms (maiitake, reishi and shiitake)
Propolis
St John's wort

Ginseng

This herb is renowned for its stimulating effect. It improves the body's tolerance to stress and is believed to possess aphrodisiac properties. Ginseng provides a natural source of steroids and boosts immunity and mental performance. Despite its stimulating properties, it is also known to have a soothing, calming effect on the digestive system.

There are three main types of ginseng. Siberian ginseng is not technically a member of the ginseng family but has very similar properties – it may be used to revitalize a run-down constitution and is particularly good for ME sufferers.

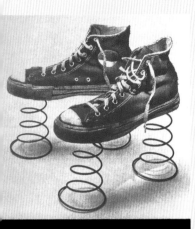

TONICS FOR ENERGY

Vitamin B
   complex
Vitamin C,
   choline
Iron
Copper
Chromium
Calcium
Magnesium
Zinc
Cat's claw tea
   with ginger
Co-enzyme Q
Ginseng
Propolis
Royal jelly

American ginseng may help calm a nervous or upset stomach as a result of work pressure or other stress.

Korean or 'red' ginseng has been used medicinally in the Far East for over 4,000 years and is thought to be the most stimulating of all the ginseng family. Menopausal women may find it helpful in controlling hot flushes.

The normal dosage is one 600 mg capsule per day; 5–10 g powder, mixed with liquid per day; or 250 ml ginseng tea per day. If you are taking a vitamin C supplement, allow two hours between taking this and taking ginseng, as this vitamin can interfere with the body's ability to absorb ginseng. Ginseng is not recommended for children, pregnant women or anyone suffering from a high temperature (through fever or 'flu, for instance) or high blood pressure. It should not be taken continuously or for more than 2 months at a time.

Glutamine

Thanks to ten years of intensive research, glutamine is the new 'superstar' amino acid being pursued by expert specialists in everything from leaky gut and ulcers to cancer, depression and rheumatoid arthritis. Illness, surgery and continued stress can depress stores of glutamine and, therefore, body functions. In the absence of this amazing amino acid, immune cells do not function correctly or even grow. 'It took researchers a very long time to consider the importance of glutamine,' says Judy Shabert, a US-based doctor, dietician and author of *The Ultimate Nutrient Glutamine*. 'With our current level of understanding it seems rather naive not to have studied glutamine more closely. It is the most abundant amino acid in the body, especially in the brain, skeletal muscle and blood. In fact, it is proving to be the most significant amino acid known.'

It is only in the last 10 years or so that we have found that glutamine is the primary nutrient for the digestive system; the primary fuel for the immune system and the brain; vital for muscle metabolism; and vital for healing and tissue repair.

As it reduces craving and addiction, as well as being an excellent healing aid, it is very effective in treating and preventing alcohol problems. In Japan most people now take it before drinking, to prevent a hangover. It is most commonly available as a powder, for sprinkling on food.

Golden rod

This plant extract has many uses, including the treatment of laryngitis and pharyngitis as a gargle, and as an anti-inflammatory in cases of urethritis, cystitis and urinary infections in general. Its carminative qualities make it useful in treating dyspepsia, but its most important use is in the treatment of upper respiratory tract infections, such as acute or chronic catarrh and, with other supplements, 'flu.

Goldenseal

This extract of the root and rhizome of the plant is useful in the treatment of all catarrhal states. A powerful tonic for all the mucous membranes, it may therefore be used for all digestive problems. Its tonic and astringent qualities also make it good for uterine conditions. It can be used externally against earache, conjunctivitis, ringworm, pruritis and eczema.

Grasses – wheat and barley

Wheat and barley grasses are cereal grasses grown in nutrient-rich soils. As they metabolize and absorb all the nutrients from the ground, they are a rich source of vitamins, minerals and fibre. In fact they are higher in fibre than bran and contain more iron than spinach. They also supply protein, chlorophyll and beta-carotene. Wheat grass has also been shown to be useful in the treatment of anaemia and high blood pressure. It is also a good liver tonic. The grasses may be eaten as vegetables or in salads, but are most often pressed to obtain their juices.

Guarana

A native plant of Brazil, this is a wonderful natural 'upper' because of its caffeine content. It helps maintain good concentration, memory and energy, possibly because its caffeine action lasts twice as long as that of tea or coffee.

Hemp seed

Hemp seed is widely acclaimed as one of the most complete sources of vegetable protein. As well as providing protein, minerals and vitamins, hemp seed is also rich in essential fatty acids. All are present in a form that is easily digested. Hemp seed is useful in reducing cholesterol and protecting against heart disease. It also stimulates the hair and nails, and encourages healthy skin.

Kava kava

Traditionally drunk at ceremonial occasions in the South Pacific islands before the introduction of alcohol, this

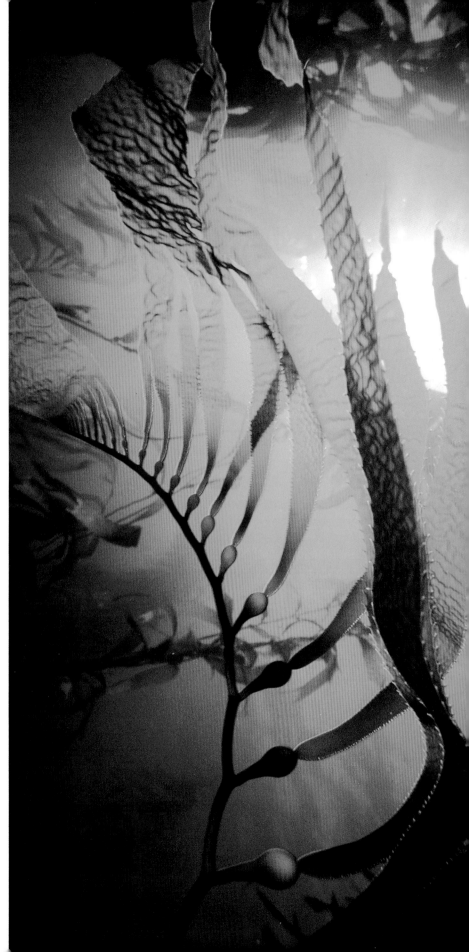

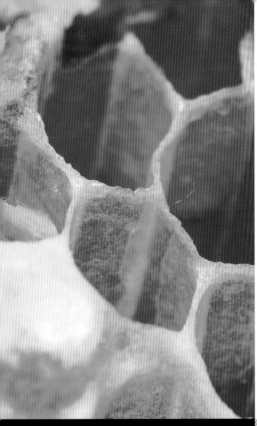

potent root extract leaves you calm, relaxed and full of optimism. The Tahitians also credit it with the power to aid concentration, promote healthy lungs and digestion, ease the joints and help you maintain normal weight.

Kelp

Kelp is a seaweed containing a concentration of minerals, such as potassium, magnesium, calcium and iron, as well as vitamins A, C, D, E and B complex. It aids digestion and soothes ulcers, as it is high in iodine. As well as in weed form, it is available as a tablet.

DAILY SUPPLEMENTS FOR HEALTHY SKIN

Multi-vitamin and multi-mineral complex (with 300 mg magnesium and 15 mg zinc)
2 x 1,000 mg vitamin C
Antioxidant complex
GLA (300 mg), evening primrose oil
Vitamin E (500 i.u.)
Fish oil or linseed (flax seed) oil

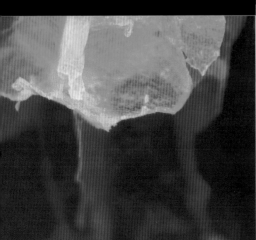

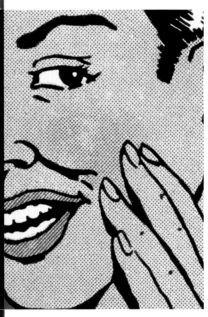

Kombucha

Millions around the world are convinced this lichen-like fungus has a rejuvenating and strengthening action. For over 2000 years the Chinese have brewed and drunk this powerful mixture of bacteria and yeast to stimulate the immune system.

The slimy pancake-like culture, not unlike a big mushroom, floats on the surface of a sweetened tea which, after ' fermentation, produces a nutrient-rich solution full of good flora and organic acids. It is fast gaining the reputation as an 'elixir of life', that can help prevent most serious illness because of its immune-enhancing properties, slow ageing, recharge your sex life, reduce the risk of cancer or the size of existing tumours, and cure arthritis!

Lecithin

Extracted from soya, lecithin's most important ingredient is phosphatidyl choline or PC, see page 196.

Linseed, see Flax

Liverite

This unique natural product, which prevents hangovers, is used by millions of Europeans, Japanese and Americans, and is catching on fast in the UK. Take 2–3 Liverite tablets before and after drinking (3 if you've been drinking excessively) and you'll wake up as clear as a bell the next day, with none of the discomfort that usually follows alcohol. It also works for overindulgence in rich foods.

Liverite has been tested in clinical trials in Germany, Italy and Japan. The researchers also found Liverite very helpful for people suffering from cirrhosis and chronic hepatitis: it showed an ability to restore the integrity of the liver cells. Yet Liverite is a completely natural supplement, made from American beef liver together with 17 amino acids, iron, potassium, vitamin B12 and lipotropic factors, etc.

Mexican yam

This root is valued for its high concentrations of steroidal saponins, including diosgenin, vital for the commercial production of both progesterone and cortisone. Wild yam root was, in fact, the pharmaceutical industry's only source of diosgenin until 1970. As a botanical medicine it is considered completely safe and non-toxic. You can apply it topically as a cream or oil, or take it internally as a supplement or tincture. It is excellent used in combination with Agnus Castus for reversing menopausal symptoms.

Milk thistle

The seed shell of this herb yields a group of flavonoid-like compounds that are excellent for restoring and maintaining liver function. The liver is an impressive hormone-filtering system and if it is congested and sluggish the delicate hormonal balance of the body is disturbed. Milk thistle features in many hormone tonics but is also used for treating cirrhosis, hepatitis, psoriasis and any form of toxicity – even emotional. Its flavonoids help protect the liver against damage from chemicals and speed up the production or regeneration of enzymes and proteins. A tea is made from a decoction of the seeds, and tinctures are also available.

Motherwort

The Latin name for this plant, *Lenourus cardiaca*, indicates its usefulness against heart problems. It is used for any heart condition that is primarily brought on by stress and anxiety, and is an excellent remedy for over-rapid heartbeat. The plant's common name also betrays its uses in the treatment of female conditions, such as menstrual and uterine flow. In the latter case, it can encourage flow where menstruation has been delayed by stress or anxiety. Menopausal women may also benefit from this herb, as it is a relaxant, and it is also used for false labour pains.

MSM

Was grandmother right to give her children sulphur and molasses? A growing body of research focused on MSM – a natural form of organic sulphur – suggests that she was. Now this nutritional supplement, which is found in rain water and has been part of the food chain since life began, is beginning to be recognized for the relief it offers to an exceptional number of health problems.

Can we really have overlooked a nutrient that offers relief to so many challenging ailments? This really seems to be the case with sulphur. MSM relieves the pain of inflammatory conditions, such as arthritis, joint pain, swelling, tenderness, osteoarthritis, bursitis and related conditions. It also appears to help ease allergies and skin, eye, digestion, diabetic and lung conditions.

People with chronic to severe allergies report substantial to complete relief of their symptoms with daily doses of MSM, and a majority of subjects with allergic asthma reported that they were able to reduce their medication by 75 per cent when taking MSM. It is available in both powder and tablet form, and there is a cream for the treatment of skin allergies.

Nettle

This 'spring' herb is thought to be an excellent natural blood cleanser and a good all-round tonic. It stimulates the digestion and generally produces a feeling of well-being. As well as the fresh leaves, it is available in tablet form.

Phosphatidyl serine

Phosphatidyl serine (PS) is unlike any other product currently available. Clinical studies have shown that it can help support brain functions that tend to decline with age. PS appears to play an important role in the function of brain cell membranes, including the conduction of the nerve impulse. As we grow older, cognitive functions can slow down; recognizing names and faces, and learning and remembering information and maintaining concentration are more difficult. Now extensive scientific research has shown that real improvement is reported after only a short course of phosphatidyl serine.

As a dietary supplement, PS provides nutrients that can positively contribute to enhanced memory, learning, concentration and behavioural balance (including negative moods and coping with stress). PS has also been shown to reduce stress hormone production. PS *was* only available from animal sources; now there is an enriched vegetarian form, derived from soya.

Propolis

The word propolis comes from the Greek for 'defences before a town'. It is in fact a resin obtained from the buds of some flowers and trees that is thought to contain a natural antibiotic, galangin. The bees collect the propolis along with the pollen and take it back to the hives. There, they spread it around to protect the hive from bacteria and viruses. Propolis is thought to be rich in nutrients and minerals. It is used in various complementary remedies to treat low-grade infections especially amongst those who do not wish to take antibiotics.

Reishi mushroom

Another 'wonder tonic' from the east, this mushroom has been the focus of much research and attention in recent years. Like royal jelly and ginseng, it is considered an important energy tonic. It stimulates the immune system and is officially listed in Japan as a substance for treating cancer. In America it is used to bolster the poor resistance of those with AIDS and is used everywhere generally for deficiency conditions and to fortify the body's natural vigour.

Royal jelly

Queen bees are known to grow to a much greater size than other worker bees and it is the consumption of royal jelly that is the reason for this. Those in the East have known of the beneficial effects of royal jelly for centuries. Royal jelly is reputed to have countless beneficial effects: it enhances your general level of well-being, stimulates your stamina and your immune system, and increases your level of energy. It has a natural diuretic action and also may help diminish the pain – and then the condition – of crippling arthritis. Indeed, the Chinese give routine injections of royal

jelly to cure arthritis. Royal jelly is also helpful in relieving allergies and asthma. Fresh royal jelly is wonderful for healing wounds and for cleaning and enhancing the blood.

Some researchers believe that royal jelly can give some protection against cancer by improving the immune system. Royal jelly can even benefit cancer sufferers by boosting resistance to the harmful side-effects of chemotherapy and radiotherapy before and after treatment.

People who swear by this tonic take a capsule regularly first thing or on an empty stomach. It may take 2–3 months before you perceive dramatic changes in your level of well-being, but converts would advise you persist!

You can also take royal jelly with honey in a liquid form which usually contains bee pollen and vitamin C. This, too, is best taken on an empty stomach, plain or as a delicious nutritious breakfast spread. Do not add it to a hot drink as this will destroy its beneficial properties.

You can take fresh royal jelly as a liquid tonic for a really fast-acting 'pick-me-up'. This form is usually packaged in a single-dose phial which is easy to use and gives an energizing effect that you feel almost immediately and which can last all day. This is not for everyday regular use, as you may get more energy than you need. Liquid royal jelly tonics are mixed with ginseng and honey, which adds to the energizing effect and the ability to fight fatigue and depression, as well as boosting both physical and mental energy. Using fresh royal jelly externally can have an excellent tonic effect on skin and hair.

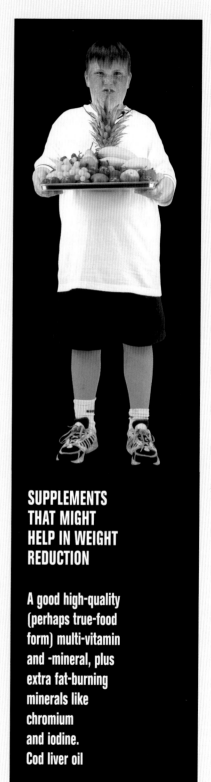

SUPPLEMENTS THAT MIGHT HELP IN WEIGHT REDUCTION

A good high-quality (perhaps true-food form) multi-vitamin and -mineral, plus extra fat-burning minerals like chromium and iodine. Cod liver oil

St John's wort

In Germany, tablets of this traditional European herb are now prescribed for depression ten times more frequently than Prozac. Research suggests that in cases of mild-to-moderate depression, St John's Wort – or hypericum – is an effective natural anti-depressant. It has been found useful against Seasonal Affective Disorder.

Sambucol

Sambucol is a natural product made from an elderberry extract and has been shown to be effective in inactivating viruses. It is derived from the black elder tree, *Sambucus nigra L.*, grown mostly in central Europe. This natural substance has rare antiviral strengths.

Proven antiviral preparations are few and far between. Even the pharmaceutical companies haven't been able to come up with an effective antiviral, with the exception of Aciclovir for herpes and the expensive and limited Interferon. Sambucol has been developed by Doctor Madeleine Mumcuoglu, a prominent French/Israeli virologist, who has patented a product combining the natural benefits of the plant with other components, like raspberry extract.

Clinically tested, sambucol has been used by thousands with spectacular results. It is a safe, non-toxic, natural product. Dr Mumcuoglu's research shows that the active ingredients in the elderberries bind with viruses before they have a chance to penetrate the wall of a normal cell. The liquid extract has been tested on numerous well-known 'flu viruses and was effective on every one.

Saw palmetto

This small North-American tree has dark red berries that are ground into a powder that is apparently excellent as an energy and sex tonic, particularly for men with impotence or prostate problems. The American Indians have a long tradition of using the berries for chronic congestion. They are also used for urinary problems.

Serotone

Serotone is a mood regulator with a calming effect. It is a natural source of 5HTP, the precursor of serotonin, the neurotransmitter involved in mood and sleep. Modern antidepressant medication, such as Prozac, increases the level of brain serotonin by preventing its removal from the system, hence the classification name SSRI – serotonin re-uptake inhibitor. One problem of the SSRIs is that serotonin is naturally supposed to be secreted by the body and by preventing it from doing so many SSRIs can cause side-effects. There is no such problem with serotone in that it helps you to produce more serotonin naturally.

Spirulina

Spirulina is a highly nutritious blue-green algae. Traditionally eaten by the Aztecs, it is a rich source of protein and more easily assimilated by the body than the protein from eggs, fish, dairy products or meat. As well as being an incredibly high protein source, spirulina is rich in a wide variety of trace minerals, vitamins, enzymes, chlorophyll and beta-carotene. Available in both powder and capsule form, this is an extremely useful supplement for people who do not follow a balanced diet, or who are on a diet, as it can also help to suppress the appetite, but at the same time supply vital nutrients.

Valerian

The rhizome and root of this plant are used to make one of the most common relaxant nervines. It is quite safe to use to reduce symptoms of stress and anxiety, over-excitability and hysteria states, and is particularly useful when treating conditions that inhibit restful sleep. An anti-spasmodic, it also aids relief from cramp, intestinal colic and period pain. It can even be used in the treatment of migraines and rheumatic pain.

Yellow dock root

This is useful in treating chronic skin complaints like psoriasis and eczema. It is also used against constipation as it has a cathartic effect on the bowel. It also promotes the flow of bile and acts as a blood cleanser; it is useful in the treatment of jaundice.

GUIDELINES FOR PITTA TYPES (see pages 11-15)

The minerals calcium, magnesium and zinc are of benefit to Pitta types, as are sea minerals and algae, like chlorella and spirulina, and wheat grass. Mint tea is also excellent for them.

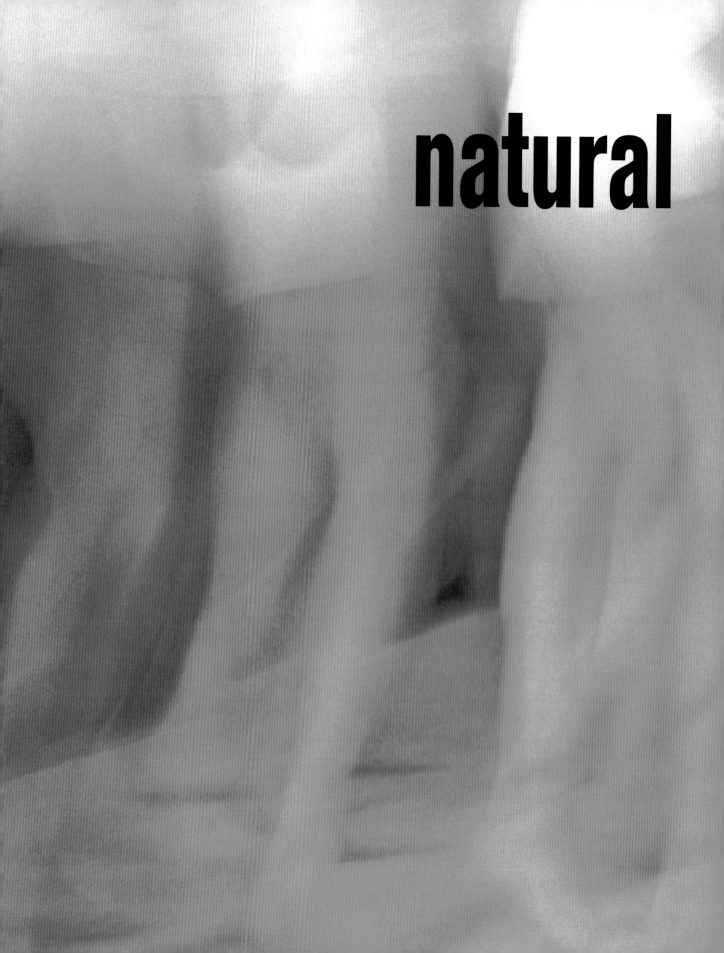

natural

exercise

As well as what we take into our bodies, the other crucial aspect of ensuring our natural health is regular exercise. As with most aspects of our holistic approach, this must be tailored to suit your own body's needs and your lifestyle, so it needn't involve joining a gym or hiring a personal trainer. All that you may need to help you restore your own balance is perhaps a few hours of gentle walking, or getting back into doing the daily two or three lengths of the pool you did until a few years ago – or even joining a salsa class. Whatever suits you best or you think you might enjoy, look at all the possibilities here, as well as assessing your current physical state, decide what exactly is the right exercise for you and then find the motivation to do it.

There is also plenty of advice on improving your posture and on how to warm up and cool down before and after exercise. This section also includes two complete exercise programmes for you to follow if you choose – one for basic stretching, strength and stamina training and another utilizing the gentle principles of yoga and associated Eastern disciplines.

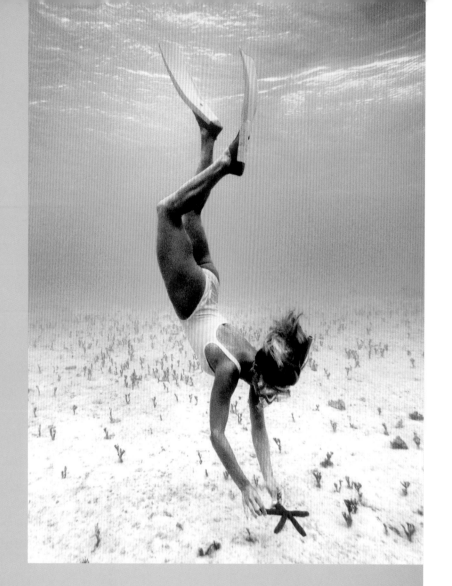

natural exercise

The natural way to a happier and healthier you is to combine a balanced whole diet with regular exercise and adequate sleep. You will then feel good and look good, making you generally more positive and able to tackle the tasks of daily living. The single best thing you can do to protect, maintain and promote your well-being and prevent serious illness, is to exercise – to stretch and move your body regularly – responsibly and within your individual needs and means.

Someone who eats junk food, sits in front of a computer all day, travels home on a packed train to snack on more junk food and then veges out in front of the television will look and feel tired, lethargic and jaded. This lifestyle actually puts a great deal of strain on the body and, strangely, the more the body is used, the better it will perform.

The human body was designed for movement. These days, unfortunately, movement can often consist simply of the short walk to the mode of transport which takes us from home to work. Even this small amount of movement can be fraught and not allow us to reap the benefits of fresh air. The society in which we live today often dictates that we actually have to allot time for exercise.

Two generations ago, without so many means of transport, or longer ago, in pre-urban society, people walked much more and generally could expect to lead much more physically demanding and active lives. Now the average person will probably rarely move at all except to perform basic functions, such as shopping for food. With such dramatic changes to our basic lifestyle, is it any wonder that the huge rise in death from heart disease and other degenerative illnesses continues, in spite of the amazing advances made in modern medicine and our understanding of disease?

The message does seem to be getting through, however. More and more people are awakening to how vital exercise is to good health and longevity. Exercise is enjoying a renaissance in the Western world and with so much choice and greater awareness people are generally turning their attention to creating a healthier lifestyle that incorporates exercise, healthy eating and attention to rest.

Unfortunately, too many of us still lead horribly sedentary lifestyles that can lead to many of the illnesses common in the modern world, including depression, stress-related conditions, and even muscular wastage in those as young as their mid-20s! Not to mention the increasing problem of overweight and obesity amongst children, who take too little exercise and watch too much TV!

There is no question that people who take exercise feel better and have more energy and vitality than people who don't. It is well known that you experience a rise in alertness for a few hours after a workout, yoga or dance class, or a good brisk walk. Exercise can help you overcome and treat depression; it raises the levels of endorphins, the body's natural opiates or pleasure hormones, that reduce the sensation of pain in the body.

The adrenal glands produce hormones like adrenalin and cortisol, the levels of which are too high in stressed and depressed people. Regular exercise keeps hormones in check and in balance, helping to stabilize your overall mood and ability to cope. There is also mounting evidence that people who suffer from too much stress or depression are much more likely to develop serious degenerative health conditions leading to disease. Anything that so dramatically reduces stress and depression as exercise and good diet do, must be a priority to integrate into your lifestyle.

WHY EXERCISE IS IMPORTANT

- Except for a healthy diet, the best thing you can do for preventative health care.
- Reduces the risk of heart disease.
- Improves your circulation.
- Helps prevent the development of cancer.
- Improves your breathing and your entire respiratory system.
- Helps alleviate symptoms of osteoarthritis.
- Strengthens your back and reduces lower back pain.
- Increases bone density.
- Reduces your risk of osteoporosis.
- Strengthens muscles, tendons, ligaments and cartilage, and stabilizes joints.
- Increases your flexibility.
- Improves your posture.
- Slows down the ageing process.
- Increases your energy.
- Helps reduce body fat level.
- Helps maintain your ideal body weight.
- Helps shift and prevent cellulite.
- Improves your digestion.
- Helps correct bowel problems, particularly constipation.
- Boosts your immune system which, in turn, makes you less susceptible to colds, 'flu and general debilitating ailments brought on by inertia.
- Improves your self-esteem and your body image.
- Reduces depression, anxiety and stress.
- Improves brain function. You really could become more intelligent or realize just how intelligent you actually are!
- Helps you look better, feel better.
- Stimulates more energy and a positive attitude to life.
- Makes you HAPPIER!

According to the Dunn Clinical Nutrition Centre in Cambridge, it could be far easier to adopt a more physical life than we think. For example, walking rather than using the car and carrying shopping home burns off nearly 10 times more calories. Losing the TV remote and walking across the room to change channels would mean that you walk three miles a year! Abandoning the duvet for real bedding will burn 15,000 extra calories just in making the bed! Of course, it is advisable to become as physically active in all areas of your life as you can, remaining mindful of how you use your body.

When taking any kind of exercise it is wise to be aware of your unique physical being and its state at that moment, and to have the courage to push yourself just enough and to know – and move within – your boundaries and limitations.

Creating your personal exercise programme

The way we approach exercise and the types of movement that appeals to us is completely individual and influenced by many different factors, be they hereditary or social conditioning, or informed by the way our family approaches play and sport. Mix that with our own unique talents, tastes and experiences and you can see why people express such different interests. It doesn't matter what kind of exercise you decide to implement into your daily regime – as long as your choices reflect your natural inclinations.

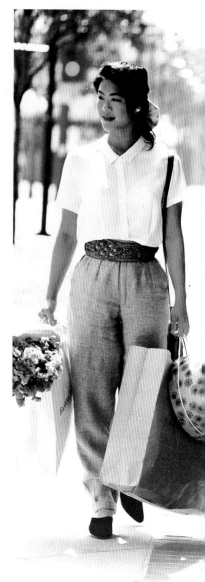

If you are taking exercise or playing sport, you are quite probably in good shape and in a healthy state of well-being, unless you simply don't know your limits and overdo it in one area without balancing in another. For example, you might be incredibly strong through intensive strength-training exercises with weights, but be inflexible and unable to run for a bus. It is important to balance your programme to incorporate all three aspects for overall fitness – Stretching, Strength Training and Stamina.

Even very fit, supple young people can push themselves too far, inflicting serious physical damage, or worse, while engaged in some physical activity. It is very important to learn to recognize your limits and the danger of pushing yourself past the point of pain in the pursuit of excellence – a hollow victory for vanity that, in the long run, will not serve you well. To prevent injury during exercise, do not overdo it – do not strain or push too far. Softly, softly is always the safest approach, especially if you are just starting to exercise again.

Walking or brisk walking and swimming are very safe, low-injury-risk exercise systems. Regular brisk walking every day is one of the best exercises you can give your body. After all, we are upright – designed physically to walk – and should do so on a regular basis to prevent any number of possible ills! For good heart- and brain-health, it is best to walk briskly, swinging your arms freely, for 10–20 minutes daily.

Remember, it is not necessary to take an aerobics class for 1½ hours every other day to reach your optimum physical health. For the many people who can't get to a tennis game, or a dance or yoga class, you can still keep fit with shorter and more frequent bursts of exercise. A lot of recent research suggests that it's just as beneficial to take 10–20 minutes a day for a brisk walk, swim or cycle, as to have a long workout at the gym a few times a week. Some experts believe a little every day is the best approach.

However, that may not be true for you. If your regular 2–4-hour-a-week session has helped you achieve an optimum level of well-being, then stay with what works for you – but perhaps every so often weaving in new ways of moving your body.

Finding motivation

When motivation fails, draw from within. If you are participating in a regime like yoga or t'ai chi (see pages 168 and 182), you will be learning gently about discipline. If not, focus on your inner self and on using the positive will within, and find the courage to continue to participate, knowing you can only benefit in the long run. If you do find it difficult to make it to a class or session and have to skip a day, it is important not to beat yourself up for it.

Instead, try to ensure that you do manage something, however small, like some gentle stretching to ensure the muscles, ligaments etc. do not tighten and shrink through inactivity. Ease out the stresses of the day with gentle neck, head and shoulder rolls and then stretch the limbs, torso and spine. About 10 minutes of stretching and mild-to-moderate activity is better than nothing at all, and will keep you on track until you can make it to your class or gym.

For many people, fitness can so often be something that other people do and the plethora of activities available can be daunting. Some even feel insecure about joining gyms or exercise classes, perhaps believing that they need to be fit before joining! They are daunted by the thought of the muscle-bound toned bodies they imagine are in attendance. This is often not the case and specialist classes for beginners abound and are the starting point for us all.

Drop-out rates are very high for first-timers at gyms, as once the initial enthusiasm has worn off it can often be difficult to maintain a programme. Others may benefit from the added incentive of commencing a programme with a friend or a 'training partner'. Often the impetus to exercise will be greatly enhanced if you are not your own sole motivator!

Keeping an exercise journal, however simplistic, is a useful tool to provide motivation. Instead of filling in what you've done when you've done it, fill out your proposed programme for a few weeks ahead. Seeing it in black and white in your diary will prompt you more readily than a hazy memory of a class or session you were supposed to attend!

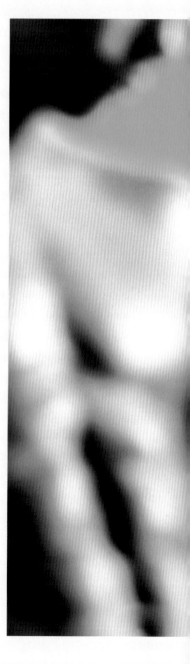

Recovery days

When exercising regularly, it is very important to allow recovery days, as the muscles continue to tone in recovery; in fact, this is when the repair work is done. It is also important not to become exercise-obsessive – a common syndrome these days. It can often be harder to allow oneself to rest for a day as the desire to make it to the gym can overshadow the need to allow the body time to recuperate. This is all part of the discipline and will only add to your overall fitness.

Of course, even on recovery days, gentle stretching after warming up is still recommended, as is walking, yoga or any activity that you find comfortable and which does not stress your muscles or heart and lungs.

It may feel like the right thing for you to jog 5 miles every day and to start training for the marathon – but starting at the beginning with gentle walking, rehabilitation and strengthening exercises would be far more sensible and beneficial. If, once you start exercising, you notice any pain or weakness in any part of your body, then you should stop or modify the exercises and get medical assistance.

With regard to cardiovascular exercise, it is essential to have a good test in order to check whether or not you are overdoing it, and potentially leading to or causing injury. A simple test that you can do for yourself is the 'talk test'. If you have difficulty talking during or immediately after exercise, then you may need to slow down and decrease its intensity.

It is important to be realistic regarding the amount of time and energy you can put into a programme. Don't set impossible goals: do something you enjoy and can stick to relatively easily, until it becomes as much a part of your daily routine as washing and eating. If your goal is to lose weight, don't go mad in the first week, exercising several hours every day and starving yourself. You will almost certainly find yourself unable to stick to such a regime and could injure yourself by pushing your body too hard too fast.

Devise a plan that fits in with your lifestyle. Increase the goals as your fitness levels increase and gradually build up to an acceptable manageable level, with the guidance of a qualified instructor where necessary. Plan to exercise for one hour, three or four times a week, and eat sensibly.

THE GOLDEN RULES OF EXERCISE

No matter what exercise or movement programme you subscribe to, there are a few important rules you need to remember. For a healthy balanced life through exercising for well-being:

- Be safe rather than sorry. When in doubt, do nothing.
- Warm up properly before exercise; cool down properly afterwards.
- To avoid injury, stretch after warming up and after cooling down.
- Allow yourself to go slowly and gently, no matter what exercise you take.
- Make gradual improvements rather than quantum leaps in your physical achievements.
- Breathe properly – evenly and deeply – when exercising, using the exhale for that extra effort or stretch.
- Never overstrain – listen to and watch yourself. Forget about the culture of competition – this is only about you and your body and no one can know better how you feel than yours truly! Work at your own level and pace.
- Be aware of your posture – shoulders down and relaxed, tummy gently pulled in.
- Do your exercises with care, control and concentration.

ASSESSING YOUR PRESENT PHYSICAL STATE

Before commencing any fitness programme it is important to identify any medical conditions or muscular-skeletal injuries or imbalances that may be aggravated by certain forms of exercise. If you have any doubts regarding your health, are a man over 40 or a woman over 45, or any of the following apply to you, then it is advisable to seek medical advice before embarking on a fitness programme.

- A history of heart problems, chest pain or stroke.

- A history of heart problems in the immediate family.

- High blood pressure.

- Any chronic illness or condition.

- Recent surgery (within the last 12 months).

- Pregnancy (now or within the last 3 months).

- A history of breathing or lung problems.

- Diabetes or thyroid condition.

- You are a smoker.

- Obesity (more than 20 per cent above ideal body weight).

- High blood cholesterol.

- Hernia or any condition aggravated by lifting heavy weights.

- Muscle, joint or back disorder, or any previous injury still affecting you.

After assessing your present physical state, the next important step is to define your goals.

don't run before you can walk

Staying motivated is a common problem for many people. In fact, only about a third of people who begin an exercise programme, typically at the beginning of the year, maintain it when results are not as rapid as they would have liked. It is a good idea to consider what incentives you might need to help you keep going, whether it be finding a fitness partner, starting an exercise log or journal, or making a realistic schedule that fits in with your lifestyle, that you can stick to and build slowly and gradually as fitness becomes an intrinsic element of everyday life.

It helps to take time to buy appropriate clothing and footwear, particularly if you are self-conscious. Wearing clothing in which you feel comfortable, and that serves the right purpose for the activity in which you are involved, is essential. Make exercise entertaining, not an ordeal, and finally make exercise non-negotiable – think of it as something you do without question, like going to work. Make it a habit.

GENERAL TIPS FOR EVERYDAY EXERCISE AND POSTURE

- Walk to work where possible.
- Get up from your desk every 15 minutes or so to stretch your back and legs.
- Check your desk positioning. Are you slouching because of a chair that's too high/too low?
- Ensure your back is supported.
- If on your feet all day, try to give your legs a break and prevent swelling in the ankles and knees – always wear very good shoes. Sit with feet up and ankles above the knees to assist in blood flow, which acts against gravity in the legs. Rotate ankles, knees and hips.
- Those on their feet and walking a lot may develop lower back problems, especially if walking on hard surfaces, like concrete and wood. Rotate hips and then lengthen spine by standing on tip-toes and stretching arms into the air.
- Driving long distances creates an imbalanced use of legs and spine – which are often incorrectly supported. Whenever possible, stop the car, get out and walk, even if only for 10 minutes every hour or so. Legs will also need stretching, to avoid tightening of ligaments or tendons.

good posture before exercise

THE GOLDEN RULES OF GOOD POSTURE

- **Feet: stand barefoot, hip-width apart, both pointing forwards.**
- **Spine: lengthen and relax, imagine a cord travelling through your crown down through body.**
- **Do not flatten natural curves at waist and neck.**
- **Lift up your head – imagine the cord pulling you up through your crown.**
- **Lengthen the back of the neck.**
- **Gently ease the shoulders down. Do NOT hold them rigidly.**
- **Shake out both arms and allow them to hang by your sides – not held rigidly.**
- **Tilt your pelvis back and forth, until comfortable.**
- **Keep knees soft.**

Good posture can help the body to function better, make you look slimmer and healthier, and help minimize stress on the spine. It also reduces the risk of muscular imbalances that can lead to injury during exercise. Good posture gives a sense of freedom, grace and ease of movement.

Posture awareness and correction are integral parts of any exercise programme. Gaining and maintaining a good posture requires a certain amount of vigilance and awareness of one's daily habits and lifestyle. Improving your posture will increase your energy levels, improve blood flow, reduce pain – for example, by helping tense tired rounded shoulders and their attendant pain, which, in turn, could have led to a crushed abdomen and, therefore, impaired use of internal organs.

As all nerves travel down through the spinal column and send messages to the brain via the medulla oblongata, a poorly aligned spine will distort the messages they carry. The body's muscular-skeletal systems will over-compensate for poor spinal alignment by tensing – potentially causing the spine to adopt a permanent, though not irreversible, curvature that will then need quite concentrated effort to correct.

Look at the way children move. Children naturally have perfect posture. To check your posture: begin by standing with bare feet hip-width apart and both pointing forwards. Good posture starts with the feet. Be aware of the feet's positioning. Is one slightly forward? One turned in and the other turned out? Correct the imbalance. This may feel uncomfortable at first, but persevere until this standing position becomes natural to you.

Next work up the legs. Be aware of any further imbalances. Is one hip sticking out more than the other? Look in a full-length mirror when checking your posture, as ingrained imbalances can often feel quite normal.

The next – and very important – stage of posture checking is with the spine and pelvis. Many imbalances in the rest of the body are caused by imbalances in the spine. If you notice anything serious, then it is best to seek the advice of a specialist. A good way to check your alignment is to place a book on your head. A basic rule of good posture is that the head, shoulders and hips should all be in the same vertical plane, in line with one another.

Tension in muscles causes 'knots' to develop and creates counter-tension in the surrounding and related areas. Therefore, a misaligned spine can affect the lungs, neck and brain – even thought processes will be negatively affected if there is excess tension in certain muscles.

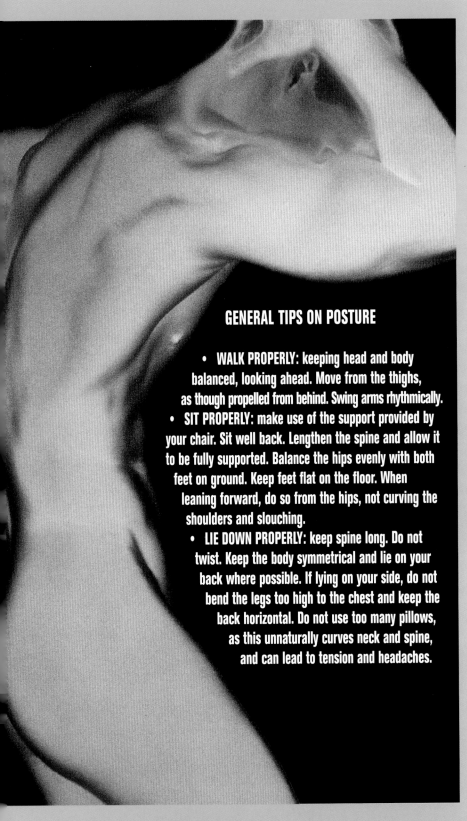

GENERAL TIPS ON POSTURE

- **WALK PROPERLY:** keeping head and body balanced, looking ahead. Move from the thighs, as though propelled from behind. Swing arms rhythmically.
- **SIT PROPERLY:** make use of the support provided by your chair. Sit well back. Lengthen the spine and allow it to be fully supported. Balance the hips evenly with both feet on ground. Keep feet flat on the floor. When leaning forward, do so from the hips, not curving the shoulders and slouching.
- **LIE DOWN PROPERLY:** keep spine long. Do not twist. Keep the body symmetrical and lie on your back where possible. If lying on your side, do not bend the legs too high to the chest and keep the back horizontal. Do not use too many pillows, as this unnaturally curves neck and spine, and can lead to tension and headaches.

All muscles and the entire skeleton, as well as all the body's internal organs, will improve from postural realignment and correction. The increased sense of well-being and energy gained from this work will encourage anyone continually to be aware of their posture, leading to new and improved habits that soon become second nature.

Once you have found the correct posture, it is important to strengthen the muscles that hold you in position, especially those in the stomach and lower back.

The most central structural part of the human body is the spinal column; it is made up of 26 articulated bones, part of a system of 33 small bones called vertebrae that are held together and supported by muscles and ligaments. Most of the vertebrae are separated by discs made of tough fibrous tissue which act as protective shock-absorbers.

The spinal column serves both as the main support to the body and a protective cover for the spinal cord, the lower part of the central nervous system, running from the base of the skull down to the lumbar region.

The spine is actually the first part of the body to be formed after conception. Indeed, possessing a spinal column with vertebrae capable of a turning movement is what distinguishes

TIPS FOR A HEALTHY BACK

- Stand straight with the shoulders relaxed and firmly supporting the neck and head, stomach held in (but not too tense or tight). Holding a firm, centred, straight but not rigid spine, neck and head is an important exercise in its own right.
- Both overarching your back and collapsing into a curved slump are bad for back health, causing strain by throwing you off balance. Your weight should be balanced between both feet.
- Sleep on a firm mattress.
- When lifting anything heavy, don't bend over from the waist or stoop down and hunch your back . Always bend the knees and get down as close to the object you are lifting as possible. Keep your back straight and use your leg muscles when lifting. Hold the object close to you when carrying it any distance.
- When carrying anything heavy, always distribute the weight as evenly as possible. Don't carry heavy loads that will strain your neck, shoulders or back. Use a cart with wheels instead.
- Make sure that your office chair provides you with the right support. Remember: you spend a lot of time in that chair!
- Those who slave before a computer for long periods should move around or stretch every 15 to 20 minutes or so.
- Get your work heights right. Stooping over a work surface too low for your height can be bad for your back.
- Do stretching exercises regularly to reach and maintain your optimum degree of suppleness.
- Always warm up before you take your regular exercise.
- Avoid being overweight – this is never easy on the back.
- Avoid wearing stilettos and over-high heels. This forces an imbalance in the alignment of your spine and throws good posture out altogether.
- Aromatherapy treatments are one of the best gifts you can give a stressed back.
- Osteopathy and cranial osteopathy are excellent for redressing the balance of a back and neck that are out of alignment.

When a man is born, he is soft and flexible;
When he dies, he grows hard and rigid.
So it is with all things under Heaven,
Plants and animals are soft and pliant in life;
But brittle and dry in death.
Truly, to be hard and rigid is the way of death;
To be soft and flexible is the way of life.

TAO TEH CHING

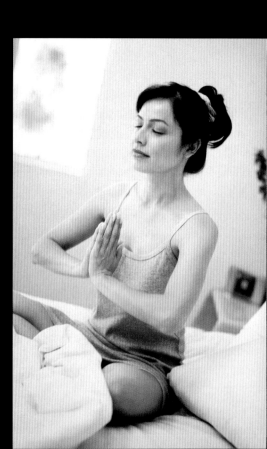

'higher animals' from the rest – hence the term 'vertebrates'. Man is the only vertebrate who stands absolutely erect and it is the distinctive characteristics of the spine that enables us to carry ourselves upright and makes us capable of an enormous range of movement.

Backache regularly affects at least 80 per cent of the population. If you are in the habit of taking exercise, you are probably in the 20 per cent of the population not suffering from some kind of back pain. Most health professionals are aware of the great value of exercise in preventing spinal problems, but getting patients to participate in a regular exercise programme is no easy feat!

Back pain is largely due to weakness in the ligaments and muscles and the spasms that result when unused bits are jolted into action! Your movement becomes restricted when unused ligaments shorten. Ligaments are sheets or bands of fibrous tissue that connect two or more bones. As you grow older, the backbone stiffens because the ligaments become tighter and shorter. This does not have to happen, however. The best way to keep your spine flexible is by keeping to a regular exercise and stretching programme that suits your needs.

Part of the reason for yoga's surging popularity in the West is that the secret is out! Yogic posture (see page 168) focuses quite considerably on spinal mobility and ligament flexibility, and many of the poses were designed specifically with the spine in mind. A key belief in yoga is that a pliable spine is the key to long life.

In the UK and the USA, back injuries are the number-one health hazard at work. Billions of pounds in work-days are lost every year due to back injuries. Many large companies are addressing this problem with screening and preventative programmes – and saving lots of money as a result. Some of them organize yoga and exercise classes at the workplace, whilst others are giving employees time off from work to attend some kind of exercise class. Still other companies arrange for massage experts to visit their premises to help staff relax and loosen the spine through massage therapy. They know that any kind of physical activity, even walking plus massage, is far more beneficial to back pain sufferers than drugs, potions or rest!

It is our couch-potato lifestyle that is responsible for all these weak and sloppy spines! At the root of the problem is too little exercise and too much stress – not to mention fashion fascism (the current vogue for stiletto heels is guaranteed to give you back problems if you wear them for more than 5 minutes after the age of 19!). Weak muscles lead to back pain. To prevent back injury, alleviate pain and restore your body's balance you must exercise to strengthen your back.

You need to exercise regularly to reap real rewards and reach your optimal spinal flexibility. Choose an activity you really enjoy. Walking, skipping, stretching, rebounding or swimming are all excellent ways to keep in shape. And of course yoga classes can really help. The choice is yours and so is the opportunity to avoid losing the flexibility and mobility a strong back provides.

warm up and cool down for safe exercise

Although often neglected, warming up and stretching the body to prepare gradually for more intensive exercise, and then cooling down afterwards, are essential ingredients of any regime and very important for injury prevention.

Try not to do any intensive stretches straight after waking up as, at this time, the muscles, joints and ligaments are especially tight. Wait for at least an hour after getting up before undertaking any deep stretches or conditioning exercises.

A warm-up should be at least five minutes long and, depending on the type of activity to be performed, should include stretches for those body parts most under stress during the given activity.

Alternatively take a brisk walk for at least five minutes. This will get the blood circulating around the body, raise the body temperature and give the synovial fluid around the joints a chance to start circulating, producing a cushioning effect around the joints and softening the ligaments ready for more vigorous exercise. If you are doing a running workout, then a good warm-up is to walk briskly or march on the spot for about five minutes, and then do stretches for the calves, hamstrings and quadriceps.

When the workout is over, it is important to cool down gradually, to bring the heart rate down to normal slowly to prevent pooling of blood in the legs. The best way to cool down is to reduce the intensity of the exercise, for example run or cycle or swim at a slower pace or walk for five minutes until breathing is back to normal and then to stretch again, usually the muscles stretched in the warm-up, holding the stretches for a few seconds longer than in the warm-up. This helps to avoid the build-up of lactic acid and lengthens the muscles, so helping to prevent muscle soreness and fatigue.

After walking on the spot in either the warm-up or cool-down, try shaking your whole body, hands, arms and legs. Then stand stationary, with feet hip-width apart and both pointing forward, keeping the knees soft and slightly bent. Keep the feet firmly planted on the floor and, without letting the area below the hips move, swing your arms from side to side, twisting the torso and loosening the spine. Continue for about 30 seconds to 1 minute.

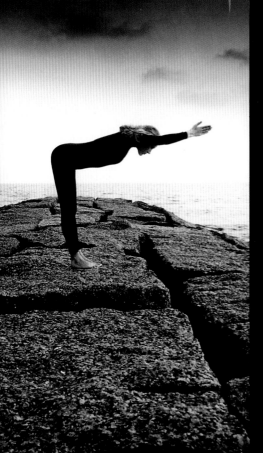

WARM-UP EXERCISES FOR THE SPINE

Head rolls

Sit comfortably with a supported back that is straight but not rigid and tense... a soft straightness. Shoulders should be relaxed and hands gently resting on your thighs. Gently drop your chin to your chest and slowly move your head all the way around, first clockwise and then, gently, in the other direction. Don't let the head roll backwards, especially if you have neck or shoulder injuries. Repeat twice. This exercise softly massages the upper part of the spine. If you feel and hear a lot of inner crackling, that's the natural by-product of a good neck-and-shoulder massage.

Knee hug and roll

Sitting on the floor, cross your feet and draw your knees to your chest, holding on to your feet or ankles in a relaxed but firm knee-hug and with your chin dropped right down and tucked into your chest. If you are comfortable and supple enough to go on to the next phase, gently roll back as far as you can go without strain and then slowly roll back up to a sitting position.

stretching, strength & stamina

Optimum physical fitness is a condition resulting from a lifestyle that leads to the development of an optimal level of a) muscular strength, b) cardiovascular stamina and c) flexibility and stretching – that is, the three 'S's: Strength, Stamina and Stretching.

As we get older, our bodies inevitably deteriorate and we realize that tasks which we used to find easy become more difficult, for example bending down to tie our shoelaces, a task that requires flexibility. To stop this gradual deterioration and to enhance our present lifestyle, it is necessary to train one's body in each of these three disciplines.

Stretching for well-being

Flexibility is defined as the range of motion of a given joint; inflexibility increases the risk of joint and muscle injury. In order to perform everyday tasks and activities, such as reaching up for a high object or bending down to pick something up, at an optimal level, one must be able to move through the motions specific to the activity with ease and fluidity. You could be very flexible in one area, even 'double jointed', but inflexible in another. You will want to attain overall flexibility. With practice, the joints can become more flexible.

Yoga, stretching and Pilates are all very good for increasing flexibility. With training, flexibility can and should be developed at all ages. Indeed, flexibility does not necessarily develop at the same rate in everyone. In general, the older you are, the longer it will take to develop the desired level of flexibility. Older people may have to work harder if they have led very sedentary lifestyles, particularly where joint stiffening has already become a problem, but perseverance always pays off. Hopefully, though, the wisdom that comes with advancing years will lend a more patient and self-loving attitude.

Stamina, or cardiovascular fitness

This describes the health and function of the heart, lungs and circulatory systems, more particularly the ability of the lungs to provide oxygen to the blood and of the circulatory system to carry blood and nutrients to tissues in the body for long periods. It is this that allows us to sustain any activity for an extended period without excessive fatigue.

There are many benefits to improving one's cardiovascular fitness or stamina. It helps lower blood pressure, strengthens the heart and lungs, increases the ability to burn body fat, helps lower blood cholesterol and gives you more energy for everyday tasks, like walking up stairs.

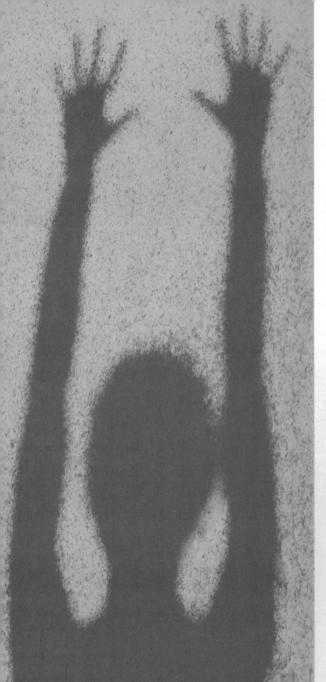

The principles of basic stamina training are fairly straightforward: at least three times a week you should move continuously and use the large muscles, such as the legs and arms, to keep the heart-rate raised for at least 20 minutes. When exercising, you should feel a little bit breathless, but not so much that you could not talk if you wanted to.

Types of stamina training

Walking, running, jogging, cycling, swimming, rowing and aerobic classes are all very good forms of stamina training, as are any sports that involve running or where the heart-rate is increased, such as football and hockey. The key is finding the activity you enjoy and which is suitable for your body type. If you wish, you can cross-train by doing several different activities. In any given week, for example, one day it could be an aerobics class, a second day swimming and a third day spent walking.

It really doesn't matter how you combine activities, as long as you adhere to the basic tenets of keeping your heart-rate elevated for 20 minutes or more, at least three days a week. Avoid over-training, however, as the body needs at least one day a week for rest and recovery. Also, try to alternate your sessions; do not do the same exercises for two or three days consecutively as you will be over-training the same muscle groups and could cause imbalance in other muscles, or strain those being repeatedly exercised.

PRINCIPLES OF BASIC STAMINA TRAINING

At least three times a week move continuously – using the large muscles, such as the legs and arms, to keep the heart-rate raised – for a minimum of 20 minutes. While exercising, you should feel a little breathless, but not so much that you could not talk if necessary.

basic exercise
programme *stretches*

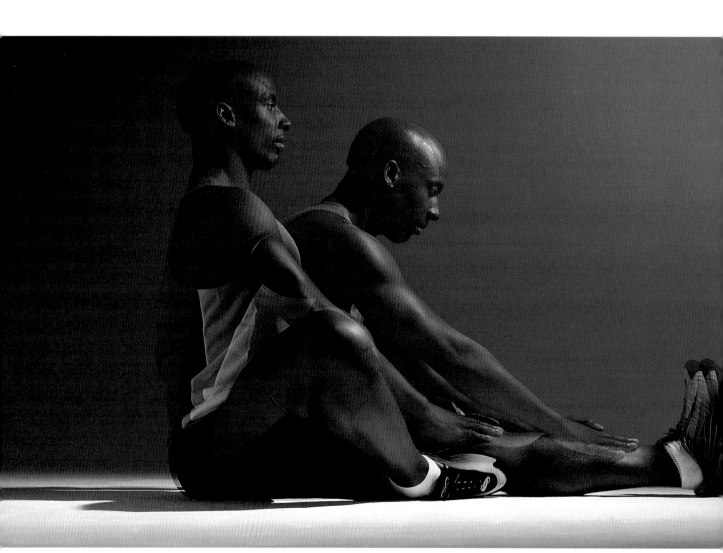

Hamstring Stretch

Stretch your left leg straight out in front, bend the right leg and lean forward from the hips as if you are about to sit down, sticking out your bottom. Rest your hands on the right knee for support, making sure both feet stay flat on the floor. Hold the stretch for 15–20 seconds, then swap sides.

Calf Stretch

From standing, bend your right knee out in front and stretch the left leg behind you – your feet should be far enough apart that you can comfortably keep your back leg straight. Both feet should be flat on the floor, with the heels firmly planted. Lean forwards, keeping the stomach and back straight, and rest your hands on your right knee. Hold for 15–20 seconds. Come back up to standing and swap legs. This exercise can also be done with hands pressed against a wall, or holding the back of a chair for support.

Lower Back Stretch

Sit on the floor with your left leg stretched in front of you and the right knee bent, so that the right sole rests against the inner left knee (left). Let the bent knee drop towards the floor to expose the inner thigh. Bend gently forwards from the hips over the left leg, keeping the back as straight as possible and bending the left knee if necessary. Hold for 15–30 seconds, then swap sides.

Posture Check and Shoulder Roll

These exercises will help to correct poor posture and relieve pressure on the spine and neck. Sit on the floor in any comfortable position – either with knees bent outwards and feet together and drawn in towards you, or with legs crossed – with the spine erect (right), as if you were sitting with your back against a wall. (Try sitting against a wall first, to test how this feels.) Keeping your stomach pulled in and the back straight, raise your shoulders slowly up towards your ears in a rolling motion, first forwards, then back, 4–8 times in each direction. Return the shoulders to their natural position, then roll the head, first to the left, then forwards, then to the right. Do NOT LET THE HEAD ROLL BACKWARDS or force it into any uncomfortable pose as this may strain the neck; allow the head's natural weight to stretch the neck and release tension in the shoulders and upper back. Repeat 8 times.

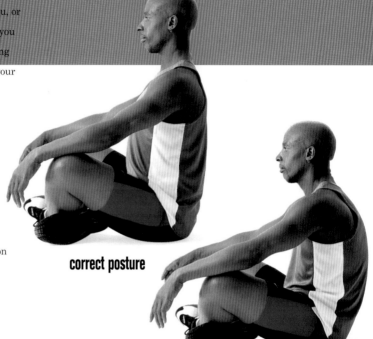

correct posture

incorrect posture

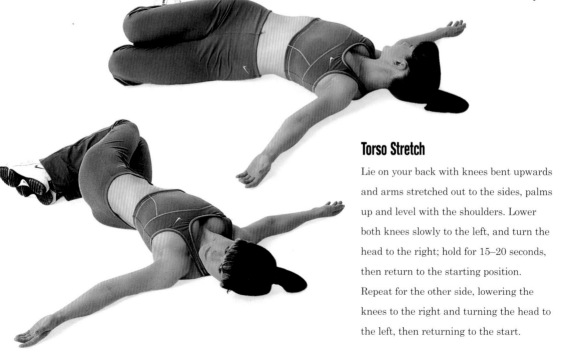

Torso Stretch

Lie on your back with knees bent upwards and arms stretched out to the sides, palms up and level with the shoulders. Lower both knees slowly to the left, and turn the head to the right; hold for 15–20 seconds, then return to the starting position. Repeat for the other side, lowering the knees to the right and turning the head to the left, then returning to the start.

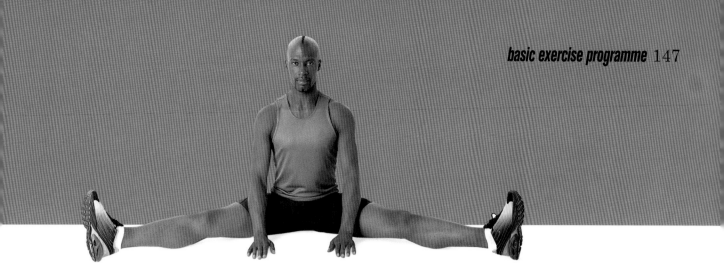

Inner Thigh Stretch

Sit upright with the legs stretched out to the sides (above), as wide as is comfortable and with the feet relaxed. If this position is uncomfortable, try this alternative (right): bend the knees and place the soles of the feet together, drawing them slightly in towards the body and letting the knees drop open and down to the floor. In either position, bend slowly forwards from the hips, keeping the back as straight as possible. Hold for 15–20 seconds, then release.

Modified Cobra

This exercise should be done very carefully if you have a history of lower back pain. Lie on your stomach with the elbows and forearms resting on the floor and tucked closely into the body. Your palms should be face down and pointing forwards, elbows roughly in line with your shoulders. As you inhale, push the floor away with the arms, slowly raising the upper torso as far as the hips – the lower abdomen and thighs should remain in contact with the floor. Hold the pose for around 5–10 seconds but release earlier if it becomes uncomfortable. (The full Cobra is pictured on page 175.)

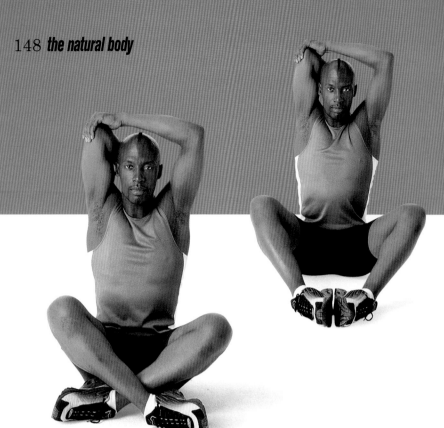

Tricep Stretch

This exercise can be done standing upright, sitting on a chair, or on the floor, either with legs crossed (far left) or with feet together and knees bent outwards (left) – choose whichever position is most comfortable for you. Stretch your right arm above your head, then bend the elbow, bringing the palm down to rest on the left shoulder blade. Grip the right elbow with your free hand and gently pull the arm to the left until you feel a gentle stretch in the upper arm. Hold for 15–20 seconds and repeat for the other arm.

Hip Stretch

Lie on your back with the knees bent and the feet flat on the floor, a short distance from the bottom (top left). Keep your left foot firmly planted and raise your right leg to rest the right foot on your left knee, letting the right knee drop open. If it is comfortable to do so, grip the the left thigh and pull it gently in towards the body, letting the left foot come off the ground (left). Hold for 15–20 seconds and repeat for the other leg.

Pelvic Tilt

This exercise is in preparation for the
abdominal strengthening exercises in the
next section, and should ideally be done with the basic crunch (see page
150). Stay lying on your back with bent knees, as in the hip stretch (below
left). Exhale and contract the stomach muscles, pressing the lower back
gently into the floor and squeezing the bottom – you should feel the stomach
hollow out slightly (top right). When you have squeezed in as tightly as you
can without straining, release the contraction and return to the starting
position, relaxing the buttocks and visualizing the stomach flattening along
the spine. Repeat 20–30 times.

Quadricep Stretch

This stretch requires some balance, so use a wall or other solid
object – maybe a chair back – for support to begin with, or even
do the exercise lying down (below). Stand with feet close
together and pointing forwards. Bend the left leg up behind you
and hold the foot with your left hand to stretch the front thigh.
If you aren't holding on for support, stretch the right arm to the
side at shoulder level for balance (right). Hold for 15–20
seconds, then release and swap legs.

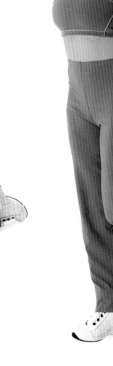

strengthening exercise

Basic Crunch

Lie on your back, knees bent and feet hip-width apart, contracting the abdominal muscles to press the lower back gently against the floor. Clasp the hands lightly behind the back of the head – don't grip too hard or you may strain the neck.

Inhale; exhale as you slowly raise your head and shoulders, keeping the abdomen pulled in tight at all times. Don't try to lift too high – if you can't control the popping-out action of the stomach muscles, you'll know you've gone too far – and resist the urge to drop back into the starting position. Don't let your feet and knees move about during the exercise, but keep them firmly in place throughout. Repeat 10–30 times.

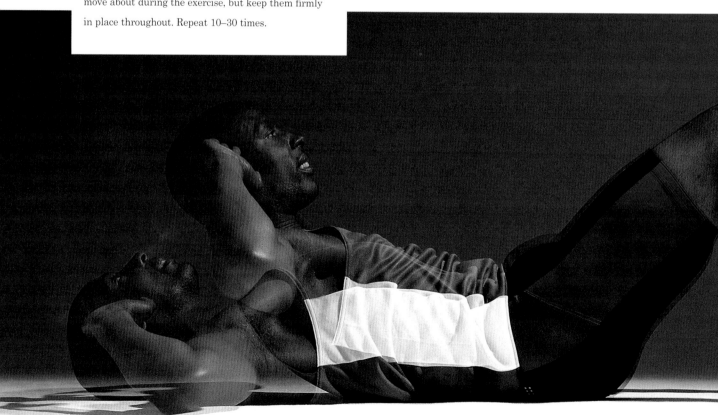

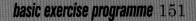

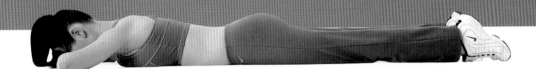

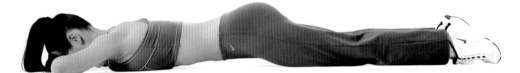

Pulling In

Lie face down on the floor with the forehead resting on the hands (palms down) and the feet shoulder-width apart (top). Inhale; as you exhale, contract the abdomen, pulling it away from the ground in a movement similar to the pelvic tilt, while keeping the rest of the body still (above). The movement is very slight – only your stomach should leave the floor – but very effective. Hold each contraction for around 10–20 seconds and repeat 5–10 times.

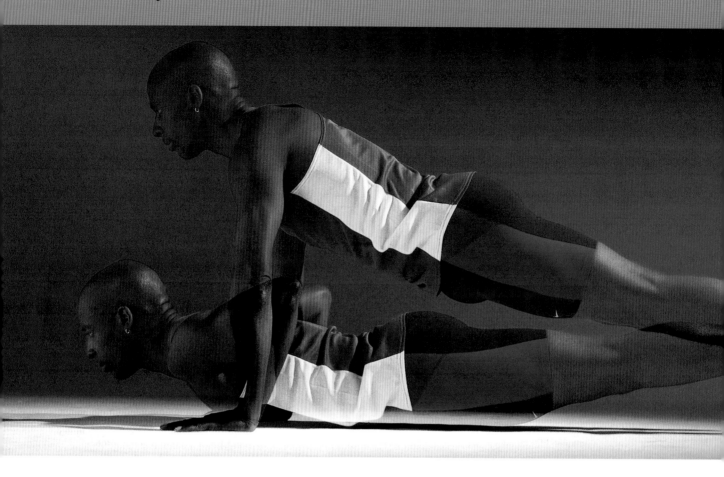

Lower Back Strengthener

Lie face down with your arms and legs extended
and palms down. Slowly raise the left arm and leg
away from the floor, without bending either and
keeping the torso in contact with the floor. Hold for
5 seconds and slowly return to the starting position.
Repeat around 5 times, alternating sides.

Advanced Press-Up

Only do this version of the exercise when you
can do the standard press-up comfortably (as
shown below). In this exercise, only the hands
and toes touch the ground, and the back should
be kept straight and the neck and spine
aligned. Lower the chest to the ground, then
return to the starting position; repeat this
process 10–20 times.

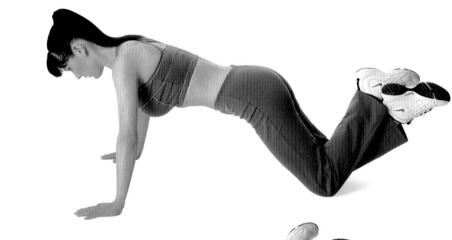

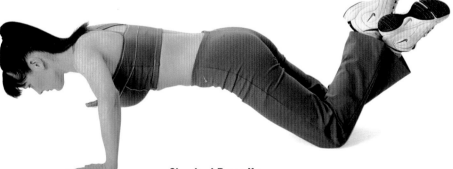

Standard Press-Up

Kneel down and rest forwards on the hands, which should be slightly
wider than shoulder-width apart. It is very important to keep the neck
and spine in line, with the back straight and stomach tucked in.
Lower the chest to the floor by bending the elbows, then return to the
starting position. Repeat 10–20 times and rest in between if necessary.

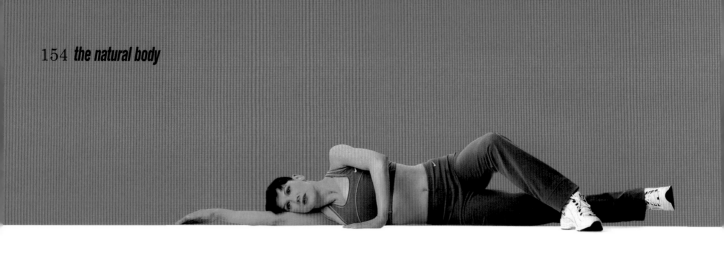

Inner Thigh Workout

Lie on your right side with
the right leg extended in line
with the body and the left knee
bent, with the foot in front of the right knee
and sole flat on the floor. Keep the stomach
pulled in tightly as you stretch the right leg
away from the hip, flexing the foot – imagine a thread
running from your hip being pulled through the heel. Raise
and lower the right leg, pausing at the top of the movement.
Keep the leg straight and don't let the foot touch the floor
during repetitions. Repeat 20–30 times, then swap sides.

Hamstring Curl

Lie on your right side, as in the inner thigh workout,
and bend the knees in front of you, so that the thighs
sit at a right angle to the torso (below). Raise the left
leg 2 or 3 inches to separate the knees and, keeping
the thighs in line and stationary, straighten the left
leg and flex the foot, without locking the knee.
Keeping the left thigh stationary, bring the lower left
leg back, heel towards your bottom, and straighten
up to the starting position. Repeat 15–30 times,
then swap sides.

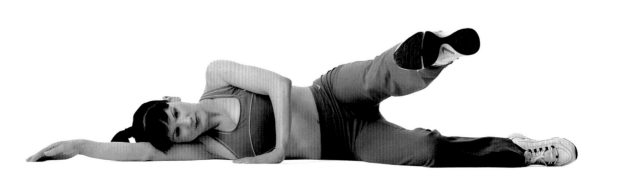

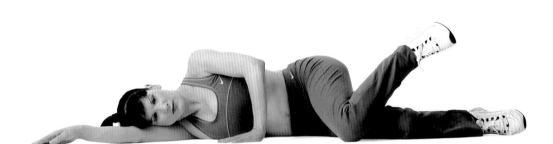

Butt Blast

Lie on your right side, knees bent up in front of the body and slightly apart (top). Lower the left knee to touch the ground in front of the right knee, then return to the starting position. Keep the movements constant and flowing and don't let the knees touch. Repeat 15–30 times, then swap sides.

Outer Thigh Toner

Lie on your right side with the knees bent, as in the butt blast (above). Extend the left leg in front of you, thighs parallel and knees slightly apart (below). Steadily raise and lower the left leg, keeping the torso still at all times. Repeat 15–30 times, then change sides to exercise the right thigh.

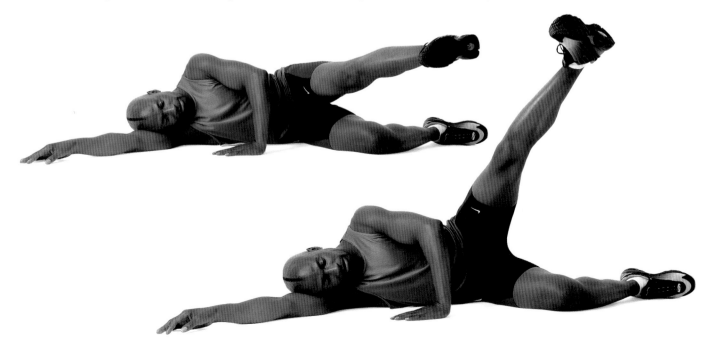

walking for a healthy heart

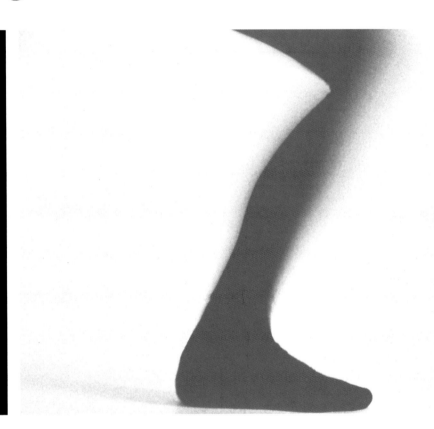

Walking is one of the best, safest and most natural forms of exercise. You can, in fact, walk your way to a healthier, stronger cardiovascular system. Walking is effective exercise for people of all ages and all states and levels of health. What's more, walking increases our sense of well-being. Think about it – we were actually designed for lengthy, regular walking.

Walking is the most underrated exercise and yet the most effective; the best starting point if you haven't moved properly in ages. One of the easiest and safest ways to get and keep fit is a brisk walk of 20 minutes three times weekly. Studies have shown that regular brisk walking can lower cholesterol levels, stimulate circulation, strengthen the heart, help control weight, reduce high blood pressure, stress and depression, prevent osteoporosis, and develop strength, stamina and endurance. New research also suggests walking is the best exercise for the brain, as it doesn't call on blood sugar for energy like aerobic exercise. As the brain is nourished by blood sugar, it much prefers a brisk walk to an aerobics class.

If you haven't taken any exercise for a while then start off gradually, strolling with a bit more determination a little longer than normal, slowly building up your endurance level. It is probably also a good idea to start walking at a fairly relaxed pace until you have warmed up, before graduating to a really brisk gait.

- Strolling walk — walking in a relaxed way, but with good posture, shoulders down, arms swinging naturally as you walk.
- Brisk walk – fitness, pace or aerobic walking: all mean pretty much the same thing, stepping up your pace and pumping your arms as you walk.
- Power walk – for a very fit, younger, experienced walker, usually working with a personal trainer. Walking with weights, carrying them in your hands and/or strapping them on your waist and ankles.
- Water walk – walking (wading) through water, either in a pool or in the sea. Walking hip- to waist-high in water is a very good low-stress, high-intensity exercise. For higher intensity, run in the water, but you will need a vest or flotation belt to keep you in an upright position.
- Treadmill walk – most gyms have treadmills, but many people are getting home versions that chart distance and speed and time the walk.

Even for walking you do need to be prepared

If you are doing a lot of serious, committed walking then you might want to buy a pair of shoes actually designed for walking. When you walk you land with 1½ times your body weight on the outside of your heels; then you roll your weight forward on the ball of your foot. A good walking shoe will allow the rolling action of the foot with ease. Older people may be more stable in a shoe with a thinner hard sole. You should also wear comfortable clothes that don't restrict your movements. In winter, wear layers that you can peel off as you warm up.

Walking is the most natural, practical, straightforward preventative exercise programme. The ultimate safe natural fitness routine, walking builds body strength, stamina and tone. It also de-stresses you – which is good for the heart and the nervous system. In your later years, it slows down the ageing process, keeping you fit, agile and mobile. Walking also helps you develop better coordination, breath control, self-esteem and endurance.

Walking should be the primary part of your fitness routine, no matter what other exercise systems, movement or sports attract you. Walk first, then run or dance or ride your bike. It's up to you – you can cycle till you're blue in the face and you still won't get all the benefits you get from a good brisk long walk. If your walking muscles atrophy, the rest of your body will soon follow. Brisk walking is the greatest form of exercise: your natural basic life-long conditioning programme, protecting your heart and enhancing your well-being.

TIPS FOR HEALTHY WALKING

- Drink water before and afterwards. If very thirsty, stop to drink during your walk.

- Don't walk right after a meal. Leave at least 45–60 minutes after eating before taking a brisk walk.

- Avoid the hottest midday hours (noon to 3.00 pm). The ideal time is morning or late afternoon.

- After a good long or brisk walk, it is a wise idea to eat some form of carbohydrate within a couple of hours to restore your glycogen levels.

- In summer, if you are taking longer walks, protect your skin with a sunscreen. You can also use your sunglasses or a visor to protect your eyes in extremely sunny hot weather.

in the swim

After walking, the next best thing you can do for your body is to swim on a regular basis. Swimming is the ultimate enjoyable safe way of exercising, providing all the aerobic benefits of, say, running and cycling without the same wear and tear on the muscles, joints and bones. It gives an excellent aerobic workout by exercising most of your major muscle groups.

The natural resistance of water strengthens and tones your muscles, joints and bones without the same risk of injury present when you exercise on land. Water is about 1,000 times more dense than air, which is why it offers considerable resistance, resulting in a 'double positive' effect on your body. It exercises opposing sets of muscles at the same time – for example, the front and back of your arms in the same movement. From a body-sculpting point of view, swimming does not encourage the bulking of muscles; in fact, with the added resistance of the water, muscles often become lean, rather like those of runners.

Just walking in water is a fantastic exercise for building up your endurance. Walk as briskly as you can in waist- or chest-high water. Swimming is your ideal exercise for a brilliant body-conditioning without the sweat.

Swimming and other water exercise are considered so much safer than working out on the ground or in the gym because water is the perfect cushion of support, allowing us to feel almost weightless. Your body is 90 per cent lighter in the water, so you are buoyant and you are safer than you would be in the gym from putting too much pressure on your joints.

The impact of cold water and the pressure of the water also promotes blood circulation in the muscles. The pulse is slowed down and there is quicker recovery from exertion than when exercising on land. Despite the exhaustion that can be experienced through exertion, the pleasant tiredness created leaves you feeling very good and invariably very relaxed.

In fact, swimming is excellent for relaxation, not least due to the enforced deep breathing necessary. Some even liken it to moving meditation, the sensation of being supported by water, the quiet, the freedom experienced by the body while gliding through the water, all add to the sense of inner calm often experienced by those who meditate. Staying focused on the swim encourages the stilling of the mind and forces out all outside influences.

The total natural support of water also usually has a very comforting and relaxing effect on your state of mind. As your mind calms down so does your whole body, improving and massaging your muscles as you effortlessly move through the water.

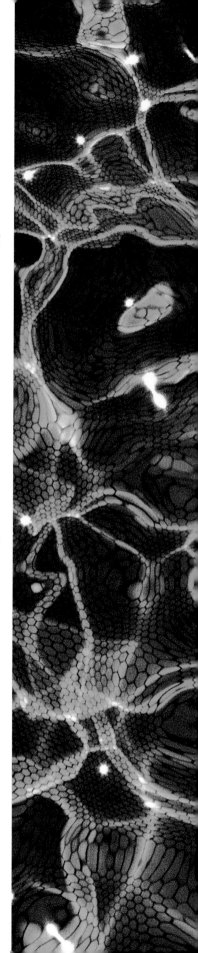

Water exercise is also excellent for the injured, the disabled, the elderly and mothers-to-be, as no additional stress is placed on your joints when moving through the water. This is the most painless way to exercise, which is why it is recommended for so many conditions. After walking, it is the best exercise for preventing degenerative health conditions, and a wonderful way of moving that enables you to maintain the well-being of both body and mind throughout your life.

Swimming can be enjoyed by people of all ages and levels of ability. Children absolutely love water from a very early age. In fact, encouraging children to find their feet in water when very young will allay any potential fears of water which may develop later on. Once children have taught their bodies how to float, there's no stopping them. Much fun can be had just splashing around and floating, or jumping in, until they are ready to take on the structure of learning strokes.

The elderly, or those otherwise less mobile, can also benefit greatly from sessions in the pool. The relaxing benefits simply of *being* in water will induce a calm state in everyone. Even if you cannot swim, working out in the shallow end can be very beneficial. Of course, people of any age can enjoy the benefits of learning to swim, even if they have not had the pleasure from childhood. Many pools will offer classes for children and adults, from complete beginners to experienced veterans.

It is important to remember that swimming is an exercise like any other and, therefore, warm-ups and stretches are just as relevant here as if you were running five miles on the treadmill. Warming up could be one lap followed by stretches, particularly of the shoulders, arms and upper back.

All warm-ups and stretches can be done in the water, and once in the water it is advisable not to get out until ready to shower, dry and get dressed again, as the muscles will cool down rapidly, which could cause problems. Remember to make sure you cool down at the end of your swimming session by slowing down in the last few laps and, again, stretching at the end of the session.

THE BENEFITS OF SWIMMING

- Strengthens the cardiovascular and respiratory systems.
- Maintains and develops bones and muscles.
- Builds stamina and endurance.
- Gentle whole-body exercise with high aerobic value.
- Increases your general level of fitness and well-being.
- Maintains flexibility and muscle tone.
- Stimulates the circulation.
- The horizontal position places less stress on your heart in respect of blood circulation.
- Gentle pressure of water on skin enhances blood circulation.
- The cardiovascular benefits are essentially the same as in running or walking, with all the major muscle groups being worked.
- Lowers blood pressure.
- Water resistance helps to build up muscle strength.
- Weightlessness in water allows one to stretch effectively, using the water's support.
- Excellent for maintaining flexibility and suppleness.
- Creates lean muscles and not heavy bulky muscles.
- Rehabilitates injured or weakened muscles.
- Speeds up the healing process.
- Relaxes and refreshes the mind.
- Good for overweight people as body is supported.
- Safe for pregnant women throughout pregnancy.
- Good for those with joint or back problems.

GENERAL RULES FOR SAFETY IN THE WATER

- Wait at least an hour after eating before swimming.
- Get out of the water if you feel persistently cold.
- Wear a buoyancy jacket if you do not know how to swim and you are going into potentially deep water. You can still exercise while wearing a life jacket.
- If you are recovering from an injury or an illness, or are very unfit or middle-aged plus, consult your doctor about the safety of swimming for you.

It is a good idea to try and vary your strokes once you have gained confidence through a qualified instructor's guidance on the best techniques for each stroke. This way you avoid overworking one particular muscle group and ensure that all muscle groups are worked in turn, creating an overall fitness programme for the entire body.

Aqua-aerobics

Water- or aqua-aerobics is another wonderful and safe way to give your whole body a really good workout, putting considerably less strain on it than with 'land'-based exercise! An increasing number of pools are now offering some type of water exercise classes. They provide a great way to get fit, keep fit and have fun at the same time.

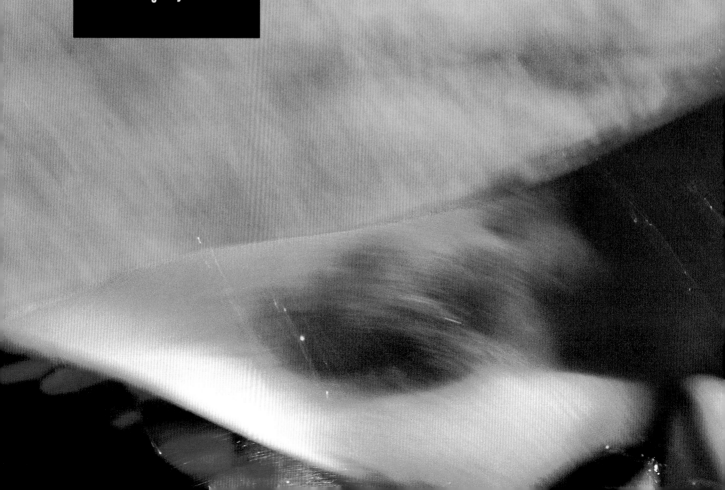

The exercise offered will normally incorporate training of the leg muscles as well as upper-body training. This form of exercise is suitable for everyone at any age and is particularly enjoyed in Britain, for example, by older people. However, more and more younger people are beginning to realize the significant benefits of aqua-aerobics.

It is particularly recommended for anyone who enjoys working out but does not like getting sweaty and hot, and who is cautious about using gyms, running, etc., for fear of joint injuries.

EXERCISE GUIDELINES FOR PITTA TYPES
(see pages 11-15)

Swimming is the ideal activity for pittas, as is walking in nature, which really calms them down.

BASIC AQUA-AEROBIC EXERCISES:

- Stretches using a handrail.
- Running on the spot in chest-deep water.
- Walking in chest-deep water.
- Running in chest-deep water.
- Using aqua weights in water to intensify training. These hand-held weights are used when jogging on the spot, walking and running, to intensify fat burning and increase the heart-rate.
- Lifting weights against water pressure increases muscular strength and toning in the arms and the sides of the body, the back, neck and chest.

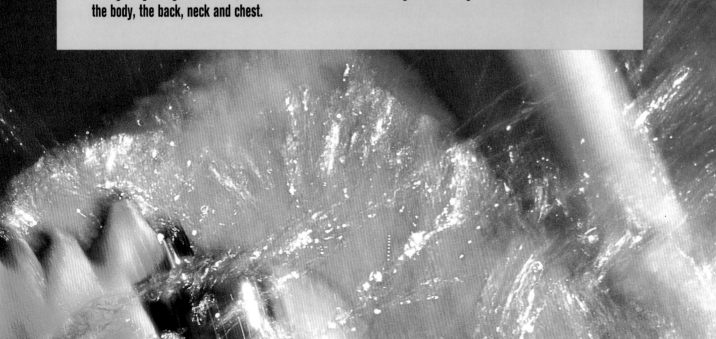

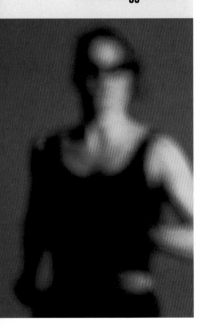

running and jogging

If the thought of getting up at the crack of dawn, donning warm and comfortable workout gear and shoes, and braving the elements for a two-mile run is a major turn-off, then think again. You can adapt running to suit your lifestyle and time-scale – and it can transform your body. The benefits of running – including boosting of the immune system, respiratory improvements and benefits to your self-esteem – simply cannot be overestimated. You also gain the benefit of being in the open air, which is something so many of us lack in our daily lives, as we are huddled into crowded public transport and stuffy offices most of the day.

Getting started

Starting off with a realistic programme will help. Keep a check on your progress and, if possible, have a fitness assessment beforehand. If you have any injuries to the bones, back, knees, ankles or feet, opt for strength-training exercises and stretches that will correct these problems. Running on hard ground may exacerbate any long-standing or recent injuries, putting you off running all together.

Start with a programme of walking and running intermittently. If you haven't run since you were at school, then begin with brisk walking. Set a goal. Even starting with just five minutes' walking, building to ten, then on until you reach your goal of, say, 30 minutes, will be more beneficial to you in the long run than trying to run a mile, finding it impossible and giving up.

When ready to start running, remember to take precautions as you would with any other exercise. Obviously it is essential that time and consideration are given to buying suitable running shoes. Most sports suppliers can advise on this.

Always warm up the muscles, particularly those in the legs, with brisk walking beforehand. Then stretch the leg muscles and the upper body for 10–15 minutes. You may prefer to alternate between running and walking, until you feel confident enough to run continuously. Wear a watch that is easy to read and run for five minutes and walk for five minutes, building up to your goal level.

Pace yourself. Don't race ahead at the beginning of your session if you are unfit or planning to walk/run a distance. If, at any time, you feel out of breath and uncomfortable, do not stop suddenly but slow down and keep moving, gradually settling into a walking pace. Stopping suddenly will be as shocking to your body as running like the wind without having trained, or warmed up and stretched.

Running technique

Hold your arms loosely by your sides, bent at the elbow. Not tight across the shoulders. The arms should move naturally in opposition to the legs, as in the swing when walking. If this feels odd at first, pay attention to it. Soon it will feel as natural as walking. When brisk walking, and in early training, bring the arm position into the walking motion. You will probably find walking becomes easier and the legs are able to stride from the hip more easily.

Be aware of your breathing. This will come naturally to you after a period but, if unused to this kind of physical activity, you might experience a tightness in the chest. Try to deepen your breathing until you are breathing rhythmically with the striding of your legs. If you begin with walking, focus on your breathing then. You will naturally breathe more deeply during exertion – training your breathing is as important as training your body and good practice during the early stages will enable you more effectively to utilize the breath when actually running. Shortness of breath can often be attributed to poor breathing techniques, such as very shallow breathing that does not allow the lungs to fill properly.

When you have finished your run, cool down gradually, slowly decreasing your pace until you are walking briskly and your breathing has returned to normal. Shake out your arms to release any tension stuck there. When you've reached your goal, do your stretches, gently holding each stretch for at least 30 seconds.

If running is your chosen cardiovascular activity, try to do it three times a week. Cross-train with other forms of exercise, including strength-training and stretching. Strength-training is vital to produce the strong leg muscles and abdominals essential for effective running.

Running in the gym is as effective and almost as beneficial as running outside. Apart from the pleasures of being in the open air, however, wind resistance and rough terrain outside can greatly increase the benefit.

Avoid any risk of injury by being sensible and seeking advice from a personal trainer, runner or another similar person beforehand.

A TYPICAL 6-WEEK PROGRAMME FOR THE COMPLETE NOVICE

WEEK 1
Warm-up; stretch.
Walk 4 mins; run 1 min.
Repeat 3 times.
Stretch.

WEEK 2
Warm-up; stretch.
Walk 4 mins; run 2 mins.
Repeat 4 times.
Stretch.

WEEK 3
Warm-up; stretch.
Walk 3 mins; run 3 mins.
Repeat 4 times.
Stretch.

WEEK 4
Warm-up; stretch.
Walk 2 mins; run 3 mins.
Repeat 5 times.
Stretch.

WEEK 5
Warm-up; stretch.
Walk 1 min; run 4 mins.
Repeat 5 times.
Stretch.

WEEK 6
Warm-up; stretch.
Run 20 mins.
Stretch.

dance is a natural exercise

TIPS FOR SAFE DANCING

- Always warm up first.
- Wear appropriate clothes and shoes.
- If you are not fit nor used to taking any exercise, take it gradually and very gently at first.
- Communicate any chronic or present health problems to the instructor.
- If dancing for pleasure at a party or night club, pace yourself appropriately.
- Drink plenty of liquids.
- If expecting to be dancing energetically for a period of time, eat slow-release energy foods (see page 43) about two hours before dancing.

The spirit of the dance is within us all. Children, on hearing music, will often move their bodies and connect to a rhythm quite naturally. Dancing is a primal and ancient form of movement that has been part of our lives from the beginning of time. There is also no doubt that dancing is a wonderful exercise, releasing and freeing not just our bones, muscles and joints, but raising our spirits.

Massively popular across the world, clubbing is a way of releasing the stresses of the week, whether at college, school or work. High-energy dancing also gives your body a great workout. But be sure to drink plenty of water and not to overdo it, as even just going out dancing can cause physical injuries, particularly in the ankles, knees and hip joints, when pounding the floor repeatedly.

There are so many dance forms from which to choose – jazz, modern, tap and ballet, or how about belly and shamanic dancing or temple dancing? Choose the one that moves and satisfies you, and to which you feel instinctively drawn.

When deciding which dance form is right for you, however, be realistic about your state of fitness, your age and your ability. Start at the beginning, learning steps and form gradually, as you build up stamina and confidence.

Shamanic dance

Free-flowing and impulse-based, shamanic dance is primal, awakening and moving sexual energy to constant rhythmic drum beats. Shamanic dance enables you to enhance the natural renewal and regenerative processes within yourself and so allow yourself to be reborn and experience elation.

Ecstatic trance dance

This dance-form, which works with techno, ambient, global and world music, is about release through euphoria and moving into higher states of consciousness. It is all about being – or discovering – who you really are, when not in competition with others or trying to be the best. You dance as each of the four elements – earth, water, fire and air – for about 15 minutes, your breathing and the music changing with the feeling the elements provoke. The session fills you with energy.

Five rhythms

This is a dance-form formulated by American dance guru, Gabrielle Roth, who says it is '...harnessing the raw power of rhythm into a part of self-realization that gives us a practice, a perspective and a philosophy that allows us to celebrate the wild, ecstatic dancer within'.

Five rhythms behaves like a build-up and breaking of a wave – from flowing, through staccato to chaos, where people really let go of stresses and their selves, turning to a lyrical stillness that takes them back to the beginning of the circular rhythmic dance-form. It is an excellent way of stretching muscles, while enhancing physical alertness and mental prowess as well as allowing free-flowing creativity. It also helps to move any ingrained stress.

African dance

This is ritualistic, earthed, vibrant and ecstatic all rolled into one. Constant drumming puts the primal self back into the fore and encourages you to move with the beats. Classes in many towns and cities teach some movements and actual ritual dance for the celebration of stages of life and seasons.

Salsa

This is a very popular form of dance, due to its vibrancy and it being just plain good fun. Dancing with a partner is coming back into fashion and is the preferred form for many. The Cuban dance is exciting and the music uplifting. The fun and laughter enjoyed in salsa are incredibly beneficial to many who may be put off exercising in a traditional way. Salsa uses a great deal of energy and is profoundly good for the soul, as well as being very sexy and releasing sexual energy.

Ceroc

This dance-form is based on traditional dance steps like two-step, cha-cha-cha and waltz, amongst others, performed to more modern music and beefed up.

Dancing with a partner makes this form of dance romantic and good fun.

Jazz dance

This popular dance-form is learnt primarily by professional dancers, although many adult education centres and dance groups cater for a wide range of abilities. It provides another great way to shape up and have fun.

Ballet

Many dance companies offer ballet classes for adult beginners! It is something that one is never too old to learn and provides an excellent discipline that maintains very high levels of fitness and suppleness. You can't expect to become a prima ballerina, but you can enjoy some of the benefits ballet dancers experience, like grace, poise, balance, well-toned muscles and a strong body.

Belly dance

Traditionally, this Middle Eastern dance-form is performed by both men and women. In America, belly dancing is recommended by doctors for the prevention or treatment of many ailments. It is useful for weight problems, toning the body, easier childbirth or PMS, reviving flexibility, self-esteem and your love life.

Temple dance

Versions of this come from most Eastern cultures, such as those in Thailand, India and China, as well as many Middle Eastern countries. Training in these ritualistic and religious dance-forms can

take many years, but the basics can be enjoyed by all. Watered-down versions of various forms of temple dance are available and often help to bring a spiritual element into one's life.

Dancercise classes

Although not widely available, these are taught in some gyms by dancers and aerobics instructors. More choreographed than traditional aerobics classes, they incorporate dance routines. They are fun and good exercise at the same time.

THE BENEFITS OF DANCING

- Builds endurance.
- Increases flexibility.
- Increases agility.
- Builds strength.
- Helps balance.
- Develops co-ordination.
- Builds confidence.
- Enhances body awareness.
- Develops overall fitness.

Overall ENJOY!

pilates

Joseph Pilates developed the Pilates system of breath and movement work about 75 years ago. He studied many forms of Eastern and Western body-work and, as he suffered from a range of disabilities, initially developed the exercises to help his own conditions. He continued studying and refining the techniques, and then began teaching what is now a well-known and very popular exercise technique. Historically the techniques were a secret known mainly to the dance world, but are now becoming more widely known and practised by a greater variety of people.

The Pilates exercise techniques, when performed regularly, constitute a complete fitness method that positively changes bodies. According to Joseph Pilates, 'In ten sessions you'll feel the difference, in twenty you'll see the difference, and in thirty you'll have a new body.'

Pilates bridges the gap between strength and flexibility training, enabling it to be incorporated into existing physical activities, whether cardiovascular, swimming, cycling or any other form of body-work. Regular practice of Pilates can significantly improve performance in all other sporting activities, as well as improving your general well-being.

Pilates combines awareness of the spine, proper breathing and strength and flexibility training. Where most forms of exercise develop muscles, Pilates is virtually unique in that it slims the muscles, making them more compact by developing slenderness rather than bulk. Regular Pilates devotees can expect to achieve a balanced body which is strong and supple, with a flat stomach, balanced legs and a strong back. Its effects, however, are more than physical, as the practitioner of this technique will feel revitalized, relaxed, confident, invigorated and more flexible, with a great and new sense of well-being.

Pilates works by assisting you in changing the way you use your body. By redressing imbalances and altering movement patterns, your body is brought back into balance. Your posture and co-ordination will be corrected and you will learn to move the way nature intended and the way that you used to move as a child before you developed poor postural habits.

With this newly learnt ease of movement, not only the muscular-skeletal system will function efficiently, but also the circulatory and lymphatic systems. In fact, every system of the body is improved through regular Pilates practice, including the nervous system, so reducing stress levels and eventually leading to a stress-free existence.

This is an exercise system that affects every part of you, down to cell level, as your body will become properly nourished, with oxygen being replenished and toxic

BENEFITS OF PILATES

- Complements other body-work and natural therapies.
- Helps prevent injury.
- Provides postural realignment and enhancement.
- Develops grace.
- Increases relaxation.
- Boosts the immune system.
- Has a beneficial effect on osteoarthritis and osteoporosis.
- Benefits knee and shoulder injuries.
- Relieves stress.
- Relieves headache and other pain.
- Purifies the blood stream.
- Permanently changes body shape.
- Provides a totally holistic system of fitness.

waste removed. Emphasis is placed on mind-body integrity, making it a truly holistic fitness regime.

Pilates is renowned for its usefulness in both injury prevention and rehabilitation. The technique is often used to rebuild and strengthen muscles after injury or strain. As it is a gentle programme, it is useful in many cases of rehabilitation, for example with lower back injury, neck and shoulder tension, even general aches and pains. Exercises can be performed without involving the injury area, as the supporting muscles are strengthened, thereby giving the injured area time to heal.

Pilates classes are held in many gyms and exercise centres throughout the country. Qualified practitioners will take you through a series of moves and breath work, correcting any errors you may make as you work into position. Every class will be balanced in its own right and through repeated attendance at class you will learn as many as 70 different exercises. Pilates instructors are very diligent in correcting errors and encouraging correct breathing during class.

Once you feel confident that you have mastered the moves and breath work, Pilates can easily be practised at home on a daily basis further to enhance its healing and physical benefits. Pilates can also be practised before gym work or other sporting activities, taking the place of a warm-up.

Pilates breathing

Breathing correctly ensures that the body receives its full quota of oxygen. Pilates breathing is called thoracic or lateral breathing. You are taught to breathe in to prepare for a movement. Breathe out, strong centre to spine, and move. Breathe in to recover. Breathe into the ribcage, therefore expanding the lower ribcage and increasing the lungs' capacity to take in more oxygen. 'Zip up and hollow' is a much-used breathing and abdominal tightening exercise used in Pilates. In it you draw the muscles of the pelvic floor up and in, and hollow the lower abdomen back towards the spine.

> 'A man is as young as his spinal column.'
> *Joseph Pilates*

> 'Above all, learn how to breathe correctly.'
> *Joseph Pilates*

THE EIGHT PRINCIPLES OF THE PILATES METHOD ARE:

- Relaxation
- Concentration
- Alignment
- Breathing
- Centring
- Co-ordination
- Flowing movements
- Stamina

yoga for keeping well

Yoga is an ancient system of mind-and-body exercises that originated in India over 5,000 years ago. Now, people all over the world are learning the simple techniques of yoga and experiencing the benefits of this holistic approach to exercise. In yoga, the goal is to balance mind and body through a series of physical, breathing and mental exercises – the word 'yoga' literally means union. Yoga's popularity in the West is increasing all the time; no surprise when you consider the high value placed on a well-honed, well-toned body/mind in our culture today.

Hatha yoga is the branch of yoga that concentrates on body postures (asanas) and movement, together with pranayama, where the focus moves to the breath. Hatha yoga practice encourages awareness of the breath as a channel through which the *prana* – the life force that makes all things possible and manifest, including the restorative practice of yoga – can flow. The very quality of the postures and breathing flow encourages the centring of our concentration within. Along with the sound of our inhalation and exhalation, we learn to listen and hear other internal sounds: muscles, joints and bones all telling us what they need. We can learn to be more aware of our inner state of being – along with the ever-demanding external state of being – the life outside our skin. Yoga can help integrate our inner and outer worlds, help us process the impact and the interface between our inner and outer realities.

Yoga is not a competitive endeavour, although some who are practising the new 'power yoga', Ashtanga, would disagree. To begin with, it's a good idea to find a qualified instructor to assist you in attaining the asanas. Instruction in correct breathing can only be given by a qualified instructor and, once enough familiarity with the asanas and breathing is attained, regular practice at home is essential. In the words of Swami Sivananda Vedanta, 'Ten minutes practice is worth more than hours of theory'.

De-stressing with yoga

Yoga is thought to be an excellent way to de-stress because it works not only on the muscles, bones and joints but also on the nervous system as well. By practising yoga we stretch and tone the body brilliantly, increasing muscle

EXERCISE GUIDELINES FOR VATA TYPES
(see pages 11–15)

Vatas are advised to get involved in yoga, T'ai chi, walking and anything rhythmic. They do have a tendency to over-exercise and should take active steps to make sure that they don't. Activities for them to avoid include aerobics and step classes.

strength and stamina and correcting posture, while learning how to relax the mind, dramatically improving our concentration, our sense of well-being and our spirituality. Asanas are designed to exercise the body while simultaneously calming the mind. Asanas have both a Sanskrit name and an English translation, and both are given here. Yoga is always done slowly and thoughtfully, concentrating and breathing into each posture. Take each pose to a point well before pain and over-exertion. Listen to your body and your breathing, taking the postures slowly and gently.

This is where the pranayama are so important – correct breathing supports and strengthens the asanas. Generally, you inhale as you begin the first phase of the posture and exhale while you expand and move into its final phase. Yoga is never competitive, but respects the limits of the individual. Never push through pain to achieve a more 'correct' asana; instead, allow the gentle unfolding of a posture to the best of your ability. In the early stages of your practice, it is always a good idea to take instruction from a professional, accredited yoga teacher. This will help you to grasp the basic principles of each pose and avoid developing bad habits.

Inverted postures

Inverted postures, where your heart is above your head, are very powerful and need to be approached with great care. Do not do these postures (asanas) if you suffer from high blood pressure or have a fever or a headache. If you have back or digestive problems consult your doctor before undertaking any but the most simple, basic forms of exercise like walking. Do try to have some proper yoga classes before attempting these postures unless you are very experienced in exercise systems and are very fit and supple. Inverted postures are so potent because the effects of gravity are reversed. The organs which are normally in the upper part of the body and usually receive a smaller flow of blood are now below. The blood pours into these organs without the least exertion of the heart, which normally has to overcome the force of gravity in order to pump blood to the organs of the neck and to the head and brain. The burden on the heart is reduced, giving it a chance to truly rest and relax.

eastern exercise programme

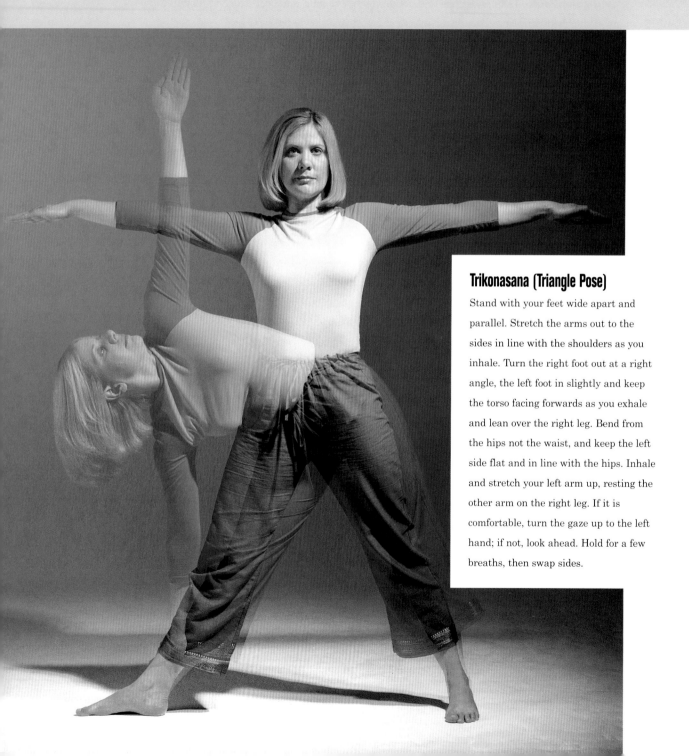

Trikonasana (Triangle Pose)

Stand with your feet wide apart and parallel. Stretch the arms out to the sides in line with the shoulders as you inhale. Turn the right foot out at a right angle, the left foot in slightly and keep the torso facing forwards as you exhale and lean over the right leg. Bend from the hips not the waist, and keep the left side flat and in line with the hips. Inhale and stretch your left arm up, resting the other arm on the right leg. If it is comfortable, turn the gaze up to the left hand; if not, look ahead. Hold for a few breaths, then swap sides.

Mountain

This is an excellent warm-up posture and is good for expanding the chest and opening the lungs. Stand up straight with the feet together and arms down by the sides. Stretch the spine by lifting up through the head and chest, but without raising the shoulders – keep them relaxed and down. Lift the thighs. Keep the gaze soft. Hold for a few rounds of complete breathing and relax.

Vrikonasana (Tree Pose)

Stand up straight with feet together and arms by your side. Inhale deeply; as you exhale, bend your right knee, drawing the foot up towards the groin and resting it as far up the inner left thigh as is comfortable. Gaze at a fixed point ahead of you to help you balance. Raise the arms above the head and press the palms together in a praying motion. Hold for a few rounds of complete breathing before changing legs and repeating on the other side.

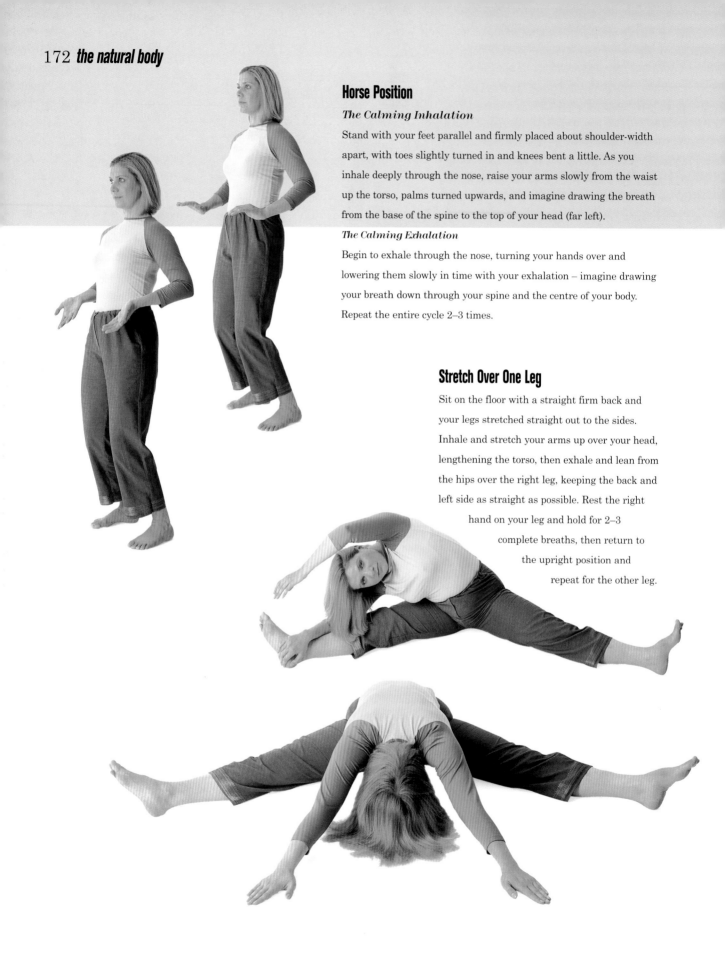

Horse Position

The Calming Inhalation

Stand with your feet parallel and firmly placed about shoulder-width apart, with toes slightly turned in and knees bent a little. As you inhale deeply through the nose, raise your arms slowly from the waist up the torso, palms turned upwards, and imagine drawing the breath from the base of the spine to the top of your head (far left).

The Calming Exhalation

Begin to exhale through the nose, turning your hands over and lowering them slowly in time with your exhalation – imagine drawing your breath down through your spine and the centre of your body. Repeat the entire cycle 2–3 times.

Stretch Over One Leg

Sit on the floor with a straight firm back and your legs stretched straight out to the sides. Inhale and stretch your arms up over your head, lengthening the torso, then exhale and lean from the hips over the right leg, keeping the back and left side as straight as possible. Rest the right hand on your leg and hold for 2–3 complete breaths, then return to the upright position and repeat for the other leg.

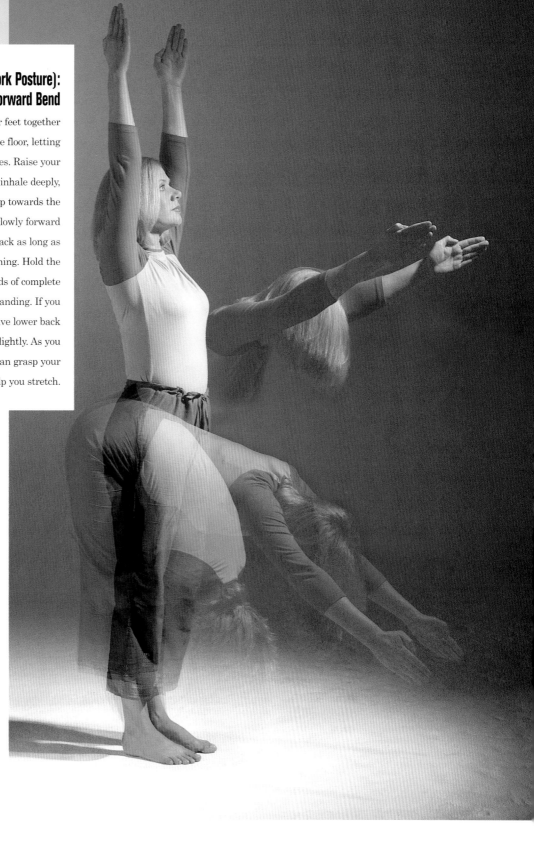

Padahastasana (Stork Posture): Standing Forward Bend

Stand up straight with your feet together and firmly in contact with the floor, letting your arms hang by your sides. Raise your arms above the head as you inhale deeply, stretching the fingers up towards the ceiling. Exhale and bend slowly forward from the hips, keeping the back as long as possible without straining. Hold the position for 3–6 rounds of complete breathing and return to standing. If you experience pain, or have lower back problems, bend your knees slightly. As you become more flexible, you can grasp your legs or ankles to help you stretch.

Spread Legs Stretch

Stay in the same upright sitting position as in the stretch over one leg pose (opposite). Inhale and place your hands on your knees; slowly exhale as you lower your head towards the floor, bending forwards from the hips and keeping your back long and straight. Hold for a few breaths. Never strain the back or legs in this posture and stop if you feel any pain.

Forward Bend Sitting

Lie on your back with the arms resting by your sides. Inhale deeply and slowly raise your arms until they are flat on the floor above your head. With the exhalation, sit up slowly, bending forwards from the hips until you can touch your toes (if you are very flexible) or grasp your ankles or calves. Hold for a few breaths. Avoid any unnecessary strain by keeping your back long and as flat as possible, and by bending your knees slightly if you feel any pain.

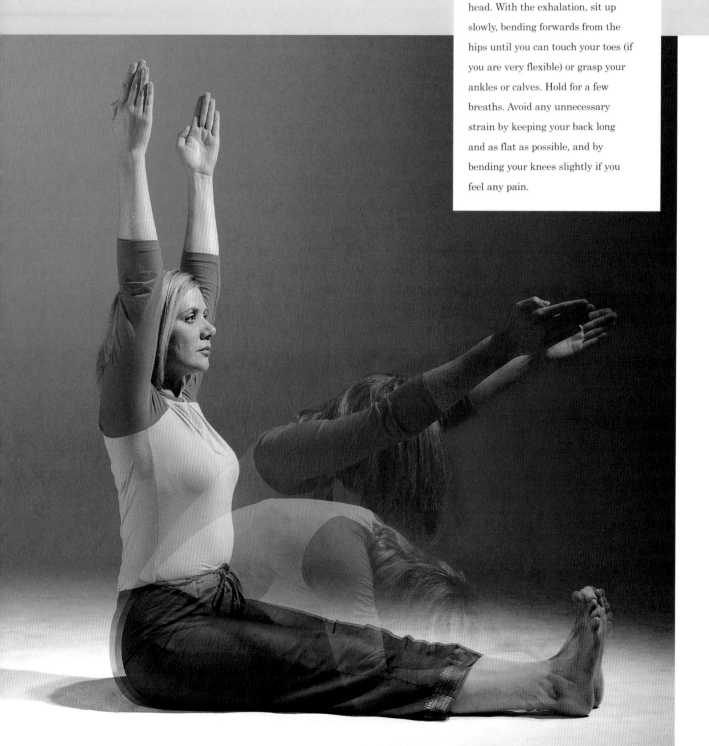

Child's Pose

Kneel with the toes touching and knees slightly apart and bend forward over the thighs. Rest the forehead on the floor to take the weight of the head. Rest the arms by the sides of your body, palms facing upwards. This is a good counterpose to the cobra, and other postures in which your spine is arched. It also helps to relieve back strain after doing inverted postures (e.g. shoulderstand).

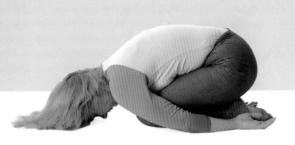

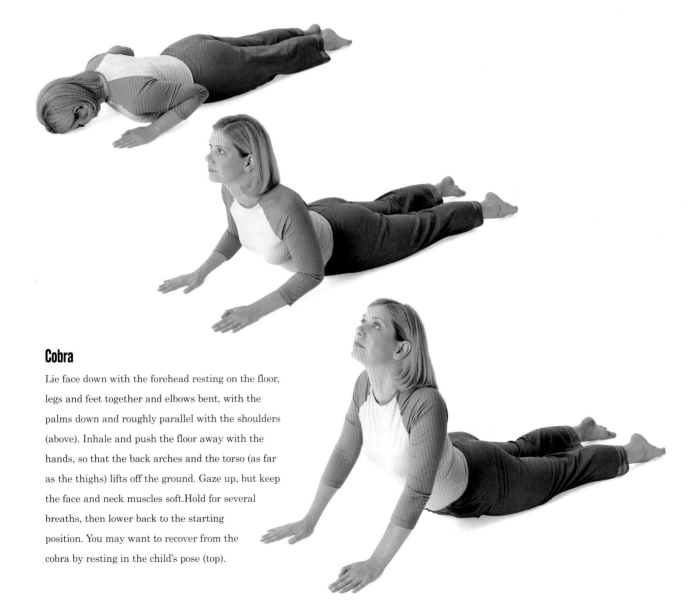

Cobra

Lie face down with the forehead resting on the floor, legs and feet together and elbows bent, with the palms down and roughly parallel with the shoulders (above). Inhale and push the floor away with the hands, so that the back arches and the torso (as far as the thighs) lifts off the ground. Gaze up, but keep the face and neck muscles soft. Hold for several breaths, then lower back to the starting position. You may want to recover from the cobra by resting in the child's pose (top).

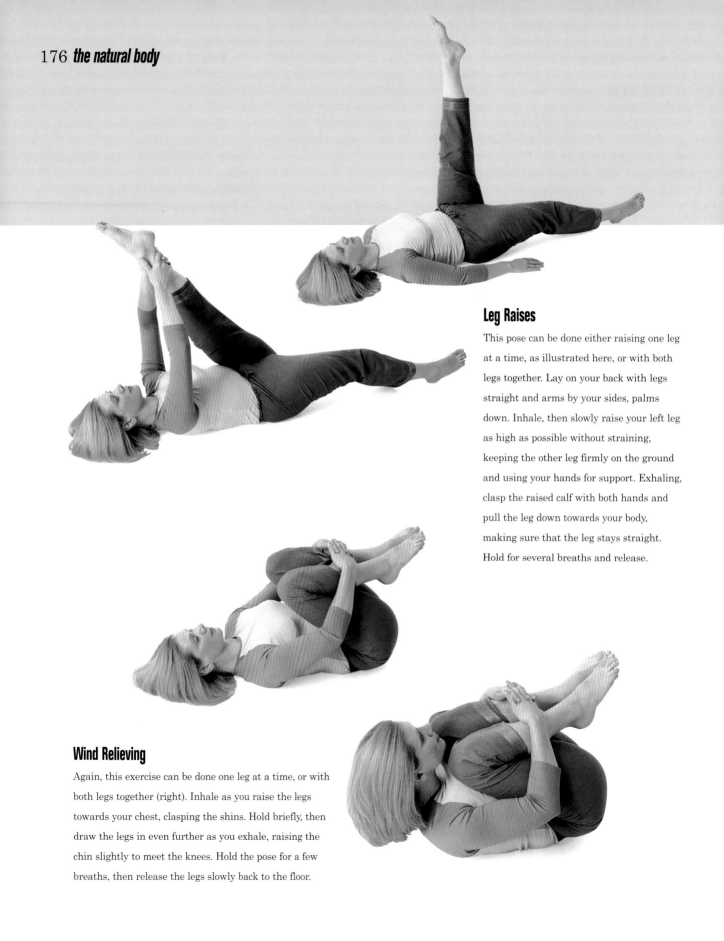

Leg Raises

This pose can be done either raising one leg at a time, as illustrated here, or with both legs together. Lay on your back with legs straight and arms by your sides, palms down. Inhale, then slowly raise your left leg as high as possible without straining, keeping the other leg firmly on the ground and using your hands for support. Exhaling, clasp the raised calf with both hands and pull the leg down towards your body, making sure that the leg stays straight. Hold for several breaths and release.

Wind Relieving

Again, this exercise can be done one leg at a time, or with both legs together (right). Inhale as you raise the legs towards your chest, clasping the shins. Hold briefly, then draw the legs in even further as you exhale, raising the chin slightly to meet the knees. Hold the pose for a few breaths, then release the legs slowly back to the floor.

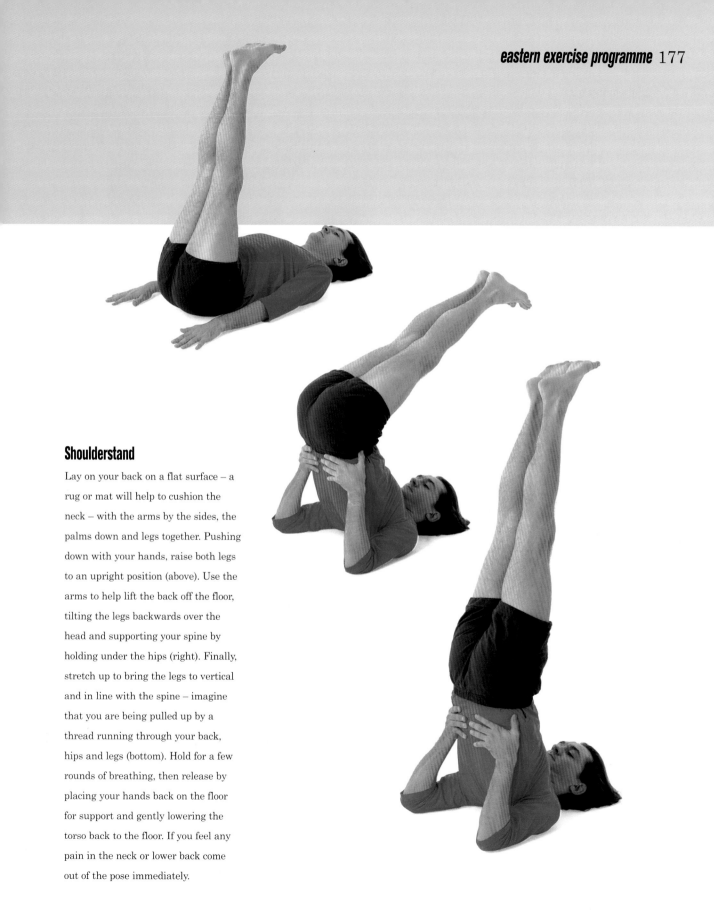

Shoulderstand

Lay on your back on a flat surface – a rug or mat will help to cushion the neck – with the arms by the sides, the palms down and legs together. Pushing down with your hands, raise both legs to an upright position (above). Use the arms to help lift the back off the floor, tilting the legs backwards over the head and supporting your spine by holding under the hips (right). Finally, stretch up to bring the legs to vertical and in line with the spine – imagine that you are being pulled up by a thread running through your back, hips and legs (bottom). Hold for a few rounds of breathing, then release by placing your hands back on the floor for support and gently lowering the torso back to the floor. If you feel any pain in the neck or lower back come out of the pose immediately.

Salute to the Sun

1 Stand upright, with feet together and weight equally balanced. Bring the hands together in the prayer position and exhale. **2** Inhale and stretch the arms above your head, arching the back slightly and keeping the legs straight. **3** Exhale as you bend forwards, placing the hands at either side of the feet in line with the toes, pressing the palms into the floor. Keep the head tucked in and bend the knees if necessary. **4** Inhale and squat down. Stretch the right leg back behind you to rest on the toes, and drop the right knee to the floor. Exhale. **5** Inhale and move the left leg back to join the right. Keep the head in line with the body, the feet together and the back straight. **6** Exhale; lower the knees to the floor and bend the elbows. Lower the chest, then the chin, to the floor, keeping the hips raised and toes curled under.

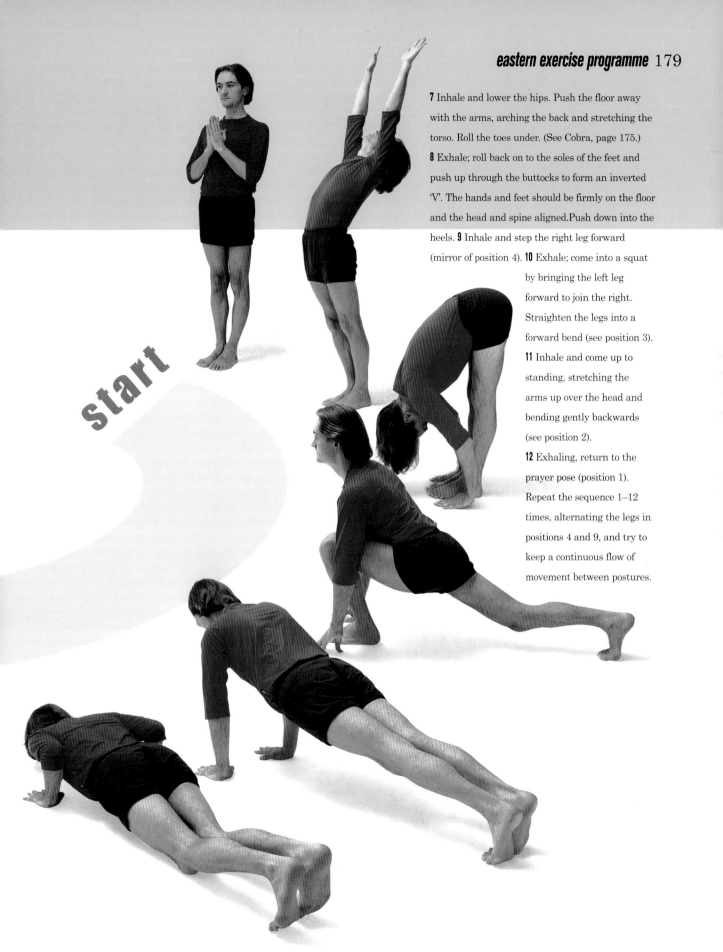

7 Inhale and lower the hips. Push the floor away with the arms, arching the back and stretching the torso. Roll the toes under. (See Cobra, page 175.) **8** Exhale; roll back on to the soles of the feet and push up through the buttocks to form an inverted 'V'. The hands and feet should be firmly on the floor and the head and spine aligned.Push down into the heels. **9** Inhale and step the right leg forward (mirror of position 4). **10** Exhale; come into a squat by bringing the left leg forward to join the right. Straighten the legs into a forward bend (see position 3). **11** Inhale and come up to standing, stretching the arms up over the head and bending gently backwards (see position 2). **12** Exhaling, return to the prayer pose (position 1). Repeat the sequence 1–12 times, alternating the legs in positions 4 and 9, and try to keep a continuous flow of movement between postures.

start

Lotus

Sit with the legs crossed, the spine erect and palms resting on the legs. This is a meditative pose, so keep the gaze soft and turned down, and concentrate on breathing deeply through the nose. Use your hands to lift the left foot up to rest on the right thigh. Then place the right foot across it to rest on the left thigh. Rest the hands palm-up on the knees (far right). If you find this position too hard, try the Half Lotus (right): stretch one leg at a time into position, hold the pose for a few breaths, then swap legs.

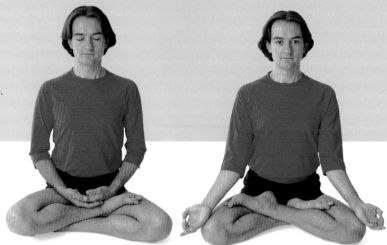

Vakrasana (Sitting Twist)

Sit on the floor with your legs stretched out in front and your back erect, and hands palm-down by your sides. Bend your right knee, drawing the leg up until the foot is parallel with the left thigh, then crossing it over. Inhale. As you exhale, twist your torso to the right, holding your right knee with your left arm and stretching your right arm out behind you. Gently turn your head to look over the right shoulder. Use your breathing to stretch up through the spine, and to gently increase the twist. Keep the spine upright to avoid strain. Hold for a few rounds of breathing, then swap sides.

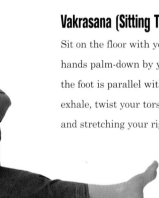

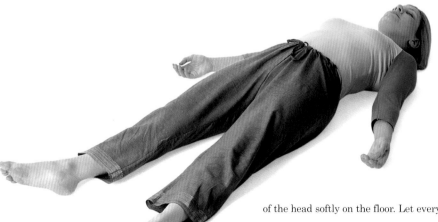

Corpse

Lie on your back on a firm surface: a rug on a hard floor, for example. Stretch the legs out straight and shoulder-width apart, rest the hands by your sides (palms upwards) and either close your eyes or gaze ahead. Rest the back of the head softly on the floor. Let every muscle relax completely. Rest in this pose for a few minutes, or as long as you need to relax, breathing deeply through the nose throughout. When you are ready, roll gently over to your right side, hold for a few moments, then sit up.

breathing for yoga

In terms of yoga, the art and science of breathing is called 'pranayama'. Breathing through the nose is a basic rule of health in the disciplines of the East like yoga. Breathing through the mouth is a bad health habit, much more prevalent in the West. It is vitally important to your health to re-educate yourself if you have the habit of shallow breathing through the mouth. Complete deep breathing through the nose will relax you on a much more profound level as well as give you the best protection from infectious diseases.

In pranayama the basis of all breathing exercise is complete deep breathing. Each breath combines 1. abdominal, 2. middle and 3. upper chest (clavicular) breathing. You inhale through the nose into your belly so that your abdomen expands as air is drawn into the bottom of your lungs. The next phase of the inhalation moves up into your middle; and your chest and upper chest area expands last. As you slowly exhale, your abdomen, middle and then your chest contract. This powerful exercise should be done 3-6 times at first. Done regularly over time it will enhance vitality and reduce your stress levels for good.

Complete Yoga Breathing

Sit comfortably, either cross-legged on a mat, in a chair or on your heels with spine firm and centred, not tense. Close your eyes, focusing on your navel, centre area. After a good exhale, breathe in through the nose, expanding first the abdomen, then the ribs, chest and collarbone, raising them as you count to 8. Then exhale through the nose, contracting the abdomen, ribs and chest and finally lowering the collarbone and shoulders to the count of 8. Repeat 3 to 6 times. This exercise induces relaxation by calming the nervous system and also oxygenates the blood and increases lung capacity.

Kumbhaka Breathing

This exercise can be done sitting, standing or lying down. The focus of your attention is on the heart area. This is the same as complete yoga breathing, but you extend the cycle by holding your breath to the count of 4 after completing inhalation and before exhalation. Always breathe in and out to the count of 8; you can extend this with practice but you should never strain and if you have a heart condition you should not do this exercise. It is very calming for the nervous system, and can regulate the pulse and an irregular heartbeat, by slowing the heart.

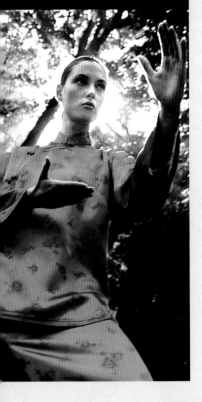

t'ai chi chuan
-'grand ultimate boxing'

T'ai chi is an ancient Chinese exercise system that co-ordinates a series of simple movements into a continuous rhythmic sequence with steady and controlled breathing. The roots of t'ai chi go back thousands of years to early Eastern philosophies, including Buddhism and Taoism, and many of the sequences are based on the movements of animals.

T'ai chi is similar to yoga in that it relaxes both body and mind, prevents tension and helps build strength and a sense of well-being. However, t'ai chi is characterized by continuity of movement, combined with regulated breathing and deep reflection, rather than a series of distinct poses. Practitioners believe this system helps to clear the blocked energy (or chi) that causes disease, and encourages a free flow of energy through the body to improve health – research at Johns Hopkins University in the USA has proved that regular practice of t'ai chi lowers blood pressure. T'ai chi is especially popular among the elderly because it improves strength and general health through low-impact exercises. With t'ai chi, you can quickly learn where you hold tension and how to release it.

As with most exercise, it is advisable to locate a teacher who is qualified in the form of t'ai chi you wish to study. Classes are widely available, and a typical weekly lesson of around two to three hours will teach you enough to practise at home. You should be prepared to study for some time to learn the movements – a full sequence can comprise between 24 and 88 postures – and learning the postures is only part of the training; it is equally important to learn how to move between the poses while keeping your balance. A session will often start with a standing meditation to release any stress accumulated during the day, followed by a warm-up to stimulate the mind and body for the sequence to follow.

qigong

Qigong is a form of t'ai chi that focuses on healing through 'energy cultivation'. Two forms of energy are activated – internal chi (qi) and external chi (qi) – through breathing exercises, movement and meditation. External chi can be emitted to heal others.

There are about 500 forms of Qigong practised around the world. Although each approach generally seeks to improve balance and awareness, there are fundamental differences between them, depending on the philosophy upon which it is based: for instance, the Buddhist form aims to release the Self through awareness; the Taoist form focuses on connecting one with nature; and the Confucian form is concerned with establishing one's place in society as a whole.

Banned in China for many years, Qigong is enjoying a huge resurgence. Practitioners around the world report on the many medical benefits of Qigong, including relief from allergies, asthma, hypertension, liver disorders, and even potentially life-threatening illnesses such as cancer.

Taijiwuxigong

A particularly interesting form is taijiwuxigong, which focuses on the daily cleansing of negative energy and posture correction. Its creator, Dr Shen Hongxun, believes bad posture is one of the main causes of disease, causing irritation of the nerves of the spinal column and damaging circulation and the metabolism. This system differs from others in that it involves a repetition of only a few key postures involving outward movements away from the body. Because of the simplicity of the exercises, it is accessible to people of all ages.

Results can be dramatic even after one session and the student is advised to remain calm and quiet for some time afterwards to avoid faintness or shock. Taijiwuxigong can sometimes induce very powerful responses, both physical and emotional, signalling a release of tension and negative energy. The result is a feeling of release from tension and an overall sense of well-being. Whichever form of Qigong you decide to do, it is important to find a qualified instructor, and to wear loose clothing in which you can move freely. Also, take a warm outer layer to help retain body heat when the class ends.

the natural mind

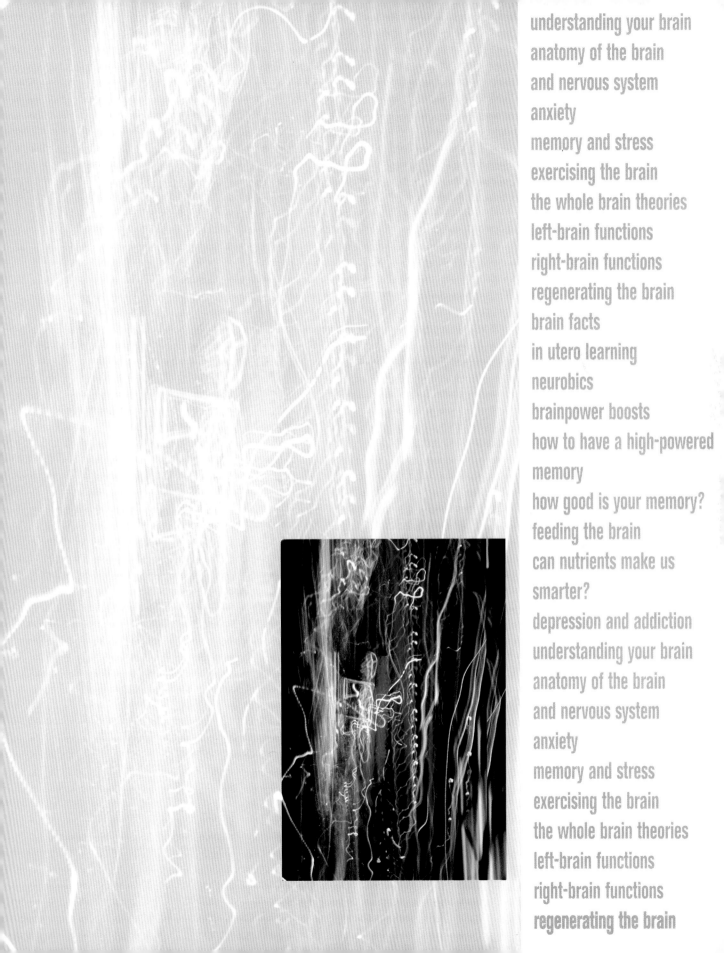

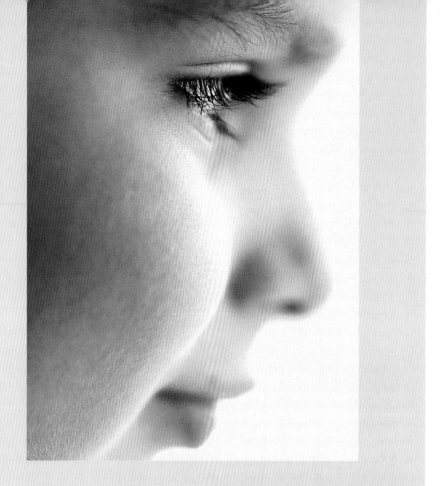

understanding
your brain

The latest scientific thinking on the brain suggests great minds are made, not born. Nurture not nature determines how agile your mind is. It is continual curiosity and learning that keeps the mind active and, like any muscle, you have to use it or lose it, and the longer you do the better the effect. Unlike other parts of the body, the more you use the brain the better it gets, the more honed and skilled it becomes... the brilliant mysterious facilitator of all we experience and perceive.

anatomy of the brain & nervous system

It is exciting and empowering to know that new scientific discoveries show you really can change your brain – that nerve endings can grow throughout life, and new brain cells can emerge. A young brain may be more malleable than one that is middle-aged but, even in our middle and later years, good and regular brain training, a sustained brain workout, can make nerve cells flourish.

World expert on the brain, Professor Susan Greenfield, of the Department of Pharmacology at Oxford University, says, 'Your brain is changing all the time. No single area of the brain is activated exclusively and solely during a specific mental task. Whole constellations of cells become active at different times and in subtly different ways, depending on what you are doing. Indeed, far more brain regions turn out to be involved than had previously been thought possible.'

The brain is our most mysterious and mighty organ, weighing no more than around 1½ kilos (3 pounds) and residing within the skull at the top of the body, capable of running the whole show without using more than a small percentage of its capacity. After decades of intense scientific research, there is still so much we do not understand about this most complex and fascinating part of the body. The command and communications centre of the body, the brain controls the nervous system, an intricate network receiving messages from the senses, processing them and then co-ordinating and directing all our actions and reactions.

The brain and nervous system work together with the glands of the endocrine system, which governs the body's hormones, to form a regulation and control system of exquisite refinement and awesome power. The home of our thoughts, feelings, sensations, perceptions, creative imagination and talents, as well as the instruction headquarters for all our body's functions, the brain's power comes from electrical energy carried in the chemical substances known as neurotransmitters.

The brain is divided into three parts – the largest is the cerebrum, where voluntary action and thought are controlled. This is the reception centre for the messages to and from the rest of the body. Speech, muscle control, vision and touch are dealt with by the cerebrum. The front lobe of the cerebrum deals with planning and complex functions; the back with vision. The second part of the brain, the cerebellum, is located behind and under the cerebrum. This is where the controls for balance and muscle co-ordination are based. The third part, the medulla, controls involuntary reflex actions like your breathing, respiratory rate, heart-rate and digestion process. The brain never sleeps – even when we do, it is still processing information from our five senses and beyond.

The nervous system includes the central nervous system, consisting of the brain and spinal cord, protected by the skull and spine, and the peripheral nervous system, which extends from the central nervous system to the rest of the body via its cranial and spinal nerve network. The central nervous system serves the rest of the body like a central computer system, receiving and analysing sensory information and then sending out the appropriate response.

Nerves conduct messages to and from the brain and around the body. The messages consist of electrical impulses that travel from one end of a nerve to the other and are then chemically transmitted to other nerves or to muscles. Motor nerves carry orders from the brain to the muscles and sensory nerves carry messages about sensations, such as itching, pain or feeling cold, etc., to the brain.

Impulses travel through the nerves, long tube-like extensions of nerve cells or neurons. Each neuron has a cell body, an axon, and branches called dendrites. The small gap which separates each neuron is called a synapse. The chemical released by each neuron as it contacts the next in the nerve chain is called a neurotransmitter. Released from the end of the axon, the neurotransmitter crosses the synapse and carries the message to the next neuron.

The central nervous system is made up of over 100 billion tiny neurons. Each is connected to around 10,000 other neurons and they are constantly sending messages to each other. All this activity takes a lot of energy and uses a high level of the body's prime fuel, glucose. The peripheral nervous system consists of the autonomic nervous system, which controls our involuntary body functions, like blinking, shivering or sweating, and the somatic nervous system, which controls the muscles responsible for willed, conscious movement.

The autonomic nervous system mostly controls the organs and glands, and is divided into the sympathetic and the parasympathetic nervous systems. Much of the time these two systems maintain a kind of balance, but the sympathetic system dominates during times of fear, delight or excitement, by stimulating the increased breathing or heart-rate required by the body's natural 'flight-or-fight' response (see page 205). Everyday functions like digestion and sleep are the concern of the parasympathetic system.

anxiety

Many people experience anxiety in one form or another. From mild to severe, from panic attack to chest pains, dizziness to breathing difficulty, palpitations to sweating, from loss of appetite to insomnia. All of these and more are symptoms of anxiety which can, if untreated or ignored, lead to more serious problems when they start affecting normal everyday life.

Normally anxiety and panic attacks are a result of emotional upset. The emotional issue should be looked at and dealt with. Vitamin B deficiency can also cause anxiety problems.

Supportive measures include:

Aromatherapy (see page 261)

Geranium, which is emotionally balancing; lavender, which soothes; frankincense, which uplifts and helps you to slow down the pace.

Nutrition (see pages 36–87)

Avoid sugar and sugary foods and drinks; avoid coffee or any caffeine-based drinks or foods; do eat foods rich in B vitamins.

Homoeopathy (see page 270)

- Arsenicum alb if anxiety worsens when sufferer is alone or in the dark.
- Calc carb if experiencing palpitations or if loss of reason is feared.
- Phosphorus if extremely anxious, worsening before a thunderstorm.
- Arg-nit or gelsemium if anxious before a key event.
- Aconitum for ailments experienced after a panic attack.

Supportive treatments include:

Acupuncture (page 260)
Alexander Technique (page 260)
Chiropractic (page 265)
Cranial Osteopathy (page 266)
Massage (pages 220–229)
Osteopathy (page 274)
Bach Flower Remedies (pages 263–264)

- Mimulus for fear with known cause.
- Rock rose for panic.
- Aspen for fear of the unknown.
- Cherry plum for fear of mental collapse.

MEMORY AND STRESS

The panic stations that go on alert when the body is stressed directly affect the amount of memory one is able to access through the retrieval system. The amygdala, which controls fear, blocks the ability of the body to retrieve stored information. Next time you need to remember something – like information for an exam – make sure you are allowing yourself the necessary tools to de-stress first before trying to access these memory banks.

Having now explored the brain in some depth, we are aware of the incredibly complex nature of this organ of consciousness. We now understand how there are two ways of knowing – two ways in which we process the same information – via the brain's two hemispheres.

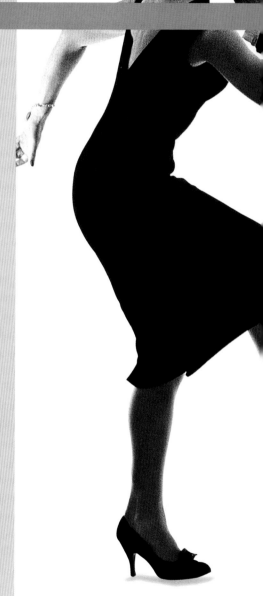

exercising the brain

The left hemisphere of the brain analyses, verbalizes, counts, plans and is rational and logical. The right hemisphere intuits, imagines, relates, integrates and freely associates. Getting to know and stimulating both sides of your brain is an important step in optimizing your creative potential.

The whole brain theories

The left hemisphere controls the right side of the body, the right hemisphere controls the left side of your body. Your nervous system is connected to the brain in a crossed-over fashion. Hence the right hand is connected to the left hemisphere and the left hand to the right hemisphere. In terms of function, human cerebral hemispheres develop asymmetrically. This is reflected in our propensity to be either right or left handed – it is the rare individual who is ambidextrous and can use both hands with the same ease and control. In recent years many experts and theorists have embraced the new 'whole brain' theories. These conclude that even though many human beings seem to be dominated by either the left (and are analytical by nature) or the right hemisphere of the brain (intuitive, creative), if the whole brain is 'switched on', all learning, healing, creating and gaining of new skills becomes easier. Open childlike enthusiasm and curiosity are rekindled when we stimulate our whole brain. Whether you are an analytical left-brain type or an intuitive right-brain person, the important thing is more integration of the hemispheres in your daily life.

According to psychologist Janet Goodrich, in her book, *Natural Vision Improvement*, more balanced use of both hemispheres 'makes for a self-realized person, who is happy, healthy and creative in a total

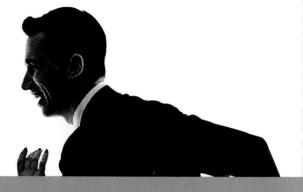

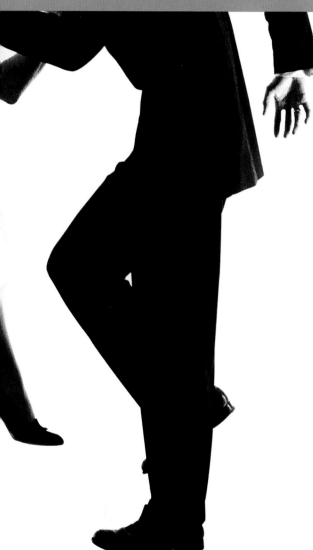

sense. When [the brain hemispheres are] integrated, we are able to see an image and describe it as well. We want to maximize the flow of energy from one side of the brain to the other and create dual dominance – full activity and interchange of both hemispheres.'

Kinesiologists as well as natural vision therapists agree on the importance of crawling in our brain's development as well as our motor development. The crawling stage begins our first autonomous exploration of the space around us. Crawling prepares us for eventually learning how to read and write 'where our eyes, hands and mind will flow from left to right across the midline of the paper'. It is during this crucial crawling stage that we first move freely from one hemisphere of the brain to the other as we move left hand in synchronization with right leg (and vice versa).

To exercise the whole brain and stimulate hemisphere integration you can simply get down on the floor and crawl like a baby. You have to have 'cross over', i.e. use alternate hand and leg movements – when your left hand moves forward so does your right leg. You could also simply march slowly in place (to music if you like), lifting the left leg and right arm at the same time, etc. See also Brainpower Boosts on page 194.

LEFT-BRAIN FUNCTIONS

Reason, logic, hearing, right-handedness, number skills, writing, time perception, details, objectivity, extroversion, tension

RIGHT-BRAIN FUNCTIONS

Emotion, intuition, ESP, left-handedness, musical skills, sight, space perception, seeing whole picture, subjectivity, introversion, relaxation

regenerating the brain

One of the most remarkable recent discoveries about the brain is that it can regenerate. If you suffer any sort of brain damage you will almost certainly be told by doctors that your neurons can't re-grow. While skin, blood and bones are all constantly replacing themselves, brain cells – so the experts have had us believe for nearly a century – just grow older.

However, according to recent research, that does not seem quite so certain any more. Last year, researchers at Princeton University in America proved the official version wrong. Using a drug originally developed to detect new cancer cells, Dr Elizabeth Gould discovered that new cells were growing deep in the cavities at the centres of monkeys' brains and then migrating up to the top layer of the cortex, which controls memory, thinking and decision-making.

This discovery is making neuroscientists rethink their theories of how the brain works and it holds out the possibility of repairing it. Within the next ten years, doctors may be able to replace cells damaged by a stroke, restore the covering to nerve fibres stripped off by multiple sclerosis and even reverse the effects of Alzheimer's.

Neurogenesis, as it is called, is throwing new light on how memories are stored. The old idea was that they were created by strengthening connections between neurons, but now it looks as if memories may be held in new cells. This explains, for instance, how memories are date-stamped – recent memories are actually stored in newer cells.

The scientists are aiming to exploit neurogenesis with all the sophisticated techniques of modern cell biology. Although it's far from perfect – otherwise no one would be permanently affected by strokes – damage to the brain does speed it up. An epileptic seizure, for instance, triggers a spurt of new growth. What is more, new cells will tend to migrate towards the site of the trouble. Currently researchers are looking to develop drugs to improve these natural processes.

Another future approach is to exploit the chemical signals that make these cells grow. As far as we know, nerve cells in the spine don't re-grow. However, take spinal cells and put them in a part of the cortex that controls memory, known as the hippocampus, and they can renew themselves. Researchers plan to grow new cells outside the body, using the chemicals that stimulate them, and then replant them when needed.

We don't have to wait for all these hi-tech approaches to deliver, however, as the good news is that we can influence neurogenesis now. Stress, for instance, slows it down. Specially treated rats, that can no longer produce stress hormones, churn out new brain cells at a much higher rate than usual. This suggests that stress delivers a double

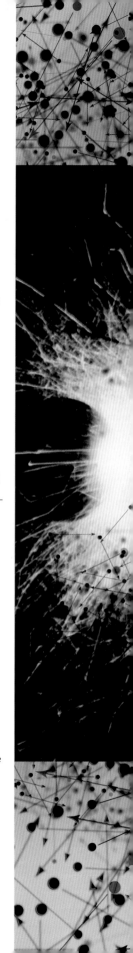

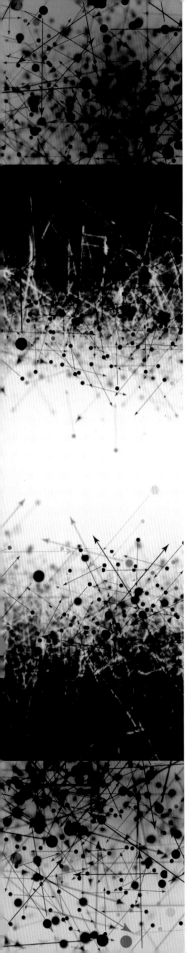

whammy: not only do the hormones involved actually kill off brain cells, they also knock out the repair system.

Until now researchers haven't really understood why Prozac cheers you up when you are mildly depressed. The secret seems to be that it speeds up neurogenesis. It has long been a mystery why Prozac, and similar serotonin-boosting drugs, don't have an effect for several weeks, since serotonin levels rise within minutes of taking them. Recently, however, scientists have found that serotonin also increases neurogenesis, which takes several weeks. Another widely available drug that seems to do the same thing is oestrogen.

You don't even need drugs to keep those new brain cells coming. Experiments by Professor Fred Gage of the Salk Institute in California, showed that rats allowed to exercise whenever they wished, rather than being forced to, and living in a spacious cage with lots of toys, grew more new brain cells. Other researchers have found that having to do vital learning tasks, like remembering where seeds are stored, also encouraged neurogenesis.

It is far too early to say how effective the hi-tech approach is going to be, although you can predict that unpleasant side-effects are inevitable. In the meantime, neurogenesis provides a fascinating new mechanism to explain why such old remedies as relaxation, exercise and keeping mentally active are all so good for the brain.

BRAIN FACTS:

Why so wrinkly? While the brain itself could be considered less than attractive, its streamlined design makes the most compact use of available surface/work-space.

IN UTERO LEARNING

Scientific evidence shows clearly that *in utero* experiences do affect the development of the brain. Hearing as an active faculty develops in the sixth month, and babies do react to stories they first heard in the womb.

Neurobics: the gym where your brain works out

Just as current research shows that cell regeneration occurs, proving that the brain is fortunately more adaptable than we've given it credit for in the past, there are ways to reverse the trend of shrinking cells, whereby growth in brain cells and in the dendrites (the connection between cells) is promoted/encouraged by learning more and interacting with new people. As you allow your own life experiences to become richer, it has a direct effect on the healthful quality of pathways in your brain.

Keep learning: where you might shy away from studying a topic you know nothing about, fight the urge to play it safe and dive in at the deep end. And when you next feel inclined to hide away, try and make it a point to meet new people every day. Acknowledging new faces and new patterns in routine behaviour, as well as expanding your knowledge, directly influence the expansion of your brain.

Professor Lawrence C. Katz, of the Department of Neurobiology at Duke

University Medical Centre in the US, has created an exercise programme for the brain he calls Neurobics. It encourages using the five senses to activate different neural pathways, and says, 'Neurobic exercises enhance the brain's natural drive to form associations – putting a name to a face or a smell with a food – which are the building blocks of memory and the basis of how we learn. Katz also says that it is important to focus your attention regularly, to make major breaks in your routine, changing the order or way in which you do things – even going to work different ways and trying to use your senses in a new way, whatever you are doing.

Brainpower boosts

Attune to the senses and stretch your sensual brain musculature: try getting dressed in the morning with closed eyes, using your sense of touch to navigate the way around the brain areas which are linked with touch.

Cross-training is not just for the gym any more: it activates both sides of the brain simultaneously: expanding the non-dominant side of the brain at the same time as working the more dominant side. As a neurobic activity: stand tall and march the legs up and down, being sure to lift the knees high. Now add elbow work: touch the right elbow to the lifted left knee and then the left elbow to the lifted right knee as you walk in place or around the room.

Other cross-crawling activities can be as simple as crossing one foot over the other when walking round the room. Cross-crawl for a few minutes before doing activities where you need your left and right brain to be working together, and see how this simple exercise adds dimension to your work.

How to have a high-powered memory

Take a look at these numbers. 3...6...5...5...2...1...2...4. Now, without looking at them again, see if you can remember them. No cheating!

How well did you do? Did you manage two? Three? Because of the way our brain works, it's a hard thing to do and yet our lives are full of numbers we need to remember – PIN numbers, phone numbers, credit card numbers – as well as names, shopping lists and appointments as well. Wouldn't it be great to be able to do away with all those notes and memos and be able to reel off your credit card number or hold phone numbers in your head?

In fact, there is absolutely no reason why you shouldn't. Look again at that number we started with, 36552124. Now look at it arranged like this 365 5212 4. There are 365 days in the year, made up of 52 weeks or 12 months of (about) 4 weeks. Bet you could remember it now, because you've taken two vital steps that make a number memorable – divided it into chunks and then connected them to something else you already know.

How good is your memory?

We all forget things occasionally, but are you really much better or worse at remembering than other people? This test will give you an idea. Answer each one with 'never', 'rarely' or 'often'.

1   Do you intend to watch a TV programme and then forget?
2   Do you find yourself wondering if you've turned off that light or the heater?
3   Do people's names slip your memory?
4   Do you find yourself forgetting points you are trying to make in a conversation?
5   When someone has just told you something, are you unable to recall all the details?
6   Do you say, 'I don't remember that' in conversations?
7   Do you fail to pass on messages?
8   Do you go into a shop and then wonder what it was you went in for?
9   Do you forget appointments?
10   Do you throw away the thing you want, say a matchbox, and keep what you meant to throw away, i.e. the used match?
11   Do you leave things behind and have to go back for them?
12   Do you do something routine, like brushing your teeth, and then find yourself doing it again?

Score 0 for each 'never', 2 for each 'rarely' and 4 for each 'often', and then add up the scores.

If your total is:
   0–20: You have an above-average memory and your life is probably well-organized.
   21–40: Your memory is average and, although there are occasional lapses, they are not serious. You could probably improve your concentration.
   41–60: You have a poor memory, but don't worry too much as it may be that you are just very busy at the moment. The more you need to remember, the more there is to forget. Try using notebooks to help you while you build up your skills.

Normally memory works best with things it can see, and the odder and more unusual the better. So to fix those phone numbers in place permanently you need a system with links, digits and pictures with a rhyme. You could have: One 'bun', two 'shoe', three 'tree', four 'door', etc. This will be your special set of connections, so spend a bit of time making each one specific and clear. Then link each number picture with an item on a list; or link the pictures so they tell a story as a way of remembering a number. So 241 might be using a shoe to bang on a door and wherever you hit, a bun appears.

The same principle works for names. Make a connection that's vivid and strange. Take the name Cindy Carson. For Cindy you might conjure up an image of Cinderella or a Sindy doll; for Carson a picture of a car driving towards the setting sun. Put them together: a Sindy doll or Cinderella in the driving seat.

feeding the brain

CAN NUTRIENTS MAKE US SMARTER?

One of the most exciting areas opening up in nutrition is the discovery that, not only can some nutrients make us more intelligent, the right ones can also improve our short- and long-term memory. Some also boost mood and energy.

How well we are able to concentrate affects practically everything we do, not just studying or taking exams. For instance, a better memory might improve our performance at work; it could also help us remember people's names, or actually get the shopping we set out for. Most people would like to be better at solving problems and planning, to fathom how to get the best rate of return for our money, for instance. Then there's mood. How many of us could say that we never get depressed, that we aren't interested in knowing how to influence how we feel?

But are these real possibilities, or just wishful thinking? Certainly pharmaceutical companies are spending a fortune on the development of smart drugs. But drugs are drugs... they are foreign to the body and it is impossible to tell what their long-term effects might be. The good news, however, is that there are natural substances, found in the body and in our food, that really can make us smarter. In fact, in many cases drug companies start with a nutrient and distort it, not because changing it makes it better or stronger, but because that's how they make their profit, as they cannot patent a natural substance.

Lecithin

Lecithin is a superfood (see page 122) that is normally extracted from soya. Lecithin's most important ingredient is phosphatidyl choline, known as PC, which is probably the body's best source of choline. Choline is needed to make acetylcholine, the neurotransmitter that is important for thought transmission, and has been shown to improve performance in intelligence and memory tests.

PC itself is the major ingredient from which all cell membranes are made. The membranes of cells are where most electrochemical activities take place, including those connected with thinking. PC is also the major ingredient of mitochondria, the energy factories inside every cell of the body, where our food is burned for energy. So PC can help us build energy and combat fatigue, as well as enhance brain power.

DMAE

Our grandmothers were right when they said that eating fish would make us brainier. Fish, it turns out, contain a nutrient called DMAE (di-methyl-amino-ethanol) that enhances memory and concentration, as well as energy and mood. DMAE, which occurs naturally in the brain in small amounts, achieves its effects by increasing the production of acetylcholine, important for memory and learning.

People given DMAE report that they feel more wide awake during the day and sleep sounder at night, often needing less sleep. After two to three weeks they commonly experience a mild state of stimulation which, unlike that produced by coffee and other stimulants, has no side-effects and no let-down when discontinued.

DMAE has also been shown to improve memory and learning, increase intelligence and raise physical energy. Powers of concentration may be considerably increased. In children it has been used to improve learning problems, under-achievement and shortened attention span. It has even helped children with hyperactivity or behavioural problems.

Perhaps this interesting nutrient's best bonus, however, is its effect on mood. Doctors and psychiatrists report that patients on DMAE are more affable, develop a more outgoing personality and show greater insight.

Pantothenic acid

Your body can't make acetylcholine for intelligent thinking without using pantothenic acid, also known as vitamin B5 (see page 95), for its assembly from choline. So if you're taking lecithin, choline or DMAE, you need to make sure you have a source of pantothenic acid as well. Pantothenic acid is also a stamina-enhancer as it is essential for making steroid hormones, including natural cortisone, which is particularly important when you're under stress.

Pyroglutamate

As people age, their memory tends to decline. This may be connected with a reduced ability to make certain substances, such as acetylcholine. When older people with age-related memory losses were given pyroglutamate, their verbal memory improved. Other research trials, with people suffering from poor memory as a result of alcohol use, found that pyroglutamate significantly improved their short- and long-term memory retrieval and also helped their long-term storage and consolidation of memory.

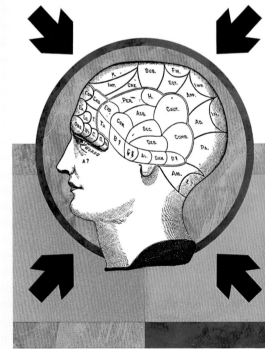

Pyroglutamate is a more potent relative of glutamine, the amino acid that can improve reduced mental performance (see page 120). It is found in large quantities in the brain, cerebrospinal fluid and the blood, and is also present in vegetables and other foods. In Italy, a form of the nutrient called arginine pyroglutamate is used to treat senility, mental retardation and alcoholism.

Niacin

Niacin, which is also called nicotinic acid or vitamin B3 (page 95), has been shown to enhance memory. It also has many other important functions. When young and middle-aged subjects were given either niacin or a placebo, the ones who got the niacin managed between 10 per cent and 40 per cent improvement on memory tests.

depression & addiction

Just below the appearance of normality, life is full of difficulty and sometimes suffering; the result, understandably, can be depression. Like animals, human beings learn that they can relieve their suffering by eating, drinking, inhaling or ingesting substances, or behaving in other pleasure-inducing ways. Some of these methods have been around for a long time and are socially acceptable, like alcohol and tobacco. Others are considered taboo, or for medical use only. Some are increasingly part of a culture of 'no limits', which uses drugs to change one's mental and emotional space. All these substances can easily become addictive, and make demands on the body. Some are relatively harmless, while others can kill you. The alternative of sinking into depression is just as dangerous for our well-being.

In the last few decades the science of nutrition has discovered that many nutrients can not only replace what is lost, but be a positive influence on our state, reducing depression and the desire for dangerous addictive substances. The hormone system and the brain, and its chemical messengers, or neurotransmitters, are the main sites of action. Three related hormone neurotransmitters are known to be important in the response to stress and mood – adrenalin, noradrenalin and dopamine. It is dopamine that is considered most closely allied with the brain's response to pleasure. For example, when laboratory rats eat, become sexually aroused, or learn an action that leads to their being rewarded, their dopamine levels increase.

If dopamine is important in depression and addiction, then what is its precursor in the brain? It turns out to be a normal fraction of dietary protein, an amino acid called tyrosine, found in animal and vegetable protein foods. The concentration in the body of the three related neurotransmitters depends on the availability of tyrosine.

In experiments undertaken in the 1960s, tyrosine levels in laboratory rats were found to be depleted during stress. However, those rats receiving extra tyrosine showed neither stress-induced depletion of noradrenalin, nor any signs of depressed behaviour. Laying up stores of these neurotransmitters could help us to cope with stress, suffering and depression. Tyrosine is also a precursor of thyroid hormones, and by normalizing the thyroid, our energy levels, appetite and mood can all be stabilized.

In 1980, Dr A. J. Gelenberg at Harvard Medical School treated a sample of depressed and drug-dependent patients with large doses of tyrosine and noted significant improvement. Later, similar results were found even when using lower doses. The normal dietary intake and use of tyrosine is about 1,000mg a day, and adding from 350mg to 1,000mg might well be enough to make a real difference. Since sex drive is also affected by dopamine, Dr Carl Pfeiffer concluded, on the basis of clinical and experimental experience, that 'L-tyrosine may decrease adrenal hyperactivity to stress, decrease appetite and stimulate sex drive.'

Reports of problems with large amounts of extra tyrosine include some schizophrenics, patients on 'monoamine oxidase inhibitors', and those suffering headaches after taking it. According to Dr. Pfeiffer, however, 'Toxicity is rare or almost non-existent in tyrosine therapy. Tyrosine is now generally recognized as one of the safe substances.' Supplementation with extra vitamin C usually sorts out any such problems.

Other amino acids can be very useful in balancing out depression and addiction. For example, L-glutamine is normally highly concentrated in the brain, where it can affect the amount of other neurotransmitters being produced, but, perhaps even more importantly, it serves as an alternative fuel. Lack of energy in the brain could be a central feature of the depression/addiction cycle, because the brain is so sensitive to blood sugar levels, and several experiments since the 1960s have found glutamine to be effective at reducing alcoholism and various other addictions.

The key to the nutritional approach is understanding how everything works together. Several vitamins and minerals have an essential role in producing the neurotransmitters and the energy required for a state of positive well-being. These include the B complex, especially B3 and B6, vitamin C, and the minerals zinc, magnesium and manganese. It is therefore quite important to add a good multivitamin and multimineral supplement, as well as some extra vitamin C, to the amino acids.

Nutrition is certainly not the whole answer to depression and addiction, but it can provide a very sound basis for a natural state of well-being that encourages recovery from these universal problems.

GOT THE PICTURE?

Our pre-frontal cortex is the part of the brain associated with perceiving the whole picture, planning ahead and using our creative imaginations. Interestingly enough, studies have shown that people with clinical depression have an overactive pre-frontal cortex.

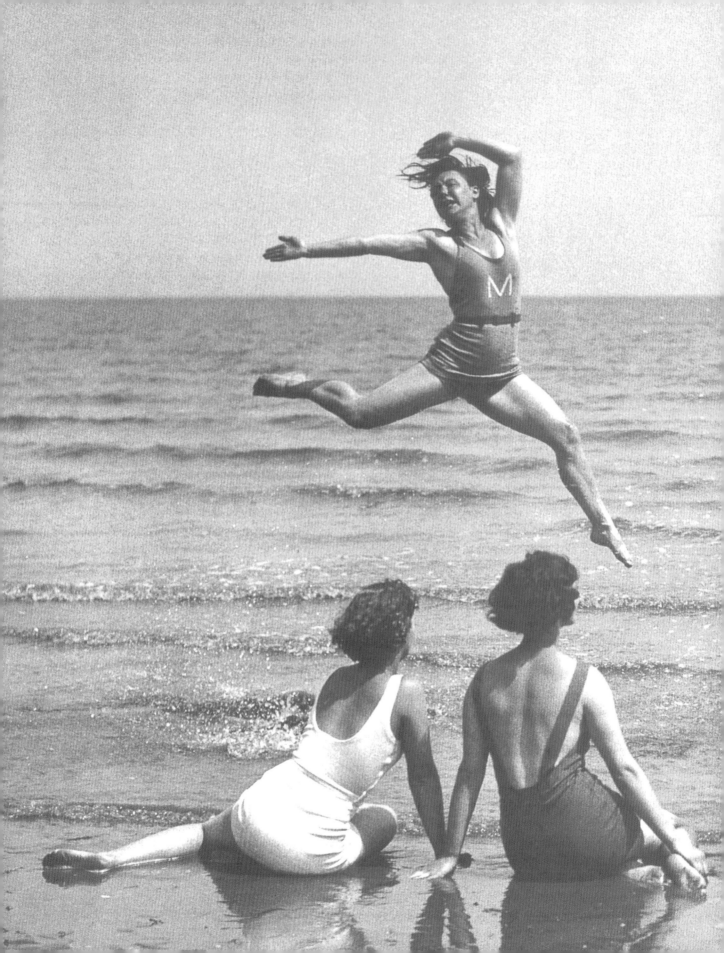

healthy mind, healthy body

The deep, interconnected and dynamic relationship between the mind and the body is rarely disputed these days. Science and mysticism have found a meeting place in measuring the effect of meditation practice on our brain waves. By slowing brain wave patterns, the rest of the body seems to follow suit, as the respiratory system, heart-rate, etc. all calm down. However, you don't have to meditate to observe or experience the mind/body relationship. Just pay attention to your own physical responses when you are very happy, sad or angry. Or have you ever noticed how tired you feel or how sensitive to physical pain you are when you are depressed? It's a real 'chicken and egg' situation – which comes first? Who knows? What we do know is that the mind has a dramatic effect on the body and the body on the mind. This is why holistic medicine makes so much sense and why treating the whole individual holds the key to a practical balanced natural health-care plan. One that each of us has to create to meet our unique needs and type.

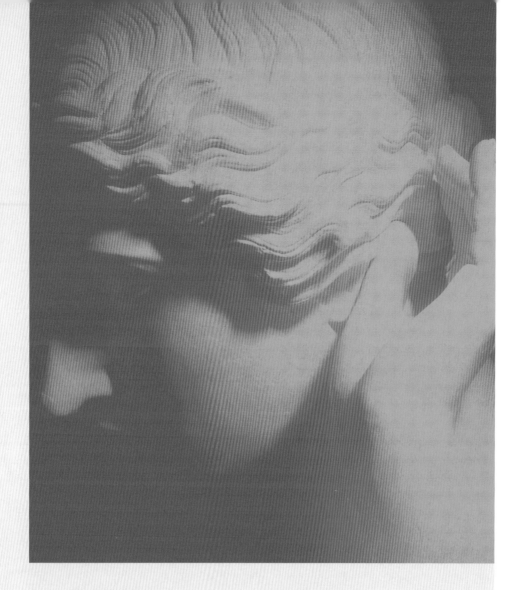

The connection between mind and body is, without doubt, the most exciting area of modern research into the causes of illness and disease and the maintenance of good health. It is now a proven fact that when you are depressed so is your immune system. More and more areas of science and medicine are increasingly being forced to give serious consideration to the mind-body relationship and its implication in the health of both your mind and your body.

your body speaks your mind

An important new science, psychoneuroimmunology, is the in-depth study of mind-body relationships and looks at interaction between psychology (the mind with all its thoughts and emotions) and the central nervous, immune and endocrine or hormone systems. Studies all over the world seem to bear out what most complementary therapists and holistic practitioners have always maintained – the whole person is much greater than the sum of all their parts. When looking at creating enduring optimum health, the interconnection of all the body/mind systems holds the vital key to our continued well-being.

The research and work of Dr Dean Ornish certainly support these findings. In a landmark study of heart disease, he proved for the first time that the clogging of the arteries – which can lead to heart attack and stroke – can be reversed without the use of drugs or surgery, but that love was the key factor in this reversal. He concluded that a sad and broken heart was as damaging and dangerous to our health as bad dietary habits or lack of exercise.

Dr Ornish believes that one of the main causes of heart problems is the profound isolation that growing numbers of people are experiencing in modern society. We are not by nature solitary creatures. Our roots take us back to extended families, the community and the tribe. Our lifestyles have changed dramatically in a relatively short span of time, however, and this has resulted in increasing numbers of people living alone, or living far away from either their family or a social network that can offer support and comfort when it is needed.

A weakened, inadequate immune system is often the result of an inadequate social support system. One indicator of the immune response is the natural killer cell activity, levels of which are more likely to be lower in people who are lonely. As Dr Ornish says, 'Looking out for No. 1 isn't enlightened self-interest. It's just lonely, and loneliness kills.' Recent research has shown that people who are usually lonely and isolated suffer more poor health and are much more susceptible to all kinds of illness, disease and general poor health.

In her excellent book, *Your Body Speaks Your Mind*, Debbie Shapiro reports on 'the link between psychological stress and physical problems as illustrated by research, cited by Dr Larry Dossey in *Healing Breakthroughs*, which states that more heart attacks occur on a Monday than on any other day of the week – and not only on a Monday but most often at 9 o'clock in the morning. No other animal suffers death more consistently on a particular day of the week. If we believe that there is no connection between the mind and the body, then what causes so many heart attacks to take place just as the first work of the week is about to begin? Certainly there are physiological reasons why death might be more likely in the morning than in the afternoon, such as higher heart rates or blood pressure, or adrenaline surging in preparation for the day ahead. There is, however, no reason why more deaths should take place on a Monday rather than any other day.'

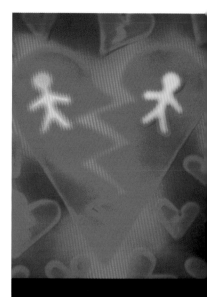

The *Journal of the American Medical Association* published evidence which showed that emotional risk factors for heart attacks might be more important than the physical – 'anger and deprivation of love might overshadow the contribution of serum cholesterol to the likelihood of a coronary.' It is therefore important to learn how to express and resolve emotional issues and conflicts.

There is a growing body of research in recent decades that demonstrates the close mind-body relationship and this mounting pile of evidence is stimulating increasing scientific inquiry into psychoneuroimmunology, PNI. Even earlier studies have shown fascinating results. Between 1948 and 1964, researchers followed the health of around 1,300 medical students who graduated from Johns Hopkins University in Baltimore, Maryland. 'While in medical school, some of the students claimed to be emotionally removed from one or both parents. After 30 years, the investigators found these same people suffered an unusually high incidence of mental illness, suicide and death from cancer.'

It is medical fact that stress has a big effect on our general and specific health and on our sense of well-being. If the mental and emotional pressures that build up inside us cannot be expressed and resolved, they are likely to find a way out through our body, usually through our weakest point – whether it is the nerves, the digestive system, the immune system or our sleeping patterns. Debbie Shapiro says of stress, 'Pushed down, it becomes illness, depression, addiction or anxiety; projected outwards, it becomes hostility, crime, prejudice or aggression.'

'It is everyday stress that affects us most deeply, by slowly grinding away at our inner reserves. The fight-or-flight response enables us to respond to danger, but it is not just major life-threatening situations that stimulate this response. Fearful or anxious thoughts do it too – the car not starting, being late for an appointment, unpaid bills, arguments with your partner, your children or your boss – all these can create a stress response.'

Debbie says Joan Borysenko, author of *Guilt is the Teacher, Love is the Lesson*, puts it well: 'The fight-or-flight response is like the overdrive on a car. It comes in handy to get us out of occasional tight spots, but if we keep the car in overdrive all the time, the wear and tear on its parts will cause a variety of mechanical problems. In people, these problems are commonly called stress or anxiety-related disorders.'

Taking the mind/body relationship another step further, the 'mind over matter' school of thought has a large body of evidence and testimony to support this idea. Here the belief is you can *think* yourself well or young. How well we feel – and even how we age – is intimately linked with our state of mind, according to celebrity ayurvedic doctor, Deepak Chopra. In his book *Ageless Body, Timeless Mind* he says

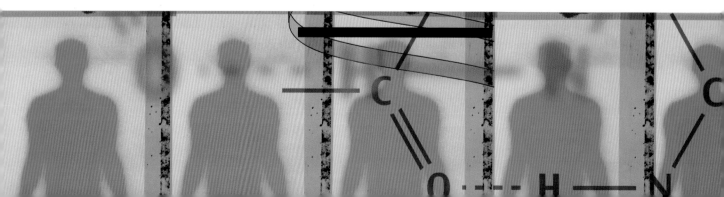

THE 'FIGHT OR FLIGHT' RESPONSE

The adrenal glands, located above the kidneys, produce the 'fight or flight' hormone, adrenalin. Adrenalin is completely vital to our survival; it stimulates all our systems, getting us prepared to flee from danger or, if this is not possible, to confront and overwhelm, or fight off, that which is a threat to us.

Adrenalin is released in response to situations which we perceive as life-threatening – whether or not they actually are life-threatening. The body immediately responds to everyday stress and tension as a threat and increases the release of adrenalin to speed up instinctive life-saving functions.

The fact that we are not actually having to run, flee or fight physically suggests this hormone is pumping through the body unused, and unchannelled except for the undesired effect of producing a heightened sense of anxiety and stress. The body then has to work harder to eliminate the by-products of this unused adrenalin, which can lead to over-taxed and exhausted adrenals.

many people lose vitality and decline in old age simply because they expect to do so.

He believes that by programming the mind to have different expectations, you can retain youthful abilities and outlook. He likes to quote one of his 80-year-old patients: 'People don't grow old. When they stop growing, they become old.' Teaching his patients how to restore all body rhythms to their intended functioning, how to calm rapid heartbeats, conquer asthmatic wheezing and stave off many other degenerative conditions is paramount to Chopra's approach and, according to him, has huge implications for ageing.

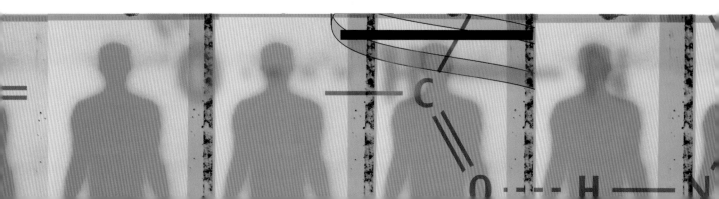

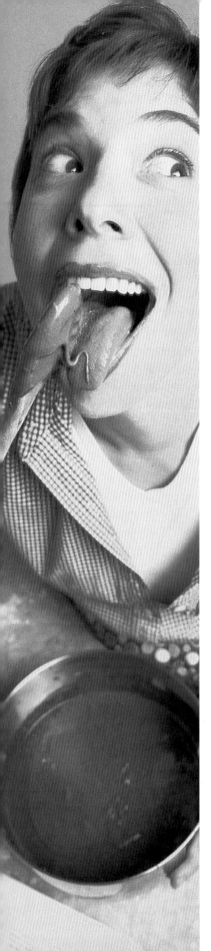

laughter and chocolate

One of the most interesting developments in the natural health field is the research into the beneficial effects of pleasure and happiness on our health. Scientists all over the world are studying the effects of pleasing experiences on the pleasure centres of the brain, and it is now a proven scientific fact – pleasure is good for you!

Happiness and humour increase our sense of well-being and help us live longer. Indulging (in moderation) in things that please you – like chocolate – and having fun in general have been proven to boost the immune system by increasing the production of immunoglobin A, which protects us against many infections, including colds and 'flus. When we're having fun, we also relax more, our cholesterol levels drop and our brainwaves change to the more calming alpha form. Another piece of folk wisdom is validated – a little of what you fancy does do you good.

Laughter is one of life's great pleasures and a primary signal of friendship. Laughing expresses our mirth and playfulness. Laughing together is a way of strengthening family and social bonds, facilitating and providing the human contact we need to survive. Laughing has many other very important physical and psychological benefits. The old adage has it that 'laughter is the best medicine' and, indeed, one study by Dr William Fry of the Stanford University School of Medicine in California clearly demonstrated how laughter boosts the cardiovascular, respiratory, muscular, hormonal, central nervous and immune systems. When laughing, we draw more air in and out of our lungs than during normal breathing, so pushing more oxygen into the bloodstream which, in turn, stimulates the circulation.

We should all laugh a great deal more, if just the act of smiling can produce demonstrably lower levels of 'stress hormones', and it has been clinically proven that laughter increases the 'feel good' hormones in the brain and the 'fighting fit' hormones in the immune system. UK psychologist Robert Holden has been organizing 'Laughter Clinics' and workshops around the world for many years. His laughter clinic in Birmingham was renowned the world over and he has managed to organize free laughter clinics for patients through the National Health Service.

The awareness of the power of laughter to enhance and help maintain our well-being is increasing, and is supported by clinical studies. These show how our heart rate usually rises when we are laughing. Studies of blood samples taken from people while they were laughing show high levels of the 'arousal' hormones, adrenaline and noradrenaline. We are more physically aroused during a good bout of laughter and, as a result, afterwards we are mentally sharper and more alert.

Laughter helps us relieve the burden of mounting daily stresses and tensions. When we laugh there is a burst of energy – physical and mental activity – followed by a cycle of relaxation, when our muscles are less tense than they were before. These alternating cycles can help prevent us becoming too stressed out about our daily problems. Laughter promotes a healthier more positive attitude which, in turn, seems to attract more positive energy, people and events to our lives.

Use it or lose it – a good sense of humour is like a muscle. The more it is used the more developed and toned it becomes. A sense of humour is a vital way of dealing with day-to-day problems. Seeing the funny side of a problem can help us manage it with ease and helps diffuse the tensions between people personally and professionally! People with a well-developed sense of fun often have fewer emotional problems than those who find it difficult to laugh – particularly at themselves.

In their book *Ultra Age*, Mary Spillane and Victoria McKee observe how 'the sense of humour is one of the first things that disappears from depressed people, and is a precious commodity to cultivate. It will not desert you with age, like your looks eventually will, and may be a truly saving grace. The ability to laugh at yourself, and even at the tragic events that touch you, can help to get you through the toughest times intact.'

One of the most popular 'mood foods' is sweet, yummy, creamy, mouth-watering chocolate. The pleasure of eating chocolate may be rooted in physiological fact as well as the psychological 'Naughty is Nice' syndrome that eating chocolate provokes. If eating chocolate pleases you it is important to allow yourself this indulgence without any guilt. The guilt is counter-productive and provokes anxiety and stress. It is important to keep your pleasures pleasurable and, therefore, guilt-free. Give yourself permission to eat good dark chocolate in the knowledge that it is good for you, is a source of protein, iron, magnesium and valuable B vitamins and, like laughter, it often triggers the release of the feel-good endorphins, the body's natural opiates.

Another reason why humans crave chocolate may be because cocoa contains tiny traces of cannabis-like compounds called endocannabinoids, and although these are not nearly powerful enough to reach 'cannabis-like intoxication', according to Italian researchers, this may help explain the enduring appeal of chocolate. Indeed, for some it may seem like an addiction. This may also be because chocolate contains theobromine, a psychoactive stimulant of the central nervous system. This may be why some people experience enhanced performance after eating chocolate.

Do watch out for addiction signals, though – a cycle of craving can result in over-eating chocolate because of the release of endorphins it stimulates. Relax and enjoy the pure sensuous delight of eating chocolate – regularly but moderately – in the knowledge it is healthy. Try to avoid the over-sugared confections, in favour of organic quality milk or dark chocolate made from more than 70 per cent cocoa solids.

A huge study of the life-spans of more than 7,000 people was carried out by researchers at the Harvard School of Public Health in Boston, USA. It concluded that regular sweet eaters outlived abstainers by around a year.

Professor David Warburton, founder of ARISE (Associates for Research into the Science of Enjoyment) observes how 'a child of 6 laughs 300 times a day, while the average adult has 50 laughs and a depressed person less than 6...'

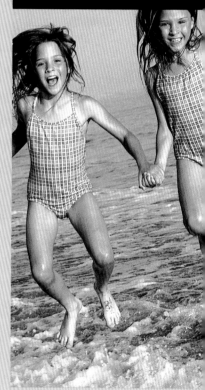

affirmations

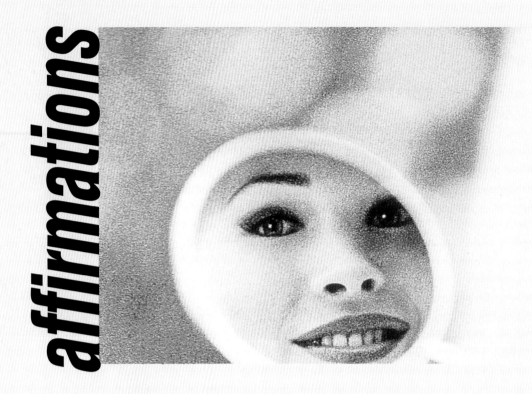

Affirmation – the repetition of a thought over and over again to embed it in the mind – is one of the principal tools of learning. There are two types of affirmations – positive and negative. Negative affirmations can start very young, even in babyhood. A baby or young child responds more openly to love than it does to anger. However, the stresses and strains of current daily life can often prohibit parents, siblings and teachers from always acting 'with love'.

Part of learning to heal and take responsibility for ourselves starts with positive thinking about ourselves. This must start with loving ourselves. It may feel strange, perhaps, or even intimidating to some, openly to admit their love for themselves, but it works. The power of positive thought cannot be overestimated.

How many times a day do you feel you have a negative thought? Countless times, possibly. 'I'll never get that done in time...', 'I'm not capable of doing that...', 'I'm useless...' to name but a few possible everyday thoughts. Switch them round. 'I am capable of achieving all that I wish to...', 'There is always enough time...', 'I'm able...' Add 'I am loving and loved – I love and approve of myself...' and you are on the way to changing those thought patterns instilled in yourself, or in your mind.

One of the most popular affirmations to offset the negative is to say, 'I love myself' – not just once a day, but 100 times or even more each day! Eventually you will feel the power of this statement. Keep it up. Check yourself. Notice any changes in your attitude as your belief in yourself starts to improve.

Catch yourself when you are feeling negative, write down what you're thinking

positive   negative

positive	negative
I can	I can't
I am worthy	I am unworthy
I have a right to be here	I don't belong here
I am loved	I am unloved
I am loving	I am unable to love
I am in the right place at the right time	I am never in the right place at the right time
I achieve all I need and want to achieve	I am a loser
I know my skills and talents are valuable	I am no good to anybody
There is always enough time	There's never enough time
I draw into my life exactly what is right	I can never attract what is worthwhile for me
I love myself exactly as I am right now	I want to change everything about myself

or feeling. Then write down the affirmative statement. How does it feel to change 'I am lazy' into 'I am productive and use my time well for me'?

You have to do a great deal of positive affirmation to combat all the negativity that usually clouds our thinking. 'I'm not good enough', 'I can't do that', 'That's not for me', 'I'm too fat... too thin... too old', 'Oh, I would never do anything like that', or those negative affirmations thrown at you by others such as, 'You're no good', 'You never do anything', 'You'd be better if you had money... got those exam results... had that job'.

It is believed that we can be unwittingly programmed to believe the 'truth' of these messages we receive very early on in our lives. They can be very damaging to us and can form the root of a failure to love ourselves that projects deeply into our teen, adult and elderly years. If we switch the negatives into positives – into the affirmative – we begin to heal ourselves and our lives of all the negative energy amassed. Such energy is useless, wasted and needs to be released. Feel the anger, resentment, fear, bitterness and guilt, and let it start to dissipate with constant affirmations.

Much illness and stress are brought on by means of such negative thought patterns. Changing your negative thoughts into positive thoughts can literally improve your health and have a knock-on effect on all those who come into contact with you. A person who truly loves themselves, unconditionally, will express this in all they do.

Getting positive

Can you look in the mirror and say, 'I love you'? Try it. This too can feel very strange, but it is certainly one of the most empowering ways of making a positive affirmation. Try to do this at least once every day, perhaps when you first wake up. Hear yourself say the words 'I love you'. How do you sound? Genuine? Embarrassed? Insincere? As you practise this affirmation day by day, make a note to yourself about how it feels to do this. It will become easier.

Try creating your own affirmations. What feels comfortable for you to say? You may need to create new affirmations every day according to your physical and emotional needs at that moment. The events of a day may prompt you to create new affirmations in the evening to be recited before you go to bed. Perhaps you are feeling stressed after a hard day. Take some time out, just a few minutes if that's all you have, to breathe deeply and focus on where in your body you are feeling that stress. Perhaps your body is giving you signals that may previously have been ignored. Create an affirmation around the stress, remembering to ensure it is positive!

Remember to be kind, gentle and patient with yourself while beginning to change your negative thought patterns. If you 'forget' one day, then begin again the next day. After many years of negative programming, it may take some time to adopt this new way of being. Encourage and praise yourself as much as you can, and enjoy feeling positive about yourself and those around you.

Positive pointers

Positively affirm yourself throughout the day. Congratulate yourself when you feel you have achieved something. Encourage yourself. Avoid panic and negative derogatory thoughts about yourself or your associates. Thinking positively requires so much less energy and enhances your own feelings of well-being. Smiling to yourself and at others is so much more positive than frowning and worrying.

If you have fears and worries, acknowledge them. Don't try to suppress them with stimulants, such as alcohol or cigarettes, or by stuffing yourself with comfort food. If they are very pressing then try to find a support group, therapist or natural therapy that really appeals to you to help you through the crisis. Do not be afraid to call on those you love to help you in times of need. Better to ask for help than to try to handle all that life doles out to you in isolation. Perhaps you, in turn, will then be able to help someone you love in their times of crisis.

Show love and appreciation to others and expect to receive it back. It works wonders for your own self-esteem and is a lovely way of creating harmonious relationships with those around you.

visualization

As discussed at the beginning of this chapter, an increasing number of doctors and scientists worldwide are acknowledging the existence of a strong mind/body connection. Today, even the most conservative practitioners accept that the mind has the power to heal, and that mental pictures are powerful tools, that can dramatically enhance or depress our sense of well-being.

Just as laughter has been proven to stimulate the immune function (see page 206), by using our imagination to visualize a particular image, we can invoke a particular response. By focusing with your inner eye on an image that symbolizes calm serenity you can lower your blood pressure, slow your breathing and generally reduce a stress response.

Mind control techniques – such as creative visualization, biofeedback, meditation and hypnosis – are some of the therapeutic relaxation methods in general use to check stress levels and redress the balance of the mind/body relationship. They help the body eliminate stress before it can accumulate and cause physical or mental disorders. All of us have within our grasp a profound and simple tool that enhances the ability to stimulate self-healing, increase energy and create a state of inner peace.

Practising creative visualization

All you need to do is make yourself comfortable, concentrate on your breathing to help you relax deeply and then let go, leaving all thoughts behind you. Then think of something that represents a peaceful calm scene; some image that evokes a deep sense of serenity. It may be a place you have visited, or an imaginary place that is your ideal.

Many professional athletes use creative visualization or 'imaging' to improve their performance. They see themselves winning or beating their own best time and often create positive outcomes with their positive belief. This mental rehearsal is sometimes called the 'inner game' by athletes. Not only physical performance, but also bodily responses can be regulated by mental imagery. Your immune system is very affected and can be regulated by mental imaging techniques. People with HIV and AIDS have had remarkable success in visualizing and befriending their few remaining 'T' cells and encouraging them to fight back, as have cancer patients scourging their wayward cells.

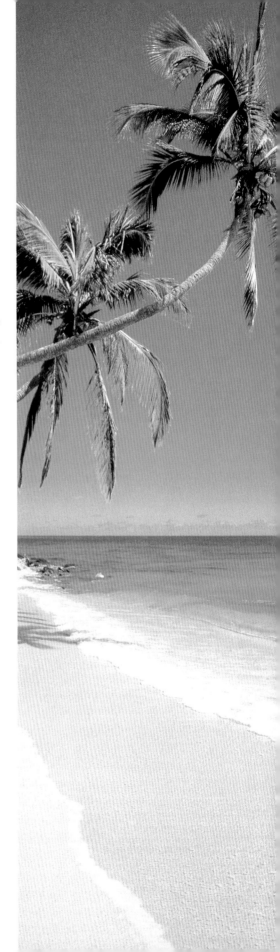

the relaxed mind

We are much more creative and intuitive when the mind is relaxed rather than tense, over-worked and exhausted. Relaxation and mind control go hand in hand, and relaxing the mind and body releases our creative and intellectual powers.

Most people agree relaxation is an integral ingredient of a balanced, healthy lifestyle, yet fail to incorporate enough of it into their daily routines. However you define it, relaxation is the antidote to stress in our lives and we need it for our survival, let alone our well-being. It is only while you are sleeping or relaxing that your body can repair and heal the damage incurred while rushing through your days. No matter what your circumstances, you owe it to yourself to take time out of your daily life for what relaxes you and helps you to unwind.

Learning to relax

Fortunately, the art of relaxation can be learned, and there is more than one path to achieving it. Relaxing is a simple habit but, like anything else, it needs to be practised regularly to get it right. Don't wait until you get near breaking point before you start, though. As well as bringing you a calmer mind, a daily relaxation programme can relieve physical symptoms, such as aches and pains, and even lower your blood pressure.

Relaxation means different things to different people... a walk in the woods, a swim or a soak in a hot bath may relax you, while a friend unwinds listening to music or playing a game of bowls. For some people relaxing in the garden with a good book and a cup of tea is the answer, for someone else it might be weeding, planting roses or building a folly to replace the old shed. A holiday on a hot sandy beach may be your idea of relaxation, while rushing down an icy mountain could be your best friend's antidote to stress. Discover what truly relaxes you and make regular time to indulge your relaxation whims – whatever they may be.

It does not matter what your personal preferences are. What matters is that you make/create the time to indulge your whims and your personal needs for relaxation, fun and creative expression. The important thing is to take time out for yourself to do the things that make you feel good and help you to relax. It's a simple message, but your life – as well as your well-being – may depend on it.

When you add up the waking hours of the day you spend doing things that please you – that enhance your life and your sense of well-being, and just make you feel happy, engaged, fulfilled – what percentage of the day do they fill? Five per cent, ten, twenty, fifty per cent? Or are you one of the rare lucky ones who fills more than half their days with pleasurable pursuits? Most of us, unless we are nourished by our work life like an artist or an athlete, really can't expect that, so 20–30 per cent would be a reasonable expectation. If your percentage is seriously below that, then make it your goal to double it over a period of a few months.

A relaxed mind is a healthy mind that encourages greater self-awareness and therefore greater self-care. Listening to yourself, your mind, your body, you will become so much more in tune with what your real needs are. Do you need to exercise? Eat more fruit? Drink more water? Sleep more? Have quiet time to yourself instead of filling every waking moment in your appointment diary so that spare time becomes an elusive commodity – if it exists at all?

Daily practice of some form of relaxation of the mind, whether simple deep breathing or an unhurried walk in the park, at a time that suits you, will enhance all this and more besides. Even coping with life's great pains, such as loss of loved ones, financial pressures, whatever, becomes easier to handle with a peaceful mind.

Next to deep breathing and intelligent eating, one of your best defences against the destructiveness of excess stress is making time for yourself. Just consider what these four words mean to you. They entail listening to your needs and giving them priority in your long list of 'must do's! Identifying the pastimes that really please you is tantamount to naming the tools for your own mental and physical survival.

The relaxed mind finds it easier to organize, prioritize and manage an otherwise hectic lifestyle. In fact, ironically, the more effort one makes to 'make time for oneself' the more likely one is to have time! Taking time to notice how you are breathing, shallowly or deeply, and correcting your breathing need only take a few short moments but can have wonderful results! If panic sets in when that train is cancelled, deep breathing will help to waylay fears. Panicking will not make the next train arrive more quickly, merely increase your heart rate and cause you stress.

If your mind is constantly rattled with thoughts and plans and reliving discussions on the telephone or movies you saw yesterday, take time to quieten and empty out those thoughts. A clear mind is a calm, relaxed mind that is more easily able to focus on the tasks in the day ahead. When the mind is peaceful, there is more room for creative, inspired thoughts and ideas to surface. Intuition is enhanced as you are more in tune with your own body and your environment. After addressing your own needs adequately you are better placed to address the needs of others, dependents you may have, colleagues, friends.

Spending time with people you genuinely love and who love you in return will enhance your self-esteem and relax you. Take the time to tell those people that you love them. Show that you care; buy flowers, gifts, make time, listen, share. Children naturally express themselves, in the moment, when happy, sad, angry, tired. We can learn so much from observing the behaviour of the children around us. They often will reflect back to us our own moods. Tension can breed tension and children will respond to like with like. Similarly a calm and peaceful state will induce the same state in those around us... the ripple effect.

TIPS FOR TIME MANAGEMENT

One of the single most important things you can do to maximize relaxation is structure your day's activities and priorities, being realistic about what can and can't be done.

- At home, organize your meals, your housework, etc., to avoid being over-stimulated by a noisy vacuum cleaner at midnight or a fast-spinning washing machine at 3 a.m.
- At work make sure you take time out for lunch. At least get away from your desk into another environment. If the weather is good, try to find a pretty spot outside to enjoy the sunshine or warm air.
- Take time for exercise.
- Take time for eating.
- Take time for play/socializing.
- Take time for support (healing treatments, counselling).
- Take time for study.
- Take time for family and friends.

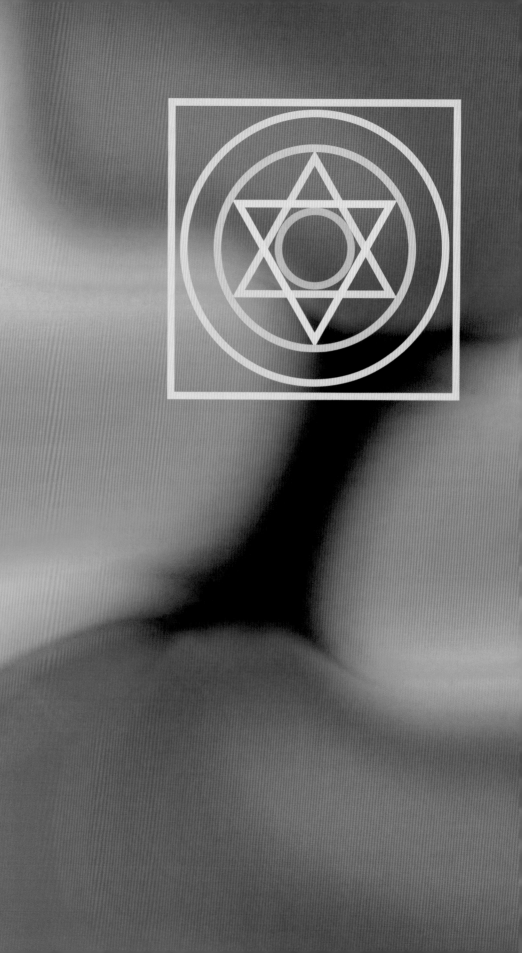

the meditative mind

Meditation teaches how to still and focus the mind. Many people learn the technique to help de-stress their mind and body, others practise meditation because it promotes a sense of well-being in both the mind and the body. Meditation is also brilliant for learning how to discipline the mind and improve attention, concentration and memory.

Common to many cultures around the world, meditation is most associated with the art of reflection as demonstrated by the Buddhist and Hindu traditions. Nowadays, however, it is widely recognized as a primary tool for stress reduction. It can help you attain a calm yet alert mind, coupled with a relaxed yet focused state of awareness.

Meditation, yoga and Eastern philosophies are often cited as a major antidote to stress, and more Westerners are turning to these techniques whether or not they subscribe to the spiritual tenets behind them. Most religious orders now offer opportunities for reflective retreats, often incorporating some of these gentle approaches to stress relief – and, particularly, time and space for spiritual contemplation or meditation. You don't have to be a Buddhist to go on a Dalai Lama meditation retreat, or a Catholic to enjoy a weekend of laughter and love with the Sisters of the Cenacle. Spiritual retreats and taking time for contemplation are not reserved for the traditions of the East alone. Today in the West, more and more people are practising these ancient techniques to benefit physically and mentally from the stress-reducing side-effects of basic meditation.

Meditation can be practised from a purely practical point of view – to help lessen the ravages of modern times on your mind and body – without in any way interfering with your personal spiritual inclinations. If anything, that part of your life will be gradually enhanced by practising contemplation.

It is one of the most effective and non-intrusive processes for reducing, controlling and removing the stress-related side effects of the very fast, pressing and quite unnatural ways in which we live in Western cultures. As the Shapiros say, 'Sitting still, doing nothing is the one and only way to give your mind a complete rest.'

Meditation is not only beneficial for the mind: it also helps to protect against stress-related illnesses, including heart disease, asthma and high blood pressure. In recent decades, it has become a way of life for millions of Westerners, as the reputation of its life-affirming qualities gains momentum and spreads – particularly in Western academic and scientific circles. Meditation is also thought to help relieve and control pain, to boost the immune system and may even be beneficial in treating HIV and AIDS sufferers. The more research into the positive effects of meditation on your mind, body and spirit, the more evidence mounts up – there is no doubt that meditation is very good for you.

'Meditation is an invaluable tool for healing – traditional yogis, who use relaxation and meditation techniques, are known to reduce their risk of cardiovascular and nervous diseases by up to 80 per cent.' Many doctors today prescribe some form of meditation.

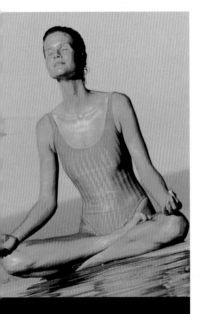

Few of us ever experience the full immensity of the mind's extraordinary capabilities. We are curious, intrigued, excited and drawn to further exploration of what we call normal consciousness. How fascinating to realize that we normally live only on the edge of a mostly unexplored territory that is as vast as the universe itself, and beyond.

What is meditation and why is it so good for you?

Meditation is primarily an experience of stillness. When thoughts drop away and there is no thinking, you enter into a quiet space. We often experience this naturally when walking in nature or sitting on a beach, looking out to sea. The practice of meditation helps us connect to this natural state purposefully – to enter fully into the present moment, giving us the chance to discover the mind, to become aware of this natural state.

The act of meditation is defined in a number of ways – 'to think over, consider, reflect, contemplate' or 'to fix the mind upon' are just a few. Meditation is about learning 'mindfulness', about entering into the present moment by observing the mind's activity. To work *with* your mind, to watch your thoughts come and go without becoming attached to them, is the most fundamental aspect of personal free will. Meditation helps us develop constructive mental habits that enhance mental and physical well-being. It teaches us how to let go of our thoughts – our 'busyness' – and just 'be', to experience our 'beingness' without thinking about anything in particular. This is what really relaxes the mind. Meditation is the space between thought.

Debbie Shapiro has these thoughts to share on the power of meditation: 'Throughout the ages, meditation has been used to enter within and explore the wonders that are there. True meditation is a fully conscious natural awareness, a mind that is clear and free. Through relaxation and meditation we unfold the vast inner world that lies hidden at the core of our being. Meditation is a process of stilling the mind and developing a completely calm mental state. Its joy is in its simplicity, in the flow of thoughts through the mind, in being in the moment.'

Clinical trials have shown that meditating regularly reduces stress. The pulse and respiratory rate slow down. If your blood pressure is too high, meditation will lower it. Your body consumes less oxygen because cell metabolism slows down. The brain's alpha waves (those associated with relaxation) increase. Meditation and yoga practice are based on learning to focus your attention and observe your thoughts. If you can master this practice, you can master anything.

How to meditate

Meditation is now taught to millions of over-stressed Westerners as a way of reaching a tranquil state of mind. Meditation can relax and refresh your body and mind. If practised properly and regularly it will do away with the need for drugs or alcohol to cope with your life. That's how powerful a tool it can be. It's simple, it's safe and it's free. It can be done anywhere, any time – but it is most easily practised in quiet peaceful surroundings dressed comfortably, without shoes, using socks or soft slippers if it's too chilly for bare feet.

The mind moves in cycles of concentration and relaxation. Meditation is about being in the moment – you just need to be still and sitting comfortably with a straight, but not tense, spine. It is good to have a quiet place in your home for meditation, where you can build up the atmosphere of peace and serenity away from

steps to meditation

1   To get the best out of your meditation, set aside space and time every day for your practice. An ideal start is 5 minutes twice a day, gradually working up to at least 15–20 minutes once or twice a day. Take the time to be quiet, to be still and be mindful of yourself in the present. Don't worry if your mind seems to leap around in endless chatter – just watch where it goes and try to instil the new habit of stillness.

2   Find a comfortable, quiet spot away from distraction, where you feel safe and warm, even if you are only meditating for 5 or 10 minutes to start with. After you have learned to meditate you will be more adept at watching the flow of your thoughts and being fully present in the moment. You may even be able to meditate in motion, while walking along a country lane, for instance.

3   The next step is to find a comfortable position for meditation, in which you can sit and relax without straining the back or legs. It doesn't have be in lotus position or cross-legged, if these are uncomfortable; a chair is fine, or on the floor with your back against the wall for support is OK too. In any pose, your back should be straight and upright, without being fixed and rigid. This helps you to maintain your concentration and steady your mind. A good way of keeping a straight back is to imagine a string pulling you gently upwards through the crown of your head (see also the 'inner dialogue' in the Alexander Technique, pages 260–261).

4   The next thing you do is suggest to yourself the release and relaxation of all your muscles and internal organs. Many people find it helpful to imagine each part of the body contracting and relaxing in turn, starting with the crown of the head and ending with the tips of the toes.

5   The next step is to steady your breath naturally by allowing your natural deep-flowing and gentle breath to emerge without force and without judgement. By first doing a relaxation exercise you should have little or no problem finding your lowered respiratory rate reflected in slower, deeper breathing. Flowing, even breathing reflects a calm, meditative inner state.

6   The 'following the breath' exercise: to begin with, try just sitting still and being aware of your complete breathing cycles – following your breath with your consciousness/attention as you inhale and exhale is a good meditation practice. The 'following the breath' exercise will help you get used to being still and focused. Mostly, we are so used to being busy all the time that we no longer find it a simple task just to 'be'. As the great mystic philosopher and author J. Krishnamurti said: 'Most of us want to have our minds continually occupied so that we are prevented from seeing ourselves as we actually are. We are afraid to be empty. We are afraid to look at our fears.'

1 Find a regular time.
2 Find a comfortable space.
3 Find a comfortable position, checking that your posture is straight and erect.
4 Allow your muscles and organs to relax to help you focus the mind.
5 Practise a gentle breathing exercise to slow down mind and body.
6 Follow your deep but gentle inhalations and exhalations.

the distractions of your daily life... a little corner for contemplating your well-being.

By observing your mind's activity you can learn to *be*. Meditation is not the same as concentration. The purpose of meditation is to let go of all your material worries, to free you to experience the vast peace of the unseen spiritual world within and around us. Concentration, on the other hand, frees your attention from all objects and thoughts or distractions to allow you to focus on one thing at a time.

To start, you need to set aside some time to practise 'being without doing', just to be with your inner reflections. To watch, observe your thoughts and then learn to detach from them and let them go, let go of all distractions. There are many varied approaches to meditation, but they all have the same goal. Each technique is a means to calm and quieten the mind by focusing attention inwards. Meditation helps us understand our mind. It doesn't always come easily at first, so practice and perseverance are important.

It helps to do some breathing and relaxation exercises before you begin, particularly if you are setting aside time for your meditation practice at the end of the day. It may then take a little bit more time and effort to clear away the day's events, but once you have you will emerge from your meditations much refreshed and recharged. Breathing is the key to meditation. Breathing exercises and generally paying attention to your breath are the most easy and natural ways to learn meditation. As soon as you start watching your breath, it takes you into your body. Try this simple exercise: breathe in to the count of one, breathe out to the count of one; breathe in to the count of two, breathe out to the count of two; breathe in to the count of three... and so on, gradually extending the length of your breaths until you reach a comfortable plateau. Don't strain; see how far you can go and try to extend that next time. This exercise helps you to focus on your breathing and to really be in the moment without distraction. Be gentle with yourself; it takes time to learn and there is no right or wrong or only one way to practise meditation.

At first you may find steadying the mind difficult enough, let alone stilling it. Don't worry – everyone experiences the 'playful monkey of the mind' and the frustration that goes with these visits! The next most important thing you must develop, after relaxation and steady natural breathing, is patience. This quality will help you to learn to meditate more than any other.

When learning how to 'sit and do nothing', beginners should bear in mind a few basic practical pointers. The three major points of attention are body, breath and mind, i.e. the 'Three Treasures' of essence, energy and spirit. An ancient Tao text states: 'Shut off the three external treasures of hearing, sight and speech in order to cultivate the three internal treasures of essence, energy and spirit.' You must acquire the art of being still before you can learn to meditate. You may be surprised just how difficult that is for many people from a Western culture. So do not be alarmed or dismayed if you are one of them. With patience and practice you will surely learn how to meditate and before long you will experience the benefits of this ancient technique.

Concentration exercise

Another excellent meditation exercise is concentrating and softening your gaze on an external object like a candle flame. This is good for learning to focus and empty your mind, helping you develop your powers of relaxation, concentration and 'one-pointedness'.

There are many different ways to meditate, both 'inner' and 'outer'. Everyone approaches meditation in their own unique way. Some use a mantra to focus and empty the mind, others use mandalas, sacred art that suggests a meditative state, and some just close their eyes and go into a very relaxed state that is meditation.

Transcendental meditation

Over the last 30 years transcendental meditation, or TM, has become one of the most popular meditation systems in the West. Many Westerners in the business world are attracted to TM because it teaches you how to reduce stress levels and promotes a sense of well-being that can greatly enhance personal and professional lives.

Deepak Chopra took transcendental meditation to a new level of popularity after his book *Ageless Body, Timeless Mind* became such a hit less than a decade ago. He helped people understand TM and how silently repeating a specific Sanskrit mantra or word can help the mind snap out of its normal patterns and move into the silent space beyond thought. Chopra said a mantra is a way of getting a direct message to the nervous system and they have been part of meditation practices in India for thousands of years. To learn TM properly you should receive personal instruction from a trained teacher.

Chanting

Chanting is a meditation technique that focuses the mind on a sound that sets up resonance in the mind/body. Mantras are repetitive sounds that you can chant over and over because of the vibration and concentration they stimulate. You become centred and serene by means of the power of the chanted word. Chanting a mantra or sounding a tone is a way to enhance 'one-pointedness', concentration and the emptying of the mind.

To begin with, certain vowel sounds are used as mantras because they have great mantric value. One of the most important and common of these is the sacred sound 'Om' or 'Aum'. The chanting of 'Om' for a few minutes at the end of your meditation practice will have a very uplifting effect. Take a deep inhalation through your nose and begin to chant 'Om' as you exhale, chanting over and over with great resonance for as long as one breath will allow. Start with the mouth open and gradually close it until you are making a low humming sound through gently closed lips. Repeat twice.

Mantras should be spoken slowly or quietly chanted with utmost concentration and attention on the meaning as they are spoken. Repetitively chanting the 'Om' or 'Aum' (O-ooo-mmmmm or ah-ooo-mmmm) often follows a hatha yoga session or ends a meditation. The 'Om' sound represents the 'universal vibration of absolute consciousness, the sound of infinity of which we cannot fathom'.

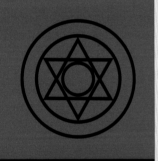

Some of the other popular sounds for chanting are 'Ra', 'Ma', 'Ram', 'Oom' or combinations of these sounds like 'Aum-ra-ma-oom' or 'Om-na-ma-ha-shi-va-ya'. You can practise more than three sounds at a time if it feels good to you, but start slowly and work your way up as you gain more confidence in your meditation practice.

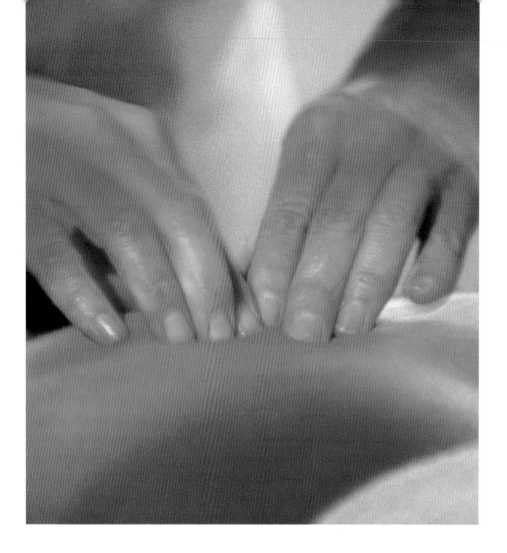

the magic
of massage

Massage is a beautiful healing art enjoyed by many today who recognize its value in de-stressing and clearing away day-to-day anxieties. Treating yourself to regular massage helps to keep stress levels at bay and goes some way towards preventing the development of illnesses that are often stress-related.

As well as being a wonderful de-stresser and a relaxing therapy, massage is also very powerful and can also be extremely provocative. During or after a massage, you may experience emotional changes – either in a very subtle way or in a striking and powerful manner – and the changes may stay with you for some time. This is because massage is brilliant in its ability to uncover emotional issues held deep in the body's tissues, either from the near past or from many years ago. This is one of the strengths of massage, its ability to aid in the healing of emotional issues.

The feeling of being gently nurtured that massage imbues us with allows us to feel in tune with our bodies in a way that perhaps many of us are no longer used to. If we are past the age when mum and dad cuddle us daily, where do we receive that nurturing touch? Massage is a wonderful way of ensuring that we continue to be nurtured in adult life and is a reminder for our bodies of those early years when we were taken care of by those who loved us.

Various forms of massage have been practised down the centuries and are now practised widely across the world. Much of the holistic massage practised today in the West, for example, finds its origins in Eastern techniques combined with Swedish techniques. Many civilizations used massage as a curative therapy and preventative treatment. In China, the massage practised there is renowned for curing all manner of ailments, from the common cold to irritable bowel syndrome (IBS), for example. In fact, any condition is believed to be a manifestation of blockage in chi along the meridians and so, by using massage to create a free flow of chi throughout all the meridians, good health is believed to be ensured.

Massage holds many possibilities for us as givers and receivers. It is communication without words. The practitioner will receive as much, if not more, information from the client during the treatment as they will in the discussions before and after. The body speaks its truth and the practitioner will detect areas of tension; if sadness is being held, if over-excitability is causing a rushing heart-beat, if pain – both physical and emotional – is being experienced. The practitioner will tune into the client and allow their hands and their intuition to guide them.

If you are aware of carrying unresolved issues that may cause disturbance for you emotionally, things you have not dealt with, such as bereavement, body/image issues (ranging from eating disorders to even abuse), abandonment issues, etc., these may come up again. This is naturally a part of your own healing process. If issues do come up, it is a sign that you are ready to deal with them. Massage is not simply a luxurious, sensuous, hedonistic pleasure. It is important and essential for us all to receive nurturing touch, caring touch. If we have not experienced this for many years, if ever, since childhood – or not even then – receiving nurturing touch could bring up a great deal of emotion for us. We may hold sadness at not having received a loving touch in our early lives; if touch has been aggressive for us, then this may, in turn, bring up other issues.

Massage is for everyone, with very few contraindications – even for pets. How wonderful does it feel for us to stroke a purring cat or a loving and devoted dog? Children love to stroke the soft fur of their pets and at any age we can reap great benefits ourselves from this experience. So why not experience it ourselves too?

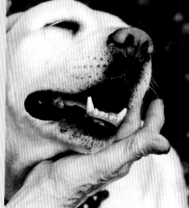

COMMONLY USED STROKES INCLUDE:

EFFLEURAGE: long strokes using the flat of the hand, which connect up different areas of the body and allow the therapist to sweep up or down the legs, for example, and which also help to induce relaxation in the client. It is also a way of 'connecting' for the therapist. During this stroke, the therapist will learn a lot about what is really going on in the client's body and any areas that may need deeper work, for example petrissage (below), to iron out those tension knots.

PETRISSAGE: small thumb circles for intensive work in areas such as the shoulders or joints.

TAPOTEMENT: very light percussion or tapping with the tips of the fingers, which may be used on the face, for example.

CUPPING: making cup shapes with the hands, trapping air inside the 'cup' to form suction, generally on fleshy areas like backs of the thighs and the buttocks. Cupping is done quickly and firmly to encourage circulation.

HACKING: (the famous technique often seen in the movies!) performed with loose wrists, the sides of alternating hands are rapidly brought down in a chopping motion over large fleshy areas to encourage circulation and disbursal of fat.

You may simply feel tired afterwards, as the process of moving through your deeply held emotions can be very draining. It is important to continue with the process of nurturing yourself and ensure that you drink plenty of water or herb teas and rest until it is time to sleep. Give yourself space and time to consider anything that has come up. If necessary, seek the help of a therapist or counsellor. Even just being with a loving partner or good friend, who will give you time and space to talk and feel your feelings, can be a wonderful complement to your healing therapy.

The person being massaged will drift into a state of what is best described as near-sleep, similar to the moments before actually going into real sleep, or like a meditative state. Fully allowing another to work on your body and to feel the trust, respect and healing that is being shared between the giver and receiver goes some way towards explaining the feeling of wholeness that massage gives. As you become more accustomed to receiving massage you will find it easier to let go and allow the processes to take their natural course.

Massage is a way of taking care of people, and of taking care of yourself. It is such a simple way to give, it seems inconceivable that it holds so much power. Massage is so much more than a relaxant and giver of health. Those who enjoy regular massage cannot fail to recognize the healing qualities that massage possesses. Massage can act as a cleanser for the entire body–mind–spirit and, once cleansing is in place, positive energy has room and space to flow into all the systems. Healing takes place on all levels, and conditions of which the client may not even be aware can be positively affected by this gentle therapy.

Strokes and movements

Holistic massage, Swedish massage, aromatherapy massage and any other types of massage that are based on any of these three forms will utilize a wide range of strokes, depending on the training the therapist has received and also on the varying needs of the client.

different types and styles of massage

Aromatherapy massage

This is generally a lymphatic drainage form of massage (see right), using long, gentle, sweeping strokes over the entire body, with the main aim being to introduce the essential oils (see page 228), blended with a very light vegetable oil into the recipient's body via the capillaries. For more details, see pages 226–229.

Chinese massage therapy

Chinese massage therapy is becoming more widely utilized in the West. Chinese practitioners spend at least three years in training at specialist centres. The treatment is both preventative and curative, and well worth experiencing. The system focuses greatly on movement of negative energy out of the meridians, so positive chi can flow freely to create balance throughout the body. The various methods of creating this balance include thumb-and-finger techniques like acupressure, firm pushing out of energy strokes and invigorating light frisking movements, for example on the top of head, to release stress and awaken you! See also T'ai chi and massage on page 225.

Holistic massage

'Holistic' is a term used to describe considering the person as a whole rather than a range of conditions. All aspects of the client are weighed and examined, including any emotional upsets and physical ailments. Holistic massage will generally follow a format that starts with the back and back of legs and ends with

the client lying on their back receiving long strokes from head to foot to aid relaxation, grounding and a sense of being back in the world after the treatment. The massage strokes themselves will be adapted to suit the needs of the individual, whether by deepening or lightening the stroking movements, for example, or spending more time on healing, holding or gentle rocking. The massage will involve many long connective strokes between the body parts being worked on and a treatment usually lasts 1 hour.

Indian head massage

This places its emphasis on stimulating the muscles and lymphatic drainage system, and alleviates anxiety and depression, migraines and sinus problems, to name but a few. It has been around for thousands of years and uses a variety of circular movements and rubbing motions around the hairline, which will make the recipient feel as though they are floating.

Kahi loa and Kahuna (Hawaiian massage)

These wonderful hands-on therapies are becoming very popular in the West. They have a deeply spiritual side, making them totally holistic and healing. Kahi loa was created by Hawaii's Master Healers and is based on the ancient Hawaiian philosophy of healing through connecting with nature. The client receives the massage fully clothed and after a

discussion with the therapist regarding their reasons for seeking treatment. They are then gently massaged while the therapist takes them on a journey into nature to a place where healing takes place for them. Kahuna body work originated in the ancient temples of Hawaii, where it featured as a part of a rite of passage. It has now been adapted to suit Western criteria of acceptability and palatability, but is still basically a transitional experience for people wishing to overcome emotional problems. The fundamental idea is that stimulation of your body permits a physical, emotional and spiritual release. Sessions usually last two hours and for this treatment you do remove your clothing. The therapist uses his or her whole arm in treatment (as opposed to primarily the hands used in Western forms) and the movements are derived from an ancient Hawaiian martial art and dance.

Manual lymph drainage (MLD)

Specialized training is required to master this extremely light, hands-on massage treatment which moves the skin across and along the lymph pathways in specific directions. Although extremely gentle, it is an amazingly powerful treatment, good for anyone congested by a bad diet, a sedentary lifestyle and exposure to pollutants. The pumping effect of manual lymph drainage increases the movement of the lymphatic system of the body, throwing its powers of cleansing, regeneration and healing into top gear. At the same time it affects the nervous system by instigating a change from the normal stressed 'daytime' (sympathetic system) state to the 'night-time' (parasympathetic system) state we use when we are asleep. This has the effect of strengthening the immune system and as it stimulates the lymph system it relaxes and refreshes you.

MLD is an excellent preventative and natural non-intrusive treatment. Even if you consider yourself to be quite healthy, manual lymph drainage treatments will increase resistance to colds, infections and 'flu. It can also firm and improve the look of the skin and has become a very popular beauty treatment as a 'natural face-lift'.

MLD also treats and prevents water retention anywhere in the body. Cellulite, swollen ankles, legs and eyes can be successfully treated, as can pre-menstrual swelling and discomfort. MLD works also on the skeletal muscles, which is helpful for those who often feel stiff after exercise. It can also lead to fast removal of the lactic acids that form in the muscle tissue, causing a rapid and pain-free regeneration of the muscle fibres.

MLD was developed in France in the 1930s by Dr Emil Vodder and his wife Estrid, treating sufferers from chronic catarrhal and sinus infections. In some places, MLD is used for oedemas following surgery and has proved to cause better wound healing by stimulating good scar tissue formation. Old scars are also much improved in appearance. MLD after plastic surgery has proven effective, as has treatment of lymphoedema after cancer treatment. See also pages 272–273.

On-site massage

This is becoming more and more popular as a way to experience the benefits of massage without removing any clothing and without having to devote more than 15 or 20 minutes of your time. This technique can be received at home or in the office, and is based around acupressure points, focusing on the head, neck, shoulders, spine, lower back and arms. It induces deep relaxation and relief from stress, and culminates with a brusque and enlivening set of movements to perk you up so you are ready to return to work relaxed yet invigorated.

Reichian massage

This was developed by Wilhelm Reich, a follower of Freud. Reich discovered that when working with his patients using a variety of physical contact techniques this enabled them to release energetic blocks and emotions held within those blocks. This belief system has been developed and is now more commonly known as 'bioenergetic therapy'. It is more often utilized by those who are also qualified therapists, as they are best suited to dealing with the often very strong emotions that come up in the client.

Rolfing

Also known as 'structural integration', this is a method of deep massage that was developed by Dr Ida Rolf, a biochemist with a background in osteopathy and yoga. Its purpose is to realign the muscular and connective tissue, achieved by the application of extremely heavy and concentrated

pressure for several seconds at a time with one knuckle, elbow or sometimes even the knuckles of a fist, often on a single point on a subject's body. The results can be startling, completely reshaping the body's physical posture.

Being rolfed is quite different from receiving a relaxing holistic massage. The sensations can be very strong, with momentary pain and exhilaration being experienced simultaneously. The 'pain' will only last as long as the pressure is being applied, about two or three seconds, and immense relief is felt instantly when the rolfer's hand is moved away. Strong emotions are often felt and people have been known to experience amazing psychological changes as well. More energy is felt when the body is correctly aligned, as the release from physical tension held in the body is eliminated.

Self-massage

Although nothing can really take the place of a full body massage given by a qualified professional, in times of need we can do a lot for ourselves. Learning the basic strokes of holistic or Swedish massage is very useful, but specific techniques – often employed with stretches – can go a long way towards reducing stress and helping you to develop a better relationship with yourself by putting the gift of nurturing in your own hands. There are many good books on this subject.

Shiatsu

This is a Japanese massage therapy practised widely there and growing steadily in popularity in the West. The word shiatsu means 'finger pressure' and the therapy was at one time practised almost entirely with the balls of thumbs, applying pressure to any or all the hundreds of points located along the meridians (energy pathways) for several seconds at a time. Shiatsu is a form of acupuncture without needles, stimulating the points with the fingertips and even the elbows. There is also a general stroking over parts of the body to stimulate a harmonious flow of energy throughout the body. The practitioner may also use gentle manipulation to stretch the meridians and to loosen joints to encourage healthy flow of energy. This helps tone up the body's energy, releasing lots of stress and tension and helping to alleviate countless symptoms and prevent many conditions.

Sports massage

With the increased interest in exercise, sports massage has become an ingredient of many avid exercisers' health programmes. It differs from physiotherapy in that it incorporates many of the techniques of Swedish and holistic massage and so aims to induce relaxation. The differences will be apparent when an injury is present; for example, torn hamstrings through over-exercising or incorrect exercising. In such cases, specific techniques are performed to enhance healing in the injured areas and exercises may be given for strengthening the surrounding areas or to reduce the risk of loss of mobility from lack of movement while healing.

Swedish massage

In this type of therapy, talcum powder is often used instead of oil, as a firmer grip is required. The practitioner will again follow a specific routine, using more invigorating movements, such as cupping and hacking, and a greater number of rotation stretches, for example on the shoulders and hip joints. It is more exhilarating than holistic massage and, although relaxing and equally beneficial, it is less meditation-enhancing.

T'ai chi and massage

In China it is commonly held that massage is a high art. The massage practitioner must learn the practice of T'ai chi (see page 182) as an integral part of his massage training. T'ai chi is a form of moving meditation, the movements of which are based on those of animals. The emphasis lies in clearing the meridians of any blockages or imbalances and ensuring a correct flow of chi, and balance of yin and yang where appropriate. This energy or chi is the same quality of energy found in yoga practice, called prana (see page 168), and is the same energy that a good massage practitioner uses.

With so much attention given to balance, gravity and grace, it is easy to see how T'ai chi becomes a relevant and integral part of massage training. It is vital that a massage practitioner is grounded, centred and free to allow the flow of chi from heaven and earth through them into their client, thus creating a two-way movement of energy. This flow of energy is like the dance that is T'ai chi: the receiver is also the giver and the giver the receiver, rather than a process of submissive receiving or focused giving.

Although it is not vital for a massage practitioner to be experienced in T'ai chi, the basic ideas of T'ai chi are undoubtedly useful. It helps protect them from picking up any negative energy from the client by providing an inner stillness and a shield around themselves, so only clear and positive energy is drawn into them and then channelled back to their client.

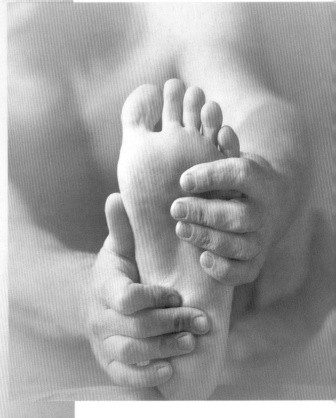

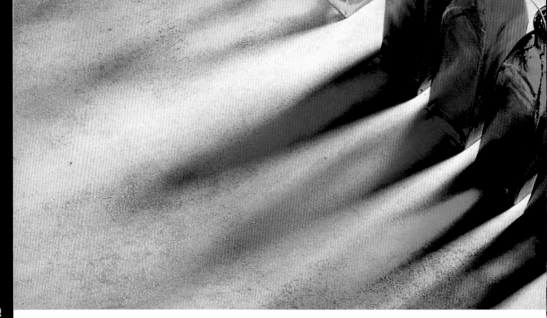

AROMATHERAPY DOS AND DON'TS

- Read all labels and enclosed instructions carefully when buying essential oils. You want to look for essential oils that are as pure as possible.
- Pure undiluted essential oils should never be applied directly to the skin, with the exception of lavender and tea tree oils, which can be applied to insect bites and other wounds; for instance, lavender is excellent for burns.
- Aromatherapy oils may already be diluted essences in a carrier oil ready for direct application to the skin. Do not dilute further until you check the instructions.

the art of aromatherapy massage

Therapeutic massage can be made an even more powerful tool by using it in combination with aromatherapy (see page 261) and, moreover, massage is probably among the most efficient means of administering aromatherapy treatment.

When essential oils are used with massage, small quantities are absorbed through the skin, the oil's healing effect then going straight into the system. For massage, essential oils are diluted in a carrier oil, such as almond, cold pressed soya or wheatgerm oil. Pure essential oils are too strong to use neat unless under the guidance of a qualified aromatherapist. Oils are very potent and should be used with care. Use around 8 drops when you are mixing with a tablespoon/10ml of carrier oil or up to 10 drops in a teaspoon of salt or milk powder (to help the oil dissolve) when using them in a warm bath.

Massage used with aromatherapy oils is generally a lymphatic drainage form of massage (see page 223), using long, gentle, sweeping strokes over the entire body, with the main aim being to introduce the essential oils (see page 228), blended with a very light vegetable oil, into the recipient's body via the capillaries. As in Swedish and holistic massage, a basic structure will be followed, starting with the back.

A more detailed medical history may be taken, beginning with a reflexology diagnosis on the feet to determine particular physical problems, and a discussion around any current or past emotional problems. Again, the oils will be chosen in an holistic fashion, with the aim of bringing about a balance of mind, body and spirit.

WHAT ARE THE BENEFITS OF AROMATHERAPY MASSAGE?

- The power of touch is so comforting and calming that difficult hospital and psychiatric patients respond positively to aromatherapy treatments. So much so that an increasing number of nurses are taking extra training in aromatherapy to complement orthodox treatment of their patients in order to help stimulate their patient's own healing process. They are in the best possible position to witness the effectiveness of this marvellous treatment.

- Aromatherapy massage is undeniably one of the most powerful treatments available to help combat illness and stress, and to maintain balance in mind/body/spirit

- Aromatherapy massage is particularly suited to anyone suffering from tension, stress and anxiety, and nervous disorders. If you are the type that gets all tied up in knots, aromatherapy – more than any other complementary therapy – helps you ease out of your tension, releasing much pent-up energy that is needed elsewhere to soothe away disturbances and help alleviate your state of stress.

- Aromatherapy has been used since time immemorial for enhancing beauty. It is said, in fact, that Cleopatra was not really beautiful but the power of the oils she used seduced her many suitors into believing in her beauty! Today an aromatherapy facial is an effective and luxurious treatment to ease signs of stress from the face and can help to ease out wrinkles.

- This is one of the most immediate, effective treatments for stress. Tensions melt away under the experienced touch of a qualified aromatherapist.

- The lymph system is stimulated, which helps your body move on and expel the accumulated toxins or 'stress crystals' that build up in the body's tissues.

some popular essential oils and their effects

BASIL

Breathing and digestive problems; stress and depression; nerve tonic; antispasmodic; mental fatigue. Basil aids concentration and a positive attitude.

BLACK PEPPER

A warming, pungent oil effective for treating catarrh, headaches, food poisoning and digestive pain; rheumatism and toothache; a diuretic; improves circulation.

CLARY SAGE

A balancing oil that can lift depression. It is calmative, nervine, treats PMT and period pain, restores tranquillity and can lower blood pressure.

EUCALYPTUS

An antiseptic, protects against colds and 'flus, can help in the treatment of wounds, relieves PMT and period pain, headaches and general muscular aches. Eucalyptus aids concentration, bronchitis and rheumatism; a natural insect-repellent and bactericide.

FRANKINCENSE

The oil of the Ancient Egyptians and burned in churches; has an uplifting and relaxing effect on the spirit, alleviates depression and helps to treat stress and skin problems. Increases immunoglobin levels, so it is excellent for the immune system and even for cystitis.

JUNIPER

Juniper and clary sage are the aromatherapists' 'clearers', used to dispel negative energy from clients. Use in an oil burner or rub a drop or two into the palms and inhale. A balancer: it can relax you while stimulating your mind and body. Treats cellulite, sleeplessness, cystitis, arthritis, is an antiseptic, diuretic, emmenagogue and a good tonic.

LAVENDER

A pharmacy in an oil; a very special and therapeutic oil that is useful as an antiseptic; it uplifts and soothes whilst relieving stress and has a balancing effect on the nerves. Excellent for treating burns and helps prevent scarring when used in a compress (under your aromatherapist's guidance).
Those with rheumatism benefit greatly from massage with this oil.

MAKING YOUR OWN SIMPLE MASSAGE OILS IS EASY:

For a body massage oil: mix 2 or 3 drops of the essential oil of choice with 1 tablespoon (5 ml) of the carrier oil of your choice (such as almond, cold pressed soya or wheatgerm). For a face oil: add 1 drop of essential oil to 1 teaspoon of carrier oil as above.

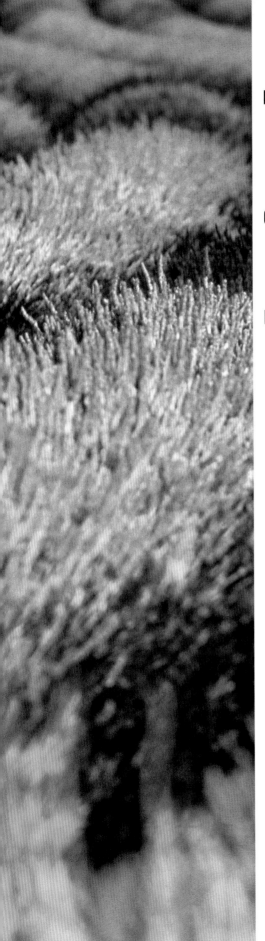

LEMON

An excellent oil for treating oily skin, acne, sluggish circulation and digestive disorders; a diuretic; emotionally uplifting, with a zinging fresh scent. Treats insomnia and nightmares, and can be used in a spray as a disinfectant.

ORANGE BLOSSOM

Orange blossom is a soothing relaxant with spectacular effects on acute anxiety attacks and stress. This beautiful fragrant oil also treats depression and insomnia, helping to release worry.

PATCHOULI

A heady, instantly recognizable aroma; patchouli is effective in treating and preventing depression. Burnt in a room it will lift despair and balance moods. An antiseptic, antidepressant used to treat dry skin and cellulite when blended with cypress, rosemary and juniper. Helps healthy circulation; an insect-repellant.

PEPPERMINT

This is a powerful oil often used in confectionery and so is a familiar smell to many of us. Extremely effective in treating digestive disorders ranging from flatulence to nausea, indigestion and heartburn to over-acidity. An analgesic; helps to treat headaches and muscular pains in general. It also helps relieve morning sickness.

ROSEMARY

A wonderful energizer; a drop or two rubbed into the palms and inhaled deeply will clear a burdened mind. Relieves mental fatigue, poor memory and is good for those studying for exams as it aids concentration. It is good for chest and lung problems and for colds, sinusitis, mucus and catarrh build-up and cystitis.

TEA-TREE

A powerful antiseptic; use around the home and in the sick room. Burn in a room for an anti-viral effect. Treats athlete's foot and insect bites and cleans wounds (under guidance); also other fungal conditions such as ring worm. Treats thrush when combined with lavender: two drops of each in a bath may relieve the symptoms. Add a few drops to cleaning products for extra protection from germs.

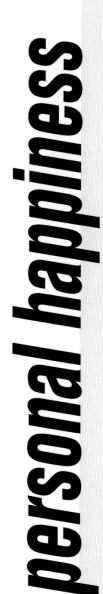

natural
pleasures

Ahhh, the bliss of being able to... ? Whatever word springs to mind when you read that sentence, stop and think... Is it possible for you to do it? What's stopping you from being able to do just that? 'My busy life!' is usually the answer. More often than not the reason we can't have a bit of what we fancy revolves around our busy schedules rather than the needs of the small voice in the back of our heads saying, 'What about me?!' If that voice is piping up louder and louder each day, it could be time to take matters away from the confines of the appointment diary and into our own hands.

In spite of our busy schedules, we're sensual creatures, who need the support and peace that time out provides. And a little bit of what we fancy... well, we all know that, in theory, it does do us good. It is, of course, one thing to know that you need a break, but what if you're working to deadlines, or you really can't take it at the moment? Perhaps you could allow yourself a small token pleasure right now. Or write an IOU to yourself, promising a special date treat when the project is finished.

If it is that the project is your life and the deadlines appear ongoing, it could be time to take an honest look at what your needs are, and perhaps why you are not allowing them to be expressed and heard on a regular basis. Delving deeper into finding out the 'why not' factor might be a precursor to making sure that next time you do allow time for more pleasures to live in your life alongside the commitments.

If, however, it truly is that this week you simply don't have time to take up the golf club or go to the cinema, then see if you can't book a few minutes by yourself simply with a cup of tea in a lovely warm bath, or even to revel in the occasional deep breath in the midst of everything.

We are the only ones who can make an active commitment to our own sanity. Once we do this, though, it need not be a lonely road. Asking for the support of friends and family can be a rewarding way of making sure you have the time to have your needs met. Sharing in this way reminds family and friends that their own pleasure bank needs to be filled on a regular basis. Enlisting the support of others means that once you have started on the path towards honouring the needs of the soul, it need not stop with one trip to the golf course or one session of meditation.

Relaxation, like happiness, works within a complex and interrelated framework of interdependent beliefs and emotions. Believing that we are worthy of taking that break, or trip to the art gallery for example, is the first step in making sure that we actually do it. Once we have agreed with ourselves that we are worthy of being able to take the important time to nurture ourselves, then finding the time is the next step.

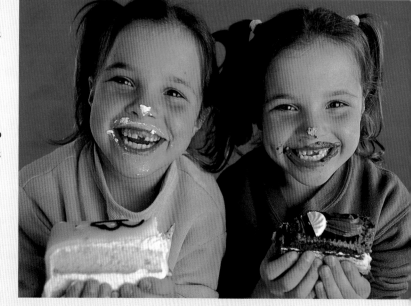

If this feels too challenging for you, or there simply aren't enough hours in the day to get all you need accomplished, then perhaps it might help if you pretend that you have promised your time to a small child who would be devastated if you didn't appear. In the quest for natural pleasures, it is also important you recognize that you are not simply committing to another task in a possibly mounting pile of things to do.

Most of us want to be happy, or happier, ever seeking the elusive elixir of happiness. The search for happiness and fulfilment is universal; what is unique is what makes us experience feeling happy and fulfilled. Happiness is so individual, subjective and relative. Freud believed the two elements of happiness were to be found in love and in work. Many studies would support that view. It is well documented that extroverts with loving family and friends are happier than introverts who have more difficulty connecting with others and who often describe themselves as unhappy, lonely or depressed. True happiness is tied up in a sense of purpose, a raison d'être, and feeling valued for your contribution, deeply interested in what you do and satisfied with the choices you've made.

We are often misguided in believing that happiness will come to us when we have achieved such and such, or acquired a certain amount of material security or fame, only to discover once we are surrounded by all these comforts and pleasures that there is still something missing, and that happiness is, indeed, the elusive treasure so many seek, so few find.

Spiritual teachers might suggest we are missing the point, creating increasingly more complex lives and then looking for, or expecting 'to find', happiness at the end of the rainbow alongside the pot of gold. We fail to find something that is not lost – so how can it be found? Perhaps it is impossible to find happiness; that in seeking to find happiness 'somewhere', we are overlooking where happiness is. We are always looking outside ourselves when, in fact, real happiness can only be found within ourselves.

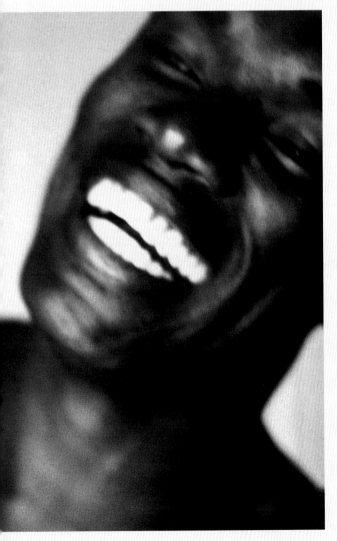

laughter is the best medicine

Really? Well, call it part of the package – since research has proved that laughing increases our physical sense of well-being by releasing endorphins that help us cope with physical pain and stresses. Laughing also has positive effects on such realities as blood pressure, heart rate, muscle relaxation and the rate at which oxygen is absorbed by the body. See more on page 206.

Happiness and the exercise factor

An approach to working with happiness in our lives at the moment is to treat happiness as if it were a muscle in need of exercise. If happiness were a muscle that needed to be toned regularly, we might take more care of it by taking it to the gym or out for walks. So if the practice of adding happiness into your life is one that is in need, then try the 'exercise' approach. Be willing regularly to 'work out' with what makes you happy. Add it to part of your routine and you'll find your experience of what makes you happy expanding.

Ingredients for cultivating personal happiness

While everyone's secret recipe for happiness is different, finding something to be passionate about is absolutely key. Get enthused about something and cultivate that enthusiasm through learning as much as possible about that subject. Make yourself into an expert about something you really love.

Seeking happiness

Be less of a critic when it comes to looking at what is 'wrong with your life' and more open to the improvements offered by what could happen if you become willing to allow more happiness in. Literally 'lightening up' helps take away the load of what is standing in between you and a natural state of being.

Auditing your happiness quotient

Are you spending too much time doing things that make you miserable because you feel you should? Be honest about what it is you actually need to get done today, and try and spend less time caught up in the errands of the day's activities and allow more time for the joys of the day's fun.

Experiencing happiness

Are you surrounded by dour faces? If you've been there recently, you'll remember that sour looks can rub off on you as easily as a smile does. If long faces are part of your current landscape and you are serious about expanding your happiness horizons, then finding different company where there is more laughter and fewer long faces can help. Surrounding yourself with those who value you and respect your worth is another crucial key in the happiness combination.

And when all else fails...

Just act yourself into the part. Sometimes the 'fake it till you make it' approach really works. If your own sense of the blues finds you living life closer to the indigo hues, then acting the part for an hour or so could just give you the lift needed to begin appreciating life again.

Why is it that some people seem to sail through difficult situations with dizzying levels of self-confidence, achieving the seemingly impossible, while others stumble along the same path just barely scraping by? Self-confidence is the reason why, and self-acceptance is crucially linked to self-confidence. But how does one get the desired package deal operating successfully together?

Difficult as it may be to do, accepting yourself exactly as you are in the moment is the most fundamental tool at your fingertips, should your desire be to move forward with an expanded sense of self-confidence. When you are brave enough to be totally honest with and about yourself 'warts and all', then you automatically free up an enormous amount of energy. If you've been wearing a mask to help you make it through the day, then much of your vital force is being depleted by the energy and concentration it takes to present a different image of yourself to the outside world.

If you're operating with a chronically low sense of self-esteem, it can crucially withhold the vitality of your life force. The capacity for real intimacy with a partner or friends also deepens when we are willing to accept ourselves as we are. The 'warts and all' approach to seeing ourselves provides the springboard for moving forwards and bringing into our lives what we actually want more of. The crucial trick is that it must be acknowledged first that we are just fine exactly as we are.

This type of self-acceptance provides the springboard, as well as the courage, from which to be able to delve deeper into personal relationships, whether they be with family, friends or with an intimate partner. Allowing a more positive sense of self-esteem is vital to uncovering deeper layers of the personal peace we desire.

Mirror work

If a confidence-building regimen is what you need, then self-acceptance exercises are the place to start. These can be as light-hearted or as deeply felt as you are willing to allow at any given moment. The simple act of looking in a mirror can bring up many feelings of frustration, coupled with an all-too-real vision of what is wrong with ourselves. We often see ourselves with critical eyes, looking for the flaws and that which we would wish to change, rather than acknowledging the brilliance that is already there, albeit perhaps lying dormant.

Stay looking at your image as you breathe deeply in and out. Allow yourself to feel love for the real image you see reflected in the mirror. Seeing yourself exactly as you are now, and not as you would wish to be perceived, can be daunting at first, but well worth it if you are willing to persevere with it.

Self-acceptance and affirmations

Affirmations (see page 208) such as, 'I am now willing to accept myself exactly as I am', when used with mirror work, can provide the spark for moving forwards in life with a new and renewed enthusiasm. Don't be surprised, though, if a welter of

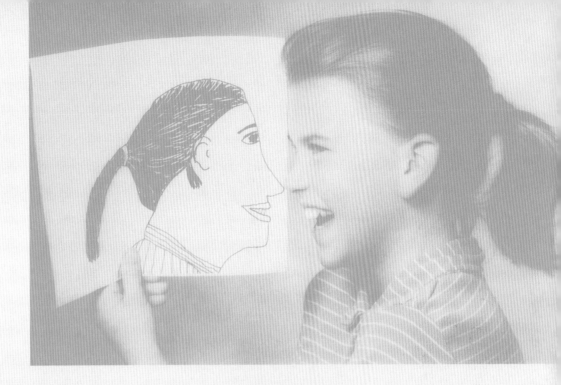

emotions and doubts come flying to the surface first. Perseverance with this work is key, and yields golden results as you move through layers of perception to finding a real and vital you.

Labelling and un-labelling

Set aside some time to allow yourself to go through your 'labels'. Take a pen and paper and go through the big 'labels' in your life, the tokens by which you identify yourself. Start with the obvious ones, like gender, age, race, religion, parents, etc., then go on to acknowledge the labels the outside world uses to identify who you are.

Next make a note of all your mental and emotional beliefs through which you experience yourself: what do you feel about things? What are you passionate about? What are your thoughts and emotional beliefs about who you are?

Now have a look at what the masks are that you use in presenting yourself to the outside world. Do you wish to be perceived as in control? At peace? Funny? Carefree? What kind of work does it take to present this to the outside world? Relax for a moment and see if you can go to what lies beyond these masks of projected image. In that state of honesty, and breathing deeply and gently, pick up a hand mirror and see if you now appear any different. Is there a more honest side of you that you've just uncovered? Is this something the outside (and inside!) world could see more of?

Now that you have established your sense of safety with this open and possibly vulnerable state, take a deep breath in and relax gently as you exhale. Move now into meditation (see page 214), and see if you can keep that sense of openness available to you throughout the meditation. As you come out of it, see if your face has retained some of that openness and honest reflection of the true you. Is it something you can carry with you more often?

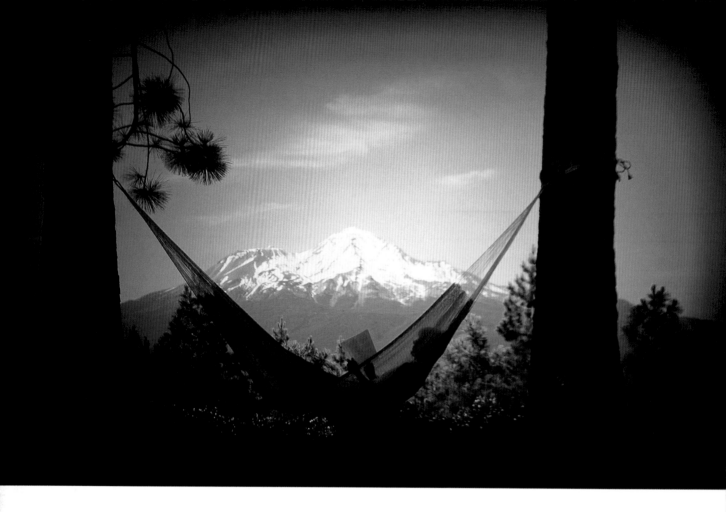

rest & sleep

We all know how crucial a good night's sleep can be if we have a full or important day ahead of us; however, simply laying our head down on the pillow a few hours earlier than normal doesn't necessarily guarantee that we'll actually be getting the rest we require. Restful sleep is, in fact, an essential building block for working with all healing modalities – be they based in natural medicine or allopathy. The long-term effects of sleep deprivation are currently being studied at some major universities in America as a long-neglected yet deeply rooted cause of many major illnesses.

If you are waking up at the same hour every night for a series of days, there could be more to it than that late-night tempting cheese platter. Chinese medicine tells us that this can mean a deficiency in a particular area, and a Chinese herbalist or acupuncturist can help to sort out these woes, and restore balance not only to your sleep but to your physical body as well.

If your problem is that you behave like there are 28 hours in a day instead of 24, then making sure that you allow adequate time for rest and sleep can prevent illnesses before they happen. Continually running our bodies down too low can leave us vulnerable to chronic exhaustion and diseases.

We spend a good third of our lives asleep, but why we do so is still a mystery. We only know for a fact that we can't do without it. Recording the brain's activity while we sleep has yielded some interesting results. There are apparently two cycles of sleep that alternate in 90-minute cycles – orthodox and paradoxical.

When we first go to sleep we fall into the orthodox mode, which is simply a resting phase for the mind and body during which our heart-rate slows, our blood pressure drops and we use less oxygen.

After roughly an hour we drift into the paradoxical cycle, in which any energy we saved during the orthodox mode is expended. In some ways, this is a similar state to being awake, but the brain's chemical balance is different. As blood flow to the brain increases, it becomes more active and we begin to dream. However, the body continues to rest: the muscles and reflexes are relaxed and only the eyes move from side to side under the lids.

Both phases are crucial to a good night's sleep and, therefore, to good health and well-being. Insomniacs should not despair, however; research into sleeping patterns and sleep deprivation suggests that insomniacs and light or irregular sleepers not only get more sleep than they think they do, but also that losing sleep is not necessarily as harmful as we might suppose. We can rest easy in the knowledge that the body nearly always compensates for it in some way.

HOOKED ON SLEEP?

Since prescription sleeping pills can be addictive, why not try a natural, non-addictive route to getting the horizontal hours you need. A glass of milk at bedtime is more than just a childhood treat; milk produces opiates that calm and soothe the body. If milk isn't for you, then a few drops of lavender sprinkled on your pillowcase can help just as well, as can a hot cup of valerian tea.

A firm mattress and a well-ventilated room are other key players in getting a full night's sleep.

Try exercising every day. Aside from helping you work through tensions that may keep you from sleeping properly, exercise has been clinically proven to reduce anxiety – one of the leading causes of insomnia.

watery delights

All of life depends on the presence of water so we should not be surprised at how valuable a therapeutic medium water has proven. Two-thirds of our body tissues are water, and water transports a lot of our body's waste products. On a daily basis, our sweat glands excrete a certain amount of water and waste matter, and one of the main benefits of hydrotherapy (water therapy) is the increased action and efficiency of the sweat glands.

Water has long been recognized as possessing therapeutic and healing qualities. The popularity of the early Roman and Turkish baths has not been diminished in modern times. People have been taking the waters for a cure throughout history and all over the world we still seek out water and spa treatments in many and varied forms.

The three hot basic baths in hydrotherapy are cold, hot and alternating cold and hot. Cold baths are invigorating and have a tonic effect, causing the small blood vessels to contract and then the dilation of the small arteries of the skin. They should not be taken for too long nor too cold, usually not less than 16°C (60°F). Young children, old people and those with any serious illness, like heart disease, anaemia and nervous conditions, should avoid cold baths.

Hot baths increase the activity and the efficiency of the sweat glands and have quite a relaxing effect. The increased perspiration promotes inner as well as outer cleansing, as the opened pores of the skin facilitate the elimination of toxins. By adding various herbal or other preparations, we can further the healing action of a hot bath. Sea salt, Epsom salts, seaweed, peat, herbs or essential oils can all be added to a hot bath to enhance its healing properties. Poor circulation, arthritis, rheumatism, muscle pains and nervous complaints all respond well to medicinal hot baths.

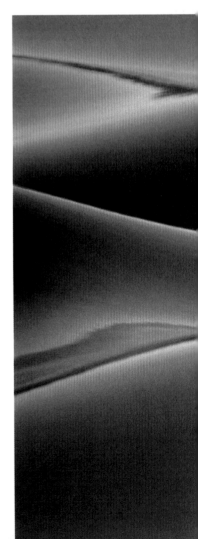

Alternate hot and cold baths or showers act like an artificial pump to stimulate blood flow and lymphatic and venous drainage. This kind of bath can quickly reduce inflammation and increase circulation and is excellent after an injury, like a sprained ankle or pulled muscle. As a general rule you should spend about 2–3 minutes in hot water followed by half a minute in cold water, repeating this 3 or 4 times and finishing with cold water.

Relaxing or lying in a bath is very different from actually taking a bath. The difference with lying in a bath is you are supposed to do nothing but relax. This is not the bath you take to scrub your body or wash your hair; this is bathing at its most therapeutic and relaxing, in the quiet privacy of your own bathroom, creating an atmosphere and ambience of peace and serenity, calming, soothing and

HINTS FOR SELF-PAMPERING:

1 Warm your towels and/or dressing gown.
2 Turn off the lights. Use a few candles, or a bowl of floating candles for light.
3 Add a few drops of your favourite essential oils to your bath, particularly the stress-reducing oils, like lavender.

warming. Calm your emotions, soothe and smooth your stresses, watch your woes float away in a bath that is as hot as you can take it. See also Hydrotherapy on page 270.

Whirlpool baths

These use small electric agitators to produce an underwater massage effect which is therapeutic for treating all kinds of ailments, from insomnia and tension to damaged nerves, joints and connective tissue.

Sitz baths

These are two baths in one, designed so that the upper part of the body, hips and abdomen can be immersed in water at a different temperature to the feet. The upper part of the bath is usually filled with warm water, while the feet are in cold or cooler water. This kind of bath is useful for treating intestinal, urinary and genital problems, as well as disorders of the reproductive system.

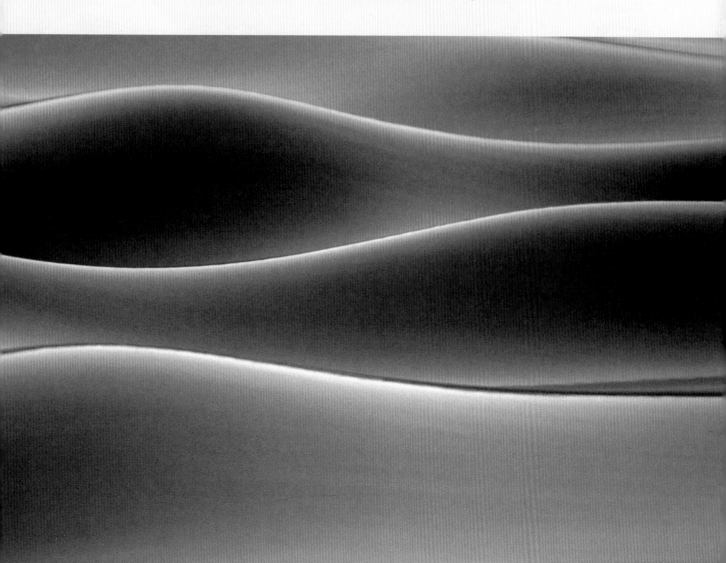

sensory delights

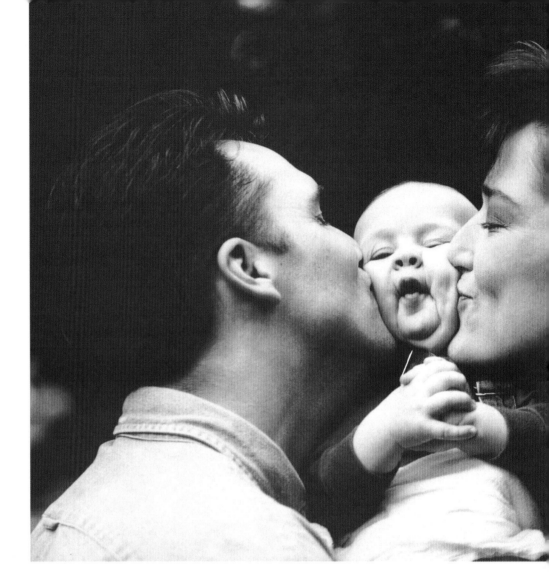

Touch

One of the greatest gifts we give ourselves and each other is the gift of touch. More than just the delight of sensuality and sensation, touch is a language that crosses all barriers, carries messages of love, of friendship and tenderness, of healing and hope. Most of us have experienced the comfort of a hug, a kiss, a hand touching our back, showing how deeply nourishing and necessary touch is to our well-being.

Touch is not only about comfort and communicating love: it is vital to the healthy function of our immune system; indeed, touch is such a primal need and primary force that it is part of what sustains us and ensures our survival. Without touch many living creatures wither, withdraw into depression and, in some cases, die.

All of us need touch and deprivation can be damaging. Research carried out in America on baby monkeys showed that the monkeys became withdrawn and unable to relate to other monkeys if deprived of touch. At worst they became psychotic! Humans who are not touched enough as children may find integration into society difficult, mixing with other people traumatic, and can even become frightened of

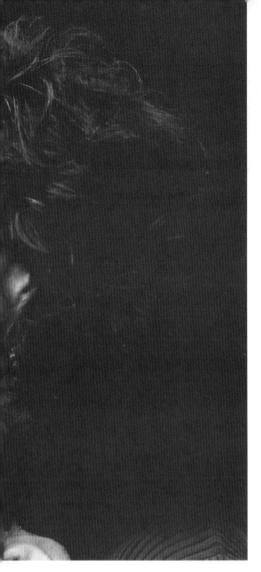

touch – unable to give or receive from others. Through the large number of wars in the latter part of the last century, which created inordinate numbers of orphans, it has been shown that those young children and babies removed from the family by the ravages of war and not having received touch became very depressed and unable to develop normal social skills and language, some even losing their will to survive.

Touch is now recognized as a powerful tool for stimulating healing, encouraging a positive immune response. It is for this reason that some hospitals and other institutions of long-term care have welcomed 'Animal Assisted Therapy'. In the UK, qualified members of 'Pets As Therapy' (PAT) regularly visit people who are ill, disabled, depressed or elderly to bring the comfort of touch, which brightens the mood along with lowering the blood pressure. Young children learn easily about love, responsibility and care-taking when small pets are put in their charge. Stroking and nurturing pets is healing and therapeutic for anyone, and the pets love it too!

Different cultures respond to touch in different ways. In the warmer Mediterranean countries it is acceptable for men to kiss on greeting, for women to hold hands and clasp arms whilst walking, and touch during conversation is effortless, warm and natural. In some cultures public displays of touch are frowned upon between opposite sexes, for example, but we often find that these cultures are vastly more tactile when in appropriate settings than we are in the West.

For centuries people have recognized how soothing, relaxing and life-affirming massage can be. How wonderful to share this experience with someone you love, your children, your partner or your friends. If touch is unfamiliar to you and would make you feel uncomfortable, start with yourself! When massaging oils or creams into your skin, notice how that feels. Massage your scalp when shampooing. This can be so relaxing and stimulating at the same time.

Of course, if you are comfortable with touch, let yourself enjoy touching other people. When speaking with friends, place a hand gently on their forearm or their back. Touch can bring people closer together in a way that words never can. Experiment with touch on loved ones. Children who are massaged or touched frequently, or have their feet rubbed, hair stroked, or backs rubbed, respond more lovingly than those who do not receive frequent loving touch. The same rules apply for us grown-ups! Take time out to touch your partner. It doesn't have to be sexual unless you want it to be. Let go and enjoy how it feels to give as well as to receive.

BANISH BOREDOM

Working with sensuality can be a pathway to heightened consciousness. Pick a sense to experience consciously and work with whenever you remember during the day.

Become a poet of the senses by playing with the crossover of sense from one recognized realm into another; for example:

• If the scent of crushed walnuts were a colour, what would it be?
• What would a taste feel like?

Working in this way is not just entertaining, it's an active way to tap into the expansive reality of the present moment. Allow your imagination to run with your senses and you will never be bored again.

sensual delights

We've all felt the sensual pleasure of slipping into a warm bath, of bare feet padding through wet grass, or the feel of sand between our toes as we run across a hot beach to a cool and waiting ocean. In an ideal world, indulgences such as these are a part of our busy lives as much as possible, but it's not always so easy to find the time.

Of course, it's easy to appreciate how blue the sky or the ocean is while on holiday, because we have travelled beyond our sensual 'familiar territory'. It is, however, equally easy to fall back into the dullness of routine once we get home and re-experience life within the limited sensuality of what we already know to be 'safe'.

Since our five senses are the tools we use to navigate our way through daily life, it can be easy enough to tune out the offerings of spontaneous and unexpected pleasures within them. Fortunately, however, working with expanding and heightening your sensuality beyond the realm of the usual can make the 'limited ordinary' into the utterly extraordinary, with just a simple shift of focus.

Our re-experiencing a completeness of sensuality can hold intimate and rewarding links with reactivating our childhood imagination and creativity. The therapeutic effects of playfully using our senses can not only help to reduce stress but can also actively enhance our personal sense of well-being.

The tangibility of touch

It certainly bears repeating that our sense of touch is hardly limited to what we experience with our hands, or at the hands of an experienced body-worker. Whether you are stuck in a rut or stuck in traffic, try and expand your sensation of what encompasses touch by regularly moving your awareness around your body. The feel of our feet in shoes, sandals or socks is just as valid a sensual experience as the obvious pleasure of letting velvet slip through our fingers, or the sensation of letting a long-awaited cup of tea nestle in our hands.

Exercise: If you decide to spend a day working with expanding your consciousness through your sense of touch, check in whatever touches your skin, as and when you remember throughout the day. What is its texture? ... its temperature? Can you enhance the experience by closing your eyes and breathing into the feeling?

Scent-ual secrets

We've all been brought back to the arms of a lover by smelling their perfume or cologne, or the arms of a mother by the hint of her powder in the air. Scents can carry emotional charges – memories waiting to be unlocked by our re-experiencing a scent we associate with them. The therapeutic effects of aromatherapy (see page

226) are well documented. It can be an equally sensual pleasure to let the play of memories that we associate with a particular scent parade before our consciousness.

Exercise: If one day you choose to work with heightening your sense of smell, try not to limit yourself, out of habit, to experiencing only the pleasant ones. Really experiencing what you think is unpleasant can sometimes be as rewarding as avoiding it. If you choose consciously to work with heightening your sense of smell, and you come across something unpleasant, ask yourself what about that scent is particularly distasteful to you. Does it hold memories of someone or something that you are perhaps now willing to let go of?

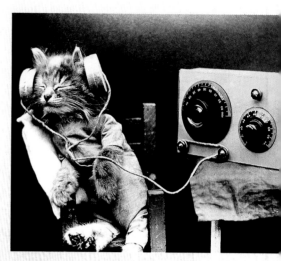

Revelling in sound

Sound is an equally fascinating sense to play with, beyond the obvious enjoyment and pleasure of tuneful music. If this is your favourite sense or 'sense of the day', what can you do right now to enhance its effect in your life?

Exercise: Even in silence, what can you hear? What sounds are outside the house, out in the garden, in the street? Do objects have a sound? Let your imagination experience what an object would sound like. See also Sound therapy on page 280.

Colour therapy

The visual effects of colour on stimulating activity within the brain are also well documented. For instance, restaurants have long been known to swathe their walls in luxurious reds as these are known to excite the appetites of diners. Other less extreme associations with the healing or stimulatory effects of colour are all around us. Allowing your eyes to travel to a leafy tree in a moment of panic or tension can significantly reduce the effect of stress on your body, not just through enjoyment of the tree's beauty, but by an active association with the healing colour of green.

Exercise: As you move through the day, try to perceive how and if certain colours affect your mood. Try wearing a colour you're not usually drawn to, to see the effect it has not only on your mood, but on the way others perceive and relate to you.

Tasting the unusual through the usual

Forget about the joys of taste being limited to the lucky gourmet's kitchen. Allow yourself to experience the delights of fresh, raw or organic food, as well as being adventurous enough to look for the wonderful in your mother-in-law's Sunday roast!

Exercise: What does your mouth taste like at this moment – when it's empty? Even 'apparently nothing' has a taste: revel in it and see what it has to offer.

the natural home & office

Today, Feng Shui is a popular part of our 'East meets West' culture, sufficiently to generate countless magazine and newspaper features. There are also many books and TV programmes dedicated to the design and placement of rooms in order to sanctify and reflect spirit, and channel the most positive energies possible for our good health, wealth, relationships and general well-being.

The basic idea behind the ancient art of Feng Shui is that every part of life is connected to, and affected by, our physical surroundings. Our general well-being, health, wealth, family and relationships are influenced by the way we arrange our rooms, our space. The orientation and placement of furniture and ornaments, water, light and space can enhance and promote 'positive energies', improving lifestyle and well-being.

Many people are reporting real and positive changes by paying attention to the principles of Feng Shui. Professional consultants of this ancient Eastern practice are almost as plentiful as interior designers, and are considered a priority for many people setting out to buy or renovate a home or professional space.

If you are feeling weighed down with lots of negative energy, you might want to have a look at a few of Feng Shui's golden rules.

Clutter is a big issue, according to Feng Shui practitioners, and the sooner we can eradicate it from the home and office environment the better. A cluttered environment confuses and can create chaotic energy. Clearing out that mess really helps if you need to 'pick-up' energy because you are tired and frustrated much of the time. Clutter in the office and house can create low blocked fields of energy, so you must throw out or put away all that 'stuff' lying around the place.

FENG SHUI TIPS

• Unclutter your space, at work and at home. Keep space clean and tidy to discourage build up of negative energy.

• The front door – the mouth of the house – must be kept clear of debris, and clean and free from dust, to encourage positive energy to flow freely into your home. The same applies to any back door you have.

• A pond full of fish in the garden or a fish tank and other water features in the house can bring good luck.

• Mirrors increase the energy of a room, but they must be placed in their optimum position. Two mirrors should not be placed facing each other. It is also best not to have mirrors in the bedroom; if you must, limit numbers and have none facing the bed!

• House plants can absorb toxic energy from electrical equipment. Spider plants are particularly notable for this effect. House plants with rounded leaves are especially beneficial.

Colour is an important aspect of feng shui. It is common knowledge that colours have a direct effect on our mood and, in many cases, even our nervous systems. More and more institutions, hospitals, prisons, and government buildings are paying attention to the colours they are choosing to paint their walls, and providing soft furnishings that are in harmony.

Colour guidelines

The blue and green end of the spectrum are the healing colours. They are soothing and calming, and so are good colours for an area or room in which you may wish to relax. If you tend to be a rather hyper type, always on the go and finding it quite difficult to relax, then try wearing the blues or decorating your living room to aid relaxation.

The yellows, oranges and warmer colours are wonderful for keeping heat and passion alive in the bedroom. They are also good for kitchens, as orange in particular will aid the digestion. The deeper reds and purples work for some people, both being warm and sultry.

For those of us who tend to err on the side of sloth, and generally seem to lack motivation, the warm, peppery, vibrant colours are amazingly beneficial in adding spice to our lives and energy to our days.

Try to avoid overloading with one colour – make use of a colour wheel, with its complementary colours. Complementary colour combinations include: blue and yellow, violet and yellow, pink and green, magenta and green, red and turquoise, orange and blue, yellow and grey (see right).

For example, orange and blue is a very popular and effective combination for an interior. Pink and green work well together, especially in a bedroom, to create an environment that is both loving and harmonic. Another variation of this would be magenta and green for a much more striking and even bolder colour combination.

Despite all these rules, it is really important to find colours that appeal to you and are appropriate for the space they are intended to enliven. Where colouring your home is concerned, your own intuition is by far the greatest tool. However, taking advice from Feng Shui experts or colour therapists is useful and can help you to make your own informed choices.

246

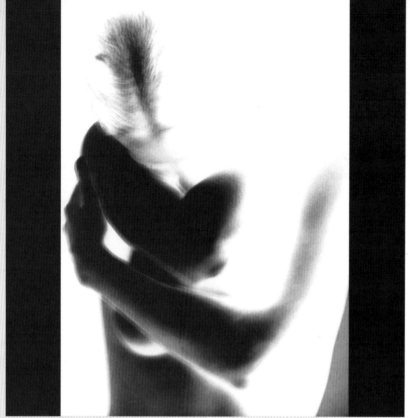

life crisis points

crisis
management

The quickening pace of life today seems inexorable and almost every adult is aware of the rapid changes gripping most communities, cultures and countries. At the turn of the last century, people got around by pony-and-trap and rarely moved far from family and friends. Their dress was modest and just about covered up the entire body. Sex and biological functions were never talked about – certainly not in mixed company. A mere 100 years later, the brave new world of the 21st Century finds us moving helter-skelter across the globe at the speed of sound, sending messages at the speed of light, while satellites thousands of miles above the earth measure our movements as well as our weather.

We are awash with gadgets and technology that tease and test us and change our lives irreversibly. The PC – in fact, the microchip and all the resulting information technology – has revolutionized our world and we are all caught up in a wave of electronic, digital wonder as we integrate ever more amazing gadgets into our daily lives. All these devices are designed to make our life easier, but they seem instead to have created a whole new level of anxiety and stress in our lives. What about all the time it takes to consult our personal organizer, reply to all our e-mail messages and our mobile phone text message boxes, deal with our Internet web site, our interactive TV?

Where does it stop and also how much of our human interaction – and therefore our relationships and intimacy – are compromised by the continual electronic demands on our time? If this wonderful life in the fast lane of the global village is so good for us, why do the seams of society appear so frayed? Can it really be true that a quarter of under-fours have their own TV set? Is it possible that this can really help these toddlers to develop their creative, communication and social skills? As the new millennium was ushered in, it was perhaps no surprise to see headlines reporting shocking rises in the number of teenage heroin and crack addicts, along with a rapidly-rising crime rate in almost every category.

Life's crisis points

If you live long enough in this world, you will undoubtedly face crises and have to work and live through them. At some time in our lives everyone must confront crisis and cope with major life changes, which shift forever our perceptions of reality and cause us to question our choices.

Bereavement, divorce, job loss, loss of home, nation or identity, ill health, an accident, acts of crime or violence – these can all trigger a state of crisis that finds one at the bottom of a pit of despair which, at that time, it seems impossible to scale your way out of. We can slip into a crisis state when more than one stressful situation occurs at the same time, like a bereavement and a job loss or a divorce and moving house the same week. Everybody has their own unique way of coping... but eventually we may all reach rock-bottom at some point and our usually dependable inner strength and resourcefulness disappears.

Negative or challenging life events provoke people, but it is usually one new item in the loss department that can set a personal crisis in motion. Sometimes it can even be a good event combined with a personal loss that tips the scales – like a job promotion that brings increased responsibilities at the same time as the death of a parent. Whatever the particular combination of factors that may provoke crisis mode in your mind and body, it is important not to deny to yourself, and close family and friends, that you are in crisis.

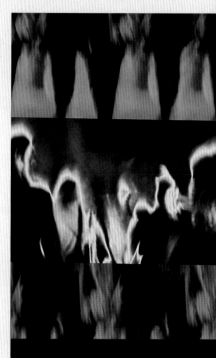

DEALING WITH SHOCK

If feeling faint, sit with your head between your knees. Otherwise, sit quietly or lie down if necessary. Don't forget to breathe or guide the person in shock to let the breath out and continue to breathe deeply, but do avoid hyperventilation. Keep warm, cover with a blanket.
Administer rescue remedy (page 264), 4 drops on the tongue or a drop on each temple and 2 drops on lips. Gently rub hands, feet or upper back to restore calm.

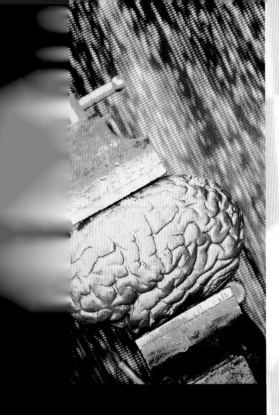

A crisis can take a big toll on your mental and physical health, and it needs to be addressed and confronted rather than ignored and denied, in order for wholeness and equilibrium to have a chance of reinstatement somewhere down the road. The important healthy self-view is an honest and courageous assessment of your state of mind and wholeness. No one knows better than ourselves when we are in trouble and need to seek help outside ourselves to restore a balanced state.

Giving yourself a good talking to is often not enough: self-counselling cannot replace the stimulation of insight that is the result of a positive counselling encounter. Too many of us plod on, ignoring our needs, symptoms and stresses until we reach a real crunch point, and a state of crisis is revealed. There are times when it is important to seek help. In the same way you would visit the doctor if you displayed symptoms of serious illness, you might consider visiting a professional counsellor or therapist if you find yourself in an emotional/mental crisis.

If you are experiencing a crisis because of the death of a loved one, there are places you can go to for help. Look for a bereavement group or counsellor in your area, to help you get over the trauma and back to your old self again. Quite often, you need only retreat from the world for a few days – to reflect and mourn in solitude – to overcome a 'mini-crisis', or have a chat with an old friend. But don't be afraid to ask for professional help if the crisis seems too big to cope with alone. It takes courage to overcome the problems we encounter in life... but it requires even greater inner strength to admit that we need help. Reach out for and demand help from one of the many sources available to you, however and whenever you need it.

RULES TO APPLY DAILY TO LIGHTEN YOUR STRESS LOAD

➡ Breathing – pay attention to your breathing; notice if it is shallow. If so, practise deep breathing. While doing this, visualize positively any 'difficult' situations in the day ahead.

➡ Eat and drink good nutritious food and liquids.

➡ State boundaries; be aware of what you can and cannot do.

➡ Sleep well, allowing enough time for recuperative, healing sleep.

➡ Plan ahead; if you will be out socializing one night, make up for it the next.

➡ Check in with yourself privately throughout the day, e.g. how are you feeling after lunch? Notice this and give yourself even just five minutes to become centred, if stressed or frantic.

stress management

Stress that is allowed to get out of control can induce a debilitating and enduring state of anxiety that destroys our peace of mind and erodes physical health and well-being. It is a well-known fact that stress contributes to several very serious health conditions if it develops unchecked.

How to take the stress out of your day

Letting go of stressful habits and replacing them with de-stressing habits is a positive step towards creating a personal programme to reduce your stress levels during the day. It is important, at this stage of your overall stress-management scheme, to make an honest assessment of the habits in your life that are creating rather than reducing your daily stress levels.

First look at the obvious ones. Do you over-commit, stretching yourself too thinly? Do you drink too much tea, coffee and alcohol, and smoke excessively? Do you bolt un-nutritious fast junk foods in between appointments, not leaving yourself enough time to digest your food? If you can answer 'yes' to more than one of the above, you have some real work (or play, depending on how you look at it) to do. De-stressing your day won't be so easy until you amend or moderate your more dangerous habits.

You can stop drinking 6 cups of tea plus 5 cups of coffee a day. Cut down to, say, 2 cups of tea and 1 cup of coffee, and replace the rest with calming herb teas, water and natural fruit juice. You can make the choice to be more disciplined concerning your negative stress-producing habits. Do you really need all that extra salt and sugar with your food for instance? Where your stress is concerned a little moderation goes a long way.

Think about your daily routine and compile a list of any stress-inducing habits or activities. Compile a second list outlining how you can start to change those habits or limit your involvement in those stressful activities – be realistic and patient and, above all, try not to create even more stress by setting targets that are unrealistic and hard to achieve. Don't expect overnight results, because it takes time to undo the habits of a lifetime. Take things one step at a time, replacing one bad habit with a good one, then moving on to the next when you feel happy with your progress. Try to have fun giving up unhealthy routines for healthy ones. After all, you'll feel better for making the change.

DE-STRESSING WITH YOGA

Yoga's powerful system of mind/body exercises can be an excellent de-stresser because it works not only on the muscles, bones and joints but on the nervous system as well. Yoga postures, called 'asanas' (see page 168), are designed to stretch, tone and refresh the body, while calming the mind. Pranayama (yoga breathing exercises, see page 168) are an integral part of yoga practice, which is one reason why it is useful for reducing and managing stress. Among the best asanas for stress are the Padahastasana pose (page 173), which is excellent for warming up, opening the lungs, expanding the chest, stretching the back of the legs and spine and 'letting go' of tensions, and the Corpse pose (page 180).

THE COMPLETE BREATH EXERCISE

This quick, seated exercise can be done anywhere, any time – at home, at work or on the move.

Sit in a chair, with your back straight but not rigid, using the chair back for support if necessary. Relax your shoulders and place your palms on either side of your abdomen. Inhale slowly though your nose, drawing your breath first into your abdomen to fill and expand it and then up though your middle and finally to expand your chest. When exhaling, contract your abdomen first and then your middle and chest. Repeat 2 to 3 times.

This is a powerful exercise and should be done in moderation at first. Done regularly over time it can enhance your vitality and help to reduce your stress levels for good.

The yoga exercises known as the Horse Positions or 'Calming Inhalation and Exhalation' (see page 172) are also very useful.

the importance of breathing properly

One of the main keys to successful stress management is your breathing. Breathing is such a primary function for our survival that we constantly take its power for granted and overlook this amazing tool with which we can regulate and stimulate our own good health.

Your automatic nervous system is responsible for your breathing process, which is why you do not need to think about it – you will breathe anyway! By understanding the very direct relationship between your breath and your brain and nervous system, you have a useful tool which can help you achieve and maintain a more balanced, positive, stress-free inner and outer life. After all, if we are feeling calm and centred, then our ability to solve problems, think more creatively and cope with the outer world is enhanced.

Breathing and relaxation are powerful tools in the daily challenge of coping and overcoming stress. Notice how your breath is fast, short and shallow when you are angry, fearful or just under everyday stress, and how you naturally take deeper, slower and longer breaths when you are in a peaceful and relaxed state.

The chest expands when we breathe deeply, helping the release of inner tensions as we exhale. By changing breathing patterns and consciously breathing deeply into the abdomen, you can create a calm relaxed state from a fraught one. Deep breathing calms both body and mind by slowing down heart rate and easing the nervous system.

The fact is the act of breathing is not necessarily the same as the art of breathing. Many people rush around, shallow-breathing their way through life and wondering why they always feel stressed, unwell and out of breath. By learning to let go of stressful symptoms, feelings and thoughts, by doing some deep breathing and using your exhalations as channels of release, you can do your body/mind some real short- and long-term good. Take a deep breath, inhaling through the nose and, when you exhale, imagine you're blowing out a candle, exhaling firmly through the mouth. Other variations on the same theme are using the 'S' sounds or a wide-open-mouthed 'AH' sound when you exhale. Repeat them two or three times.

It may seem too simple to be true, but the reality is our breathing holds the key that can unlock the stranglehold of stress and teach us invaluable lessons on how to cope

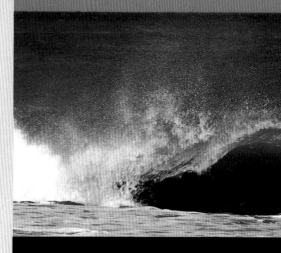

with the inevitable stresses most of us face in modern life.

Through breath awareness and conscious relaxation you can take control of all aspects of your health and enhance your ability to cope with life's increasing pace. The importance of understanding how useful your breath is in stress control, of how to breathe well and breathe deep cannot be overemphasized. Deep breathing also enhances concentration, releases tension and eases pain.

By learning simple breathing exercises and by becoming more mindful of the art as well as the act of breathing, you can do a power of good for your mind and your body. Try steady deep breathing three or six times, while you give yourself the inner direction to 'LET IT ALL GO', letting go until you return to your own rhythm of calm, quiet breathing (through the nose with the mouth closed).

Breathing and brain waves

The developing technology of biofeedback and electroencephalograph machines has demonstrated the direct relationship between breath and brain. An electroencephalograph measures brainwaves and biofeedback machines allow us to monitor the state of our mind. There are four major types of brainwaves: alpha, beta, delta and theta, each associated with a different level of mental activity.

Alpha – When you are awake and in a very relaxed state, listening to music or just closing your eyes, your brain emits alpha waves. Breathing is slow and easy. This state can be induced by meditation or hypnosis, and makes you highly receptive.

Beta – When you are awake and attentive, your brain remains in beta mode during periods of intense concentration or anxiety, even if your eyes are closed. When you are alert, busy, walking, talking, writing a letter, reading a book or operating under pressure, all theses activities require beta-type brain waves.

Delta – Slower than the other waves, delta waves are usually generated during sleep or coma. Some neuroscientists believe delta waves act as the brain's defence mechanism. The brain often emits delta waves when endangered by disease or injury.

Theta – When a yogi is able to lie comfortably on a bed of nails or can walk on fire without feeling pain or heat, his brain is in theta-wave emission. Theta waves usually suggest a deep trance, a state when sensations of pain are dulled. Their slow frequency is associated with drowsiness or dreaming. Slow theta waves also occur during periods of creative thinking.

IONIZERS

Have you ever noticed how invigorating it is to breathe mountain and sea air? How clean and fresh the air is after a thunderstorm? How well you feel after a walk in such air? This is because the air is charged with negative ions, which are refreshing and stimulating.

Fresh air is rich in negative particles, where city or industrial air contains little or none. The conditions in modern houses and offices in modern cities – particularly the electrical gadgets we surround ourselves with – destroy negative charges and account for the rising rate of asthma, chronic respiratory infections and allergen reactions.

If you fall into this category, you may find an ionizing machine helpful. Ionizers are electrical devices that produce a steady stream of negative ions when switched on. They help restore the balance of positive and negative ions in the air around you. Small machines cost around £30–60 and can be found in electrical goods and health food shops as well as chemists and department stores.

RELAXATION TIPS

When you feel tension mounting, do 3 rounds of complete deep breathing, remembering to inhale and exhale through the nose and to listen to your breath as it journeys through you.

Take a hot bath by candlelight, with soothing music in the background. Add bath salts or aromatherapy oils, like lavender and camomile.

Take a sauna, jacuzzi or whirlpool bath after a swimming or exercise session. Pamper, relax and rejuvenate yourself – book an appointment with a qualified aromatherapist.

Lie down with a special cooling eye pack, listening to gentle music, for 15–20 minutes.

Learn to 'catnap'; just closing your eyes for 10–15 minutes can really refresh you, be it in the office, on the train, on a bus or sitting in your favourite armchair at home. Just close your eyes, let go and relax – turning off to everything while you rest.

Have a foot, head, neck and face massage.

Take a walk in a favourite place, be it a park, woods or beach that you love. Or just close your eyes and imagine you are there, taking in fresh invigorating air with every inhalation.

relaxation technique

In spite of how essential relaxation is to well-being, many people do not really know how to relax. For a fuller treatment of the subject, see The Relaxed Mind on pages 212–213. The following yoga-based exercises will also help you learn some of the subtleties of relaxation.

This first relaxation exercise is very good for releasing some of your physical and mental tensions. Lie down on your back, feet shoulder-width apart, arms relaxed, a little away from your body, palms turned upwards. Close your eyes and take a few deep breaths, following your breath's journey with your conscious attention as you inhale and exhale through the nose. Make sure some of those breaths get into your belly and, while you are exhaling, imagine all your tensions flowing out of your body with each outgoing breath. You can also do a version of this sitting at your desk or in a traffic jam.

Another excellent relaxation exercise to do while lying down with your eyes closed uses creative visualization and affirmations (pages 208–211) to relax you completely. First do at least 3 rounds of steady deep breathing through the nose, and then just move naturally into a calmer natural breathing rhythm of your own, observing with your inner awareness your breath's journey. Listen to your breath.

Become aware of your head and neck, maybe gently move your head from side to side a few times and relax back into the centre. Inhale deeply and then, as you exhale, give yourself the inner direction to release and let go of all tension you are holding in your head and neck. Feel the tensions flow out and away as you exhale.

Next move your awareness into your shoulders, arms, hands and fingers. Perhaps flex or tense them a few times and let go, then breathe into them and, as you exhale, imagine all the tension you hold in that region flowing away. Then move your attention down through your chest, middle and abdomen, breathing into these areas and releasing all tension as you exhale. You may need 2 or 3 rounds in a particular area to let go of all the held tension. Continue downwards, through the pelvis, hips and buttocks, thighs, knees, legs, feet and toes.

By learning the art of relaxation you can do more to ensure your future good health and well-being than any tonic. Reducing your stress levels is something only you can do for yourself and the single most important contribution you can make to your healthy future.

On waking, greet the day and thank the night

Drink water.

Gentle stretching exercise (qigong, yoga or simple stretches).

Cleansing and substantial breakfast.

Take time to consider the day ahead.

Make lists or plan movements. Create a realistic structure within which to work, allowing flexibility.

Cleanse the body

Take stimulating showers or relaxing baths.

Create a harmonious environment at both home and work

Be aware of lighting — harsh hot lighting can cause headaches.

Try to take time to be in natural light every day.

Be aware of your comfort levels — if seated most of the day, is your body (particularly your back) well supported? Be aware of your posture, being hunched over a keyboard can cause stress in the back and poor circulation in the hips and legs. Try to walk or stretch away from your desk for a few minutes every half-hour.

Travelling

If driving in frustrating traffic jams causes you stress, can you take the train? Allow plenty of time.

Read, focus on deep breathing or meditate while travelling (it is possible, even if crushed and standing!)

Listen to healing music on your personal stereo at low volume.

Walk to the station or to work, where possible.

Breathe in fresh air each day and notice nature and the cycle of the seasons.

State your boundaries

Can you really work every day until 7.00 pm or later, when you have a lovely home you'd much rather be in? Be realistic about what you can and cannot do. It is important to treat each other respectfully, we all deserve consideration. Kind words of encouragement or praise do much to enhance self-esteem and create a pleasant ambience in the workplace. Too much criticism and rudeness only serves to create disharmony and, therefore, increases stress in the individual and the workplace. Constructive criticism works wonders when given politely and with positive advice.

Work and social life

Most people enjoy socializing with their work mates.

Offer, or encourage your employer to arrange, sporting facilities and/or bring in natural health therapists who can work during lunchtimes.

Encourage get-togethers for relaxation and letting off steam.

Social and family life

Make time to socialize with yourself! You deserve some time for yourself. What do you enjoy doing? It may be reading, walking, thinking or just luxuriating in a very long bath. Whatever it is, you deserve it.

Make time to be with those you love and who love you, your family and good friends. A few hours spent in the company of loved ones works wonders for boosting morale. Laughter and shared experiences are all 'money in the bank' for your own health. Look at your diary. Do you have NO TIME? Reassess, and try to make time for yourself, family and friends. It is worth the effort. You are worth the effort. Positive experiences boost the immune system, your health generally and that of those around you.

Time management

Structure your day's work and be realistic regarding what can and cannot be achieved... what takes priority.

At home, organize your meals and your housework to avoid being over-stimulated by a noisy Hoover or dishwasher at midnight, or tapping away busily on a personal computer at 3.00 am in the morning.

Be sure to schedule in time for *you*. Your work will be enhanced the more you take care of yourself. You will get more done in less time once you have created harmony where there might have been chaos.

At work, make sure you take time out for lunch. At least get away from your desk into another environment. If the weather is good, try to find a pretty spot outside to enjoy the sunshine and warm fresh air.

Try to exercise at least 3 times a week

Choose a sport or physical activity that you really enjoy. (See Natural Exercise, pages 126–183.)

Stretch daily to ensure your body retains its flexibility

Breathe deliberately (see pages 16–19)

Enjoy eating

Have meals with your family. Don't grab a snack on the move. Sit down to relax and enjoy food. Eat healthy, nutritious food, allowing yourself indulgences when you feel the urge! Even if you are eating alone, pleasure yourself. Chew slowly, continuing to breathe and make the process of preparation and eating a sensuous pleasure. It is!

Make time to support yourself when in need

In times of crisis, seek help wherever possible. You may benefit from any number of complementary therapies or hands-on treatments. Massage and aromatherapy are notably useful therapies for dealing with the stresses of everyday living. Treat yourself... you are worth it. For treating specific problems, find out what you need. Osteopathy? Homoeopathy? Acupuncture? Any of the wonderful therapies listed on pages 258–281? For any problems of a non-physical nature, seek help. Counselling, psychotherapy, support groups... find whatever suits you and your needs, and allow yourself the space and time to be well.

Rest and sleep

Sleep is an essential ingredient in the stress-free day/lifestyle. A good eight hours, or whatever is your particular requirement of peaceful and healing sleep, will work wonders in helping to keep your stress levels at bay in the day that follows.

Ensure you give yourself sufficient time to 'wind down' an hour or so at least before bedtime.

Don't use any stimulants, like tea, coffee or spicy foods, or anything that may keep your mind alert and therefore awake.

Don't watch TV, especially anything that will make your mind work overtime, in the last hour before bed.

Thoughts

Thinking positively requires so much less energy and enhances your own well-being. Positively affirm yourself throughout the day (see pages 208–210). Congratulate yourself when you feel you have achieved something – encourage yourself. Avoid panic and negative derogatory thoughts about yourself or your associates. Smiling to yourself and at others is so much more positive than frowning. If you have fears and worries, acknowledge them to yourself and, where possible, to another. It is true that a problem shared is a problem halved. Another person witnessing your worries helps prevent the worry getting out of hand and driving you out of your mind!

Don't suppress your fears with stimulants and comforters like alcohol, cigarettes or comfort food. If those fears are very pressing, then try to find a support group or therapist or natural therapy that really appeals to you to help you. Do not be afraid to call on those you love to help you in times of need. Better to ask for help than to try and handle all that life doles out to you in isolation. Perhaps you, in turn, will then be able to help someone you love in their time of crisis.

Show love and appreciation to others and expect to receive it back. This works wonders for your own self-esteem and is the perfect way of creating harmonious relationships.

why therapy?

Up until about 50 or 60 years ago it was very unusual to live more than a few feet – let alone miles – from closest family and friends. People usually ended up living their entire lives in close familiar groups, turning to an elder in the family or close community for advice and counsel during periods of personal devastation. Now we're lucky if we live in the same country – let alone city – as our nearest and dearest. The post-war, post-technological revolution of the last century has given rise to the mobile society – people seeking a living across the globe, rather than just across the country.

The rise and rise of nuclear families, expanding urban cultures and, in many cases, increasing isolation, might account for the growing use of counselling or psychotherapeutic support during periods of intense emotional pain in our lives.

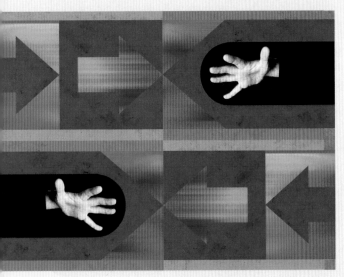

Where once we may have turned to the church or a village elder for support, we now seek help from the modern map-readers of the maze of existence we call 'modern life.' Talking therapies have replaced the tribal hearth. A new language has developed in the last century; a language that depicts the twists and turns of an individual psyche as it journeys from birth to death and endeavours to explain the many experiences and levels of consciousness. As well as learning to cope with changing circumstances catalyzing turning points in our lives, another underlying motivation for therapy is the quest for meaning in our lives, while facing and coming to terms with our own mortality and limited 'tenure of being'. See more on various types of psychological therapy on pages 275–277.

Counselling

Counselling is often more short-term than therapy and will be focussed on one area - for example, bereavement or careers. Counselling provides a space for the client to be heard, otherwise often lacking in today's world. Counselling aims to assist the client in releasing pain, dealing with difficulties associated with life stresses and coming to know themselves better and to be more self-loving and so more outwardly loving.

What is Humanistic Counselling?

The humanistic approach to counselling developed in the years just before the Second World War, to become a widely recognized therapeutic approach by the '50s and '60s. Carl Rogers, one of the 'fathers' of Humanistic Counselling, was very familiar and experienced with the development of Analytical Therapy (see page 276).

In humanistic counselling great emphasis is placed on feelings – getting more and more in touch with, and honest about, one's feelings. The counsellor needs to be working on his/herself as well as working with the client. Utilizing his/her own unique collage of skills, techniques, feelings and knowledge to empower the client to make the sometimes difficult and scary journey within. The humanistic counsellor listens, reflects, mirrors, empathizes, respects and nurtures, and by establishing a safe, caring environment, the client may be encouraged to explore, unravel, discover, have hope and dig deeper within to find those inner resources that will lead to understanding, resolution and transformation.

It empowers the client because the humanistic counsellor communicates genuine care and respect for the client, and their empathy and non-judgmental attitude create an environment in which the client can feel safe and understood. Carl Rogers refined his approach and his view of a more humanistic psychology, observing his own evolution by stating, 'in my early professional years I was asking the question, How can I treat, or cure, or change this person? Now I would phrase the question in this way: How can I provide a relationship which this person may use for his own personal growth?'

Family counselling

The importance of the family in our development as whole and well individuals is recognized as a basic truth by family counsellors/therapists as well as analytical psychotherapists, etc. That is not to say that supreme strong blooms may not blossom from a very disturbed non-nurturing early environment. It is possible that some individuals are so strong and evolved as to survive the worst possible starts in life. In most cases, however, a disturbed and distressed client will have some difficult challenging relationships within his/her family and these will need to be explored and addressed if the client is to discover and create relief and resolution of their problem.

Transpersonal psychotherapy

Transpersonal psychotherapy takes a holistic approach and represents a reintegration of mainstream psychological theory with spiritual enquiry and research into the mind–body relationship. It incorporates many of the principles of accepted psychological streams but aims to provide a more spiritual perspective. The client is encouraged to develop trust in their instinct and intuitive powers, and in their power to self-heal. Transpersonal psychotherapy is particularly good for those searching for an ongoing process of self-awareness, and who perhaps feel that the structure of a typical Freudian psychotherapy session, for example, is too rigid. Meditation is commonly used by transpersonal psychotherapy practitioners to clear and create 'sacred space' in the all-important therapeutic relationship. Clients who are struggling with the integration of spiritual and material values particularly benefit from this branch of psychotherapy.

natural

Over the past 25 years, a slow-but-sure revolution in attitudes towards health has been taking place. The public has begun to awaken to the fact that modern 'orthodox' medicine does not necessarily hold the only key to perfect health and that hospitals are not always sanctuaries of healing. While most people accept that current advances in medical and surgical skills are staggering, they are not always without side-effects, risk and failures. The discovery and regular use of antibiotics and vaccinations have wiped away many diseases that used to ravage the population with uncontrollable epidemics, yet in their wake have emerged stronger and more deadly bacteria and viruses – 'super-bugs' that are able to resist and overpower even our strongest drugs.

therapies

At the same time, the second half of the last century saw more people travelling to far-off shores than ever before. Air travel circulates people and 'bugs' at sound-barrier-breaking speeds and at no other point in history have our immune systems been so sorely taxed and tested as in these environmentally challenging times. The modern world isn't necessarily a safer or healthier place, in spite of our amazing scientific and technological feats.

In the light of all this it has dawned on large numbers of the populations of 'first world' industrialized nations that it is perhaps a foolish thing to abnegate all responsibility for one's own health and well-being, when all around us we see casualties of bad health habits – or even bad luck – that even modern medicine cannot cure. The general public has become increasingly educated, aware and concerned about the effects of orthodox medicine on them, their children and even their pets. Many have become disenchanted with the medical profession or their GPs, with regard to the treatment of common ailments with antibiotics and other strong drugs that often create a whole set of other symptoms while curing or alleviating a particular complaint.

The information revolution has meant that we are generally far better educated about our minds and bodies than the generations before us. We understand how important a healthy immune system and nervous system are to our health, and that we cannot possibly keep fit unless these systems are in good working order. We also now understand that 'prevention is better than cure' and that no one is better placed to ensure our good health and continued well-being than ourselves. We now understand that each of us is in the front line when it comes to our own health – that the way we treat our bodies on a day-to-day basis determines our state of health and well-being in both the short and long term.

Perhaps this is why there has been such a tremendous increase of interest in alternative medicine and natural therapies: from nutrition and herbalism to homoeopathy and aromatherapy, people are flocking in droves to practitioners of these 'holistic therapies', who do not just simply treat the symptoms but who try to determine the cause and also endeavour to treat the whole person.

Guidelines to using natural therapies

- Always consult a fully qualified practitioner recommended by the Society or Institute holding a register of qualified practitioners in each field.
- Always follow instructions carefully when self-administering natural medicine.

Acupressure

Acupressure is a combination of finger pressure and acupuncture (see below) and is considered by some to be the forerunner to acupuncture. Acupressure comes from China and from Japan and is still used widely in homes there today by many families. See also Acupuncture and Shiatsu.

Acupuncture

Acupuncture is an integral and highly respected part of traditional Chinese medicine, with a history spanning the last 4,500 years. The theory behind acupuncture embraces the concept of chi, the life force in your body, in the air you breathe or the water you drink – an invisible but all-powerful, all-sustaining energy, the unseen force all around and within us. This is a basic tenet in the system of thought that created one of the most powerful natural medicine therapies in the world.

According to this line of thought, dual flows of energy exist in the body; the Chinese call them yin and yang. Duality, the manifestation of opposites – opposing but complementary forces – is reflected everywhere in life: positive and negative, masculine and feminine, creative and receptive, day and night, sun and moon, for example. The first in all these pairs is considered yang and the second yin. The Chinese believe that balancing the opposing energies is the path to well-being, wholeness and good health throughout life.

They teach that vital energy – chi – circulates along 'meridians' throughout the body. There are 14 main meridians, paths or channels of vital energy. The acupuncturist assesses the condition of your internal energy grid by feeling two radial pulses on the arm near your wrist, by checking your tongue and many other visual clues, and listening carefully to what you have to say as well as considering your entire health history. In this way the practitioner can assess the condition of the meridians and detect any disturbances or serious imbalances in your body. There are dozens of different variations in the pulses

and an experienced acupuncturist can distinguish all the differences and assess why they are there.

Once the therapist locates the meridian that needs rebalancing and then chooses the actual points – there are hundreds of acupoints along the meridians – a needle is inserted in that point to stimulate or soothe the energy in order to redress the balance of chi. The acupuncturist usually places needles in a few points, leaving them for various lengths of time or twirling them, depending on your symptoms and condition. This is not nearly as painful a procedure as it sounds. In fact, at its worst, it is only mildly uncomfortable. Acupuncture produces very immediate, dramatic results in some cases, and in others it may be a gradual movement back to balance and well-being.

The use of acupuncture for pain relief is renowned. In many Chinese hospitals general anaesthesia is replaced with acupuncture anaesthesia for numerous major as well as minor operations. The needles placed in specific points, many in the ear, enable patients to endure surgery while fully conscious without the dangers or side-effects of general anaesthetic and without pain. It is also well documented that drug addicts do not experience any physical craving for their drug while under the influence of acupuncture anaesthesia. Increasingly, acupuncture is recognized as an invaluable, important diagnostic and therapeutic treatment.

Some conditions that acupuncture has been demonstrated to treat effectively: anxiety, arthritis, asthma, bronchitis, colds and 'flu, depression, dermatitis, diabetes, digestive problems, eczema, headaches, high blood pressure, infertility, impotence, lumbago, migraine, psoriasis, respiratory conditions and infections, stress conditions.

Alexander technique

The Alexander technique was created at the turn of the century by an Australian actor, Frederick Mathias Alexander, who had chronic voice problems and

endeavoured to find out why in order to save his career. Alexander sought medical help, but to no avail. He continued to lose his voice on stage, and recover it when resting. He realized that he had to discover why, so he studied himself in the mirror acting out a stage role and noticed how the position of his head changed, as did his breathing, while he delivered his lines.

Frederick felt how his throat tightened and his head lowered as he prepared to project his lines. He became aware of the effects of stress on his neck, throat and vocal cords, and began to make conscious corrections, and observations to support his radical new 'view' that mind and body are connected and interdependent, always affecting one another. He eventually evolved a whole new language of mind-body relationship – a new way of looking at the effects of negative patterns and bad habits on our mind and our body.

Look at yourself now. How are you sitting? Are your legs crossed? Are you collapsed back in your chair? Lower back unsupported? Do you throw your head back when talking, like Alexander, or forward when walking? By studying himself in the mirror Alexander had discovered the importance of a balanced, open, relaxed and full approach to body/mind health. By correcting negative, compensating patterns of attitude and physical movement, we can treat and prevent all sorts of conditions.

Alexander realized that unless you discovered the root cause, the unconscious bad habit behind your ailment, treatments would only alleviate the symptoms temporarily. All his experiences and observations thereafter seemed to confirm to Alexander that most of our common health problems are caused or exacerbated by a lifetime's accumulated bad habits. The Alexander technique teaches you how to improve your health and prevent disabling conditions through conscious movement, stillness and better posture.

An Alexander teacher or practitioner would describe what they do as 'an educative process with preventative and therapeutic consequences'. It is the most subtle and gentle manipulative body therapy around! It retrains you to use your body in a healthy balanced way and promotes a way of awareness. You experience an awareness of the alignment of your skeleton on a whole new level and achieve an 'inner dialogue' with it that allows optimum relaxation and equilibrium in your bones and your muscles and your mind. You allow release by gentle suggestion and persuasion.

The technique can teach you how to recondition your body/mind responses and how to unlearn bad habits through observation, self-empowerment through suggestion, allowing yourself to be wholly conscious of yourself and how you use and treat your body. Simple things like getting in and out of a car or getting up from a sofa or sitting down in a chair – movements we do all the time, some with more ease and grace than others, but all usually with little conscious thought about how we are moving and using our body.

A bad habit like crossing your legs or a slouching posture, with your weight on one leg more than the other, are so long-standing and unconscious that they feel absolutely natural and easy to you. The Alexander teacher gently guides you through very subtle adjustments and positions, whether standing, sitting or lying down, to encourage correct co-ordination, posture, poise and alignment. You simply learn how to change harmful positions into healthy ones, how to use your muscles with maximum effect and minimum effort and strain. If you or anyone close to you suffers rounded shoulders or an overarched back, the Alexander technique will help improve your spine and skeletal/muscular system through this gently manipulative treatment.

The Alexander technique is widely recognized today and AT teachers are employed in many prestigious institutions of the arts like RADA and the Royal College of Music, because it has such a beneficial effect on posture, voice, breathing function and ability to manage stress and

tension. AT gives you the opportunity to learn some very simple yet powerful health secrets. The importance of posture and carriage on your well-being should not be underestimated. The Alexander technique teaches you how to release the body's power through balance and equipoise of posture.

This technique is an effective treatment for: all postural problems, rounded shoulders, stooping posture, overarched back, backache, shortened or tight neck, tight throat, headache, RSI (repetitive strain injury), breathing and respiratory conditions, voice problems, stress-related conditions, arthritis.

Aromatherapy

In modern terms, this touch therapy, which combines soothing strokes, lymphatic drainage massage and gentle deep muscle massage using essential oils of plants and flowers, is only a little over half a century old. Yet there is irrefutable evidence that many thousands of years ago, oils were regularly used in the ancient temples of Egypt, Greece and Rome for their healing and comforting qualities. Today, we have rediscovered the beneficial effects that can be induced by inhaling the potent fragrances of plants and flowers, or applying them to the skin. Interestingly, research is currently being carried out by members of Newcastle University's Medicinal Plant Research Centre to discover whether *Melissa officinalis* (lemon balm) is beneficial to patients suffering from moderate to severe dementia.

The more recent history of this therapy leads us to France before World War II when a cosmetic chemist called Rene Maurice Gattefosse discovered the positive effect on the skin of a number of essential oils with which he was working. This led him to research further the efficacy of essential oils for treating medical skin conditions. Gattefosse also noticed the antiseptic and antibacterial qualities of some essential oils and he is credited with the term we use today to describe this healing tradition, aromatherapy.

Aromatherapy as practised today is a combination of creating highly concentrated essential oils, potent plant extracts that contain its 'essence', and applying the appropriate oils, generally by means of massage techniques that can be either relaxing or stimulating, depending on your needs (see pages 226–229).

It is highly likely that the system of aromatherapy developed in response to the recognition of the therapeutic and mood-altering powers of fragrances. Cells in the nose send rapid messages to the brain when they detect a smell, which relays the information around the body, depending on the type of fragrance detected. Essential oils each possess varying properties (see pages 228–229); furthermore, one plant can even produce more than one type of oil. For instance, neroli oil comes from the flowers of the orange tree and orange essential oil from the fruit peel.

Blending of oils plays an important part in an aromatherapy treatment, and for use at home too. Oils can be divided into three main categories: uplifting, balancing and calming. An aromatherapist will try to create a blend that is pleasing in aroma to the client; if the client doesn't like the blend, then the oils are the wrong ones. Blending can be surprising, even startling, with mixtures like lavender with ginger for a warming, relaxing, circulation-improving winter mix.

Aromatherapy is one of the most important components of a health programme and regular treatments will help to encourage an experience of sublime well-being in a way few other therapies can.

Warning: essential oils are for external use only and should not be taken internally. There are a very few oils that may be prescribed by your doctor or aromatherapist for internal use; in any case, never treat yourself internally.

Autogenic training

Extensive research into a simple exercise system called autogenic training (AT) has demonstrated that this is a relaxation technique that can help banish stress forever! AT has proven an effective catalyst for the whole healing process. Its biggest plus point is that people immediately feel better, calmer and able to cope. AT helps the body cure itself by eliminating the effects of excessive stress that are so threatening to our well-being.

AT was developed by a German neurologist, Dr Johannes Schultz in the 1920s in Berlin. It grew out of his observations and use of hypnotism in his own practice. The technique's reputation quickly spread around the world and today is established as one of the most brilliantly effective, simple, harmless techniques available to the seeker of a truly stress-free life.

AT can significantly relieve tension, pain and insomnia, and lessen anxiety. It helps prevent heart attacks by lowering both blood cholesterol and blood pressure. It has been used in the treatment of all manner of ailments – sufferers from asthma, diabetes, infertility and migraine have all been helped by learning this simple exercise technique. It is now recognized by many doctors and nurses, as well as holistic natural medicine practitioners, and by many in the business world too – indeed some airlines use AT to help their staff combat sleep problems and jet-lag.

AT teaches you how to focus your attention through a simple series of mental exercises. No wonder many professionals use it to reduce stress, improve concentration and communication and decision-making skills.

The three basic components of AT are:

• The art of passive concentration, quietly allowing your mind to focus on your body and learning how just to watch your breath.
• Repeating words or phrases to target certain parts of your body, inducing feelings of relaxation, heaviness or warmth, for instance.
• Using one of three basic postures that help you relax and let go of the outside world while you do passive concentration or repetition exercises. Firstly, the Reclining position, where you lie on the floor or a bed in a totally relaxed position (like the corpse

pose in yoga, see page 180). Secondly, you can sit comfortably in a chair, preferably an armchair, with your arms resting on the chair or on your thighs. Finally, you can do it on the edge of a hard chair, with your back, neck and head hanging forward in a kind of a slump position.

Eventually, you don't need to do all the steps; you just need to think of the exercises to suggest and evoke the stress release response. However, you do need to learn the technique from a qualified therapist. It doesn't usually take more than about eight sessions to master the technique and acquire a treasured tool for a healthier life. There are private clinics and courses specializing in AT. You can find autogenic training on the NHS through some hospitals. Also some psychologists and psychotherapists use AT in their work.

Ayurveda

Ayurveda is the oldest system of natural medicine in the world, and has been practised in India for over 5,000 years. It is a holistic system that seeks to treat the whole person, by examining your entire lifestyle, the ways in which you express yourself and your nature, as well as hereditary and environmental factors. Ayurveda strongly emphasizes the connection between the individual and nature; it aims not only to treat disease and improve your general quality of life, but also to bring you into harmony with nature. Ayurvedic treatment methods include diet and nutritional changes, herbal remedies, exercise, meditation, aromatherapy, internal cleansing and detoxifying, among other therapies, all of which can help restore your well-being by promoting balance and harmony. Your unique needs and individuality are always considered, as your path to good health and optimum well-being is highly personal.

Ayurveda is still the main form of medicine in India and is gaining a great deal of recognition in the Western world in recent years. A Sanskrit word, ayurveda has two roots – *ayur*, which means 'life' or

'daily living' and *veda*, which means 'knowledge', and can be interpreted as 'science of life'. It is a medical system which emphasizes that all beings come out of nature; if we are all integral parts of the universe, we therefore have a responsibility to our source. Living a balanced life in accordance with the laws of Nature lets us fulfil this primal responsibility.

Ayurveda evolved at the same time as yoga and meditation, and is quite connected to both of these in many of its treatments and programmes. It seeks to create harmony by balancing the five elements – earth, water, fire, air and the ether from which the entire material world is composed – in the doshas – the bodily 'humours'. There are three forms of dosha, Vata, Pitta and Kapha, and each person has their own unique doshic mix (known as prakruti), although most of us have one or two dominant doshas. Internal and external change may throw your doshas off balance and restoring this balance is the aim of ayurveda (see also pages 11–15).

The Vata dosha is a combination of the ether and air elements. People with the Vata physique tend to have dry hair and skin, a light frame, little body fat (they are often underweight) and an active metabolism. They may have bad circulation and prefer warm weather. Vata people are quick-witted and creative with lots of ideas. They are often restless. When out of balance they tend towards irritability and, in extreme cases, nervous exhaustion.

The Pitta dosha is a combination of the fire and water elements. The Pitta person has a medium frame, soft, warm and often fair, pink or red and freckly skin. They have a strong appetite and possess a sharp mind and a quick wit. They are busy and like to achieve a lot. They are clear, sharp and precise. When out of balance, they can be angry, judgmental and fiery. They are usually very intelligent and love knowledge and reading.

Kapha represents the earth and water elements. A Kapha person has a tendency to gain weight due to a slow metabolism and digestive system combined with a strong appetite. They often have a pale or white complexion, thick, lustrous hair and big eyes, and walk and talk at a slow, steady pace. Kapha people can often be slow to grasp an idea, but have an excellent long-term memory and are loyal and caring. When out of balance they can be greedy and possessive.

The degree to which a person possesses different proportions of energies accounts for individual diversity. Despite this variation, however, doshas tend to collect in certain areas, causing illness: Vata energy accumulates in the colon, and nervous system, Pitta in the intestines, skin, eyes and liver and Kapha in the stomach, joints and mucous membranes. When a severe blockage of energy occurs, the affected area can become weakened, and susceptible to bacteria and viruses.

There are a number of possible causes of energy imbalance, including heredity, environmental factors and bad habits. Behaviour, however, is the biggest determinant; in other words, how you choose to live your life directly affects your well-being. Ayurveda describes behaviour by classifying human temperament into three constitutions, which describe an individual's basic qualities, as well as the way they react to their environment. The first, satva, represents purity and clarity of perception; rajas denotes over-excitement, ambition and aggression; finally, tamas indicates inertia, sloth and materialism. A Kapha person with tamasic tendencies, for example, takes little exercise and overeats, and their health will suffer accordingly.

By examining the patient and questioning them about their medical and family history and behaviour patterns, by feeling the skin and key parts of the body and listening to the heart, lungs and intestines, the ayurvedic practitioner makes a personalized diagnosis based on the needs of the individual. Tongue diagnosis is a highly specialized practice used in ayurveda: areas of the tongue are thought to correspond with other body

parts, so examining and touching the tongue provides an extra perspective on possible health problems. A practitioner will recommend a combination of the many ayurvedic treatments to rectify a dosha imbalance – perhaps lifestyle and nutritional changes specific to the condition, herbal remedies and detoxifying and cleansing rituals (known as panchakarma). Meditation and yoga may also be suggested, or even marma therapy: ayurvedic acupuncture. According to Indian ayurvedic doctors, marma points are the 107 'junction boxes', where nerves and muscles meet, around the body. While marmas are clear and balanced you remain in good health and are strong enough to prevent illness. If, however, your marmas become unbalanced or clogged, your health and state of mind start to suffer. The job of the ayurvedic practitioner is to bring a person's constitution back into balance.

Bach flower remedies

An English doctor of medicine and bacteriologist, Dr Edward Bach, developed a series of 38 flower treatment preparations – made from a wide variety of plants and wild flowers – to treat not our physical ailments directly but our mental attitudes instead, as he thought this would have a direct bearing on our ability to heal our bodies' problems and imbalances.

Dr Bach trained at University College, London, at the beginning of the century, later gaining a Diploma of Public Health at Cambridge in 1913. He began his career in London's Harley Street in 1915, where he practised homoeopathy as well as orthodox medicine. Dr Bach strongly believed there was a natural cure for every ailment. Even during his medical training, Dr Bach recognized the importance of a positive state of mind in the healing process. He noticed how patients with a fearful, worried, depressed mental state made slow progress when recovering from serious illness; whereas those of a more cheerful, hopeful and determined, positive mental state seemed to recover much more quickly.

Dr Bach believed a practical approach to helping the sufferer overcome a negative attitude was the course to pursue when trying to treat the cause of ill health. Negative thinking was the root of most physical and emotional problems as far as Dr Bach was concerned. After pursuing a number of branches of conventional medicine, as well as doing research in bacteriology, he discovered the work of Hahnemann, father of homoeopathy (see page 270), and Dr Bach became a homoeopath. Working in the laboratories of the Royal London Homoeopathic Hospital, he successfully developed remedies for temperament types and achieved excellent results in treating emotional problems.

His approach was totally holistic and ahead of its time, like that of Hahnemann, who so impressed him. The basic principle he embraced was 'treat the patient and not the disease'. Bach then decided to seek out a more direct simple approach to treating the whole person. He wanted to find a harmless cure that could restore hope and peace of mind to sufferers. He believed that the trees, plants and flowers must hold the natural key for anything that ails us! He retreated to the country suddenly in 1930 to seek the information he needed.

He became very attuned to nature and quickly developed a keen intuition about the healing qualities of different flowering plants. Over a seven-year period, Dr Bach identified 38 harmless tree, plant and wildflower remedies that were prescribed to treat a patient's state of mind – from depression and anxiety to severe depression and uncertainty – and not a particular physical ailment.

He divided his 38 remedies into seven groups to treat despair, fear, insufficient interest in life, loneliness, over-concern for the welfare of others, over-sensitivity to influences and ideas, and uncertainty.

The Bach flower remedies are still prepared at the Bach Centre in Mount Vernon in Wallingford, using the original methods devised by Dr Bach. Perfect flower heads are used and instantly placed into bowls of spring water in which they are left for three hours in bright sunshine. This process is considered to 'potentize' the water, meaning the water takes on the elements of the flowers placed within it. The potentized water is mixed with equal parts of brandy for its preservative qualities and this mixture is put in stock bottles, which are readily available in chemists and health shops today.

The following are some remedies and the states of mind they are used to treat:

Agrimony Suffering a lot internally, but keep it hidden

Aspen Fear of unknown things

Beech Arrogant, critical and intolerant

Centaury Weak-willed, subservient, easily used

Cerato Lack of self-confidence, asks advice

Cherry Plum Fear of going mad, losing control or causing harm. Violent tempers

Chestnut Bud Fails to learn by experience, repeats mistakes

Chicory Over-possessive, selfish, attention-seekers

Clematis Absent-minded, dreamy, escapist mentally

Crab Apple Self-dislike, feels unclean – cleanser

Elm Temporary inadequacy

Gentian Depression with known cause, easily discouraged

Gorse Depression, everything seems pointless

Heather Obsessed with own problems

Holly Jealousy, suspicion, revenge, hate

Honeysuckle Living in the past

Hornbeam Procrastinators

Impatiens Impatient

Larch Depression, inferiority, expects to fail

Mimulus Fear of known things

Mustard Deep depression without reason

Oak Brave, plodders, determined

Olive Exhaustion, mentally and physically

Pine Guilt, self-blame

Red Chestnut Fear for others

Rescue Remedy A combination of cherry plum, clematis, impatiens, rock rose and star of Bethlehem used for shock, trauma, accidents, emergencies, first aid, external and internal

Rock Rose Terror, panic

Rock Water Self-demanding, self-denial

Scleranthus Indecision, mood swings

Star of Bethlehem Shock

Sweet Chestnut Despair, no hope left

Vervain Fanatical, tense, over-enthusiastic

Vine Ambitious, tyrants, demanding, unbending, seek power

Walnut The 'link' breaker, for times of change

Water Violet Reserve, pride, reliable

White Chestnut Persistent thoughts, mental chatter

Wild Oat Helps define goals

Wild Rose Apathetic drifters, unambitious

Willow Bitter, resentful

Bioenergetics

Bioenergetics works directly with the dynamic link and interaction between our body and mind. Physical and psychological techniques combined with bodywork exercises help to locate the physical resonance of a stored trauma within the body. Bioenergetic work allows for these conditions or memories of trauma to be safely brought to the forefront of the body/mind consciousness. Bioenergetic work not only safely accesses these traumatic states but assists in successfully reintegrating and healing them.

Wilhelm Reich was an Austrian associate of Freud who identified the energetic and kinetic force in the body as being sexual in nature. Reich labelled this energy 'orgone'. His work formed the basis for Alexander Lowen's system of bioenergetics, which emerged fully in the 1960s.

Bioenergetic work helps one to become aware of how one's habitual stances are the effect of one's negative attitudes and emotional states. Extreme states such as anger and fear have a direct effect on posture, as well as on the way we move and breathe.

Initially the first consultation with a bioenergetic practitioner is on a one-to-one basis. Thereafter the work is done in group sessions. Exercises can include work in grounding, animal games and breathing work.

Grounding: In bioenergetic work how you stand and what your relationship with the earth is like is of vital importance. Group participants are encouraged to find different ways of interacting with the ground, from stamping to tiptoeing. Feedback is shared back to the group whereby other participants say how they responded to these exercises.

Animal games: By choosing a favourite animal to identify with, and mimicking its stance and behaviour patterns, vital information about how a person operates within his or her relationships can be revealed. This work, done in groups, provides stimulus for acting and reacting to each participant's animal choices.

Breathing: How we function within emotional states directly affects our breathing patterns. Learning to breathe efficiently helps stabilize the body's energy flow, so participants are shown how to breathe correctly. This may seem very basic, but its importance in dealing with a variety of emotional states can't be overestimated.

Bowen technique

The Bowen technique is a gentle hands-on therapy that is useful in promoting healing where long-term muscular pain has been inhibiting the client's lifestyle. Although it does involve active bodywork, Bowen work is not a type of massage.

The treatment comprises a specific series of vibrational movements applied to muscles, tendons and connective tissue, performed in a fixed sequence. The aim is to disturb the muscles and soft tissue, as well as the energetic body surrounding the physical. After three or four of these movements, the client is left in peace to process the last section and allow for the body to be receptive to the next sequence.

The treatment was developed by Tom Bowen, an Australian, who established it as a recognized therapy between the 1950s and the 1970s. Now practised worldwide, the Bowen technique is useful in treating cases of chronic or acute musculo-skeletal pain, and in the healing and regeneration of tissue as a result of sports injuries.

A Bowen technique treatment lasts for approximately 45 minutes and is performed with the client wearing light clothing.

Chinese Oriental medicine

Chinese medicine, like ayurvedic medicine (page 262), is an ancient form of healing. There are several aspects to it, two of which have become popular in the West, acupuncture/acupressure and Chinese herbal medicine. Traditionally Chinese medical practice has been one of prevention. You saw a doctor and, as long as you lived by his guidelines, you paid him to keep you well. If you got sick it was his problem – he had to fix it and you stopped paying.

Chinese herbal medicine stems, as all ancient and traditional herbal medical practice, from the gradual evolution of knowledge over millennia about the effects of plants on human health. However, unlike in the West, where older forms of treatment are considered by modern doctors to be outdated and irrelevant to the twentieth and twenty-first centuries, in China great reverence is expressed for the treatments that have evolved over thousands of years.

Chinese herbal medicine is not only an ancient and historical form of medical treatment, it is the dominant form of prescription therapy today in China. There are now more than four thousand herbs that have been studied and that are used, singly or more often in combination, in Chinese medicine. In addition, Chinese doctors will prescribe foods that should be eaten and foods that should be avoided, activities that should be done and those that should be avoided. To a far greater extent than Western doctors, they are concerned about the total well-being of the person, involving both therapy and lifestyle.

Chinese doctors study the writings and teachings of medical practitioners going back to the earliest documents. These documents contain details of both acupuncture procedures and the principles of Chinese medicine and, although written several thousand years ago, are still relevant today. Thus knowledge of the action of herbs is detailed, extensive and precise, and the practice is essentially devoid of unwanted side-effects. This is in sharp contrast to Western medicine, in which the sad

tendency to deride the old methods goes hand-in-hand with acclaim for the modern, new and often unproven drugs, many of which have adverse side-effects, effects that are considered worth the perceived benefit of the main action of the drug.

The Chinese consider that each person has their own individual balance of the yin and yang energies (see Acupuncture, page 260) and their own individual balance of the five elements, earth, water, wood, fire and air/metal. If these balances are disturbed, ill health will result. Conversely, it is the job of the traditional Chinese practitioner to maintain this balance and to restore it when it has been lost and poor health has resulted. Each element is also associated with specific characteristics, like colour, smell, flavour, sound and so forth.

Chinese herbal medicine has grown in popularity in the West, starting in the eighties and increasing in the nineties and on into the new century. There are now many people practising Chinese herbal medicine. However, unless they have been fully trained over many, many years within the Chinese system and fully enter into and appreciate the Chinese philosophy, it is probable that they are only practising a part of this art of therapy. (See more on pages 109–113.)

Taoism states that we, as humans, are a microcosm representing the macrocosm and that everything, and every small part of everything, contains within in it a reflection of the whole. Thus Chinese practitioners believe that they can come to an understanding of the whole of you by studying a part of you. This is seen in the West by the study of reflexology where, by studying the feet and the pressure points on them, information can be gleaned about the whole body (see page 278).

For this reason a session with a Traditional Chinese Medicine (TCM) practitioner may involve a study of parts of your body seemingly unrelated to your presenting problem. They may look closely at your face, mouth and tongue, your skin, nails and hair. They may listen to your voice, your breathing and to other sounds

you make, such as those stemming from the digestive system. The nature of urine and stool are important. You will also be asked many questions, almost certainly more than when seeing a Western doctor, and many of the questions may seem strange and unrelated to your problem as you see it.

A major part of a diagnostic work-up in TCM is the taking of pulses. You may consider you have only one pulse, but TCM practitioners identify a large number of pulses and will almost certainly take three pulses (shallow, medium and deep) at three points on each wrist. Having looked, having asked the questions and listened, having felt the pulses, they will then put all this information together and determine your state of balance of yin and yang, of the five elements, and of the chi or energy flowing in your body. They will then decide on the appropriate form of treatment. This will almost certainly involve lifestyle modifications; it may well also involve acupuncture treatment. It will almost certainly involve the use of a number of herbs. Your prescription, taken to a Chinese herbal pharmacy, would be prescribed weights of a variety of dried herbs. These would be combined and you would be told to infuse them and drink, as a tea. Commonly the flavour is unpalatable.

Chiropractic

Chiropractic is arguably one of the 'oldest' of the modern alternative therapies, having been founded in 1895 by Daniel David Palmer, who successfully treated a man who had become deaf after a back problem. Daniel David Palmer was a 'magnetic healer' and his first such patient was his office cleaner. Palmer discovered some of the small bones in the cleaner's spine were misaligned. After manipulation, the cleaner's hearing was successfully restored.

Palmer then went on to found the Palmer School of Chiropractic, from the Greek *kheir*, meaning 'hand' and *praktikos* meaning 'practical'. 'Displacement of any part of the skeletal frame,' he said, 'may press against nerves, which are the channels of communication, intensifying or decreasing their carrying capacity, creating either too much or not enough functioning, an aberration known as disease.'

Chiropractors aim to correct any disorders of the joints and muscles – especially the spine – primarily by joint manipulation. By working on the muscles, joints, ligaments and tendons, and focusing on spinal function, the chiropractor can treat a range of conditions. Relieving pain by joint manipulation is their main aim.

Chiropractic differs from osteopathy as osteopathy works on a joint indirectly by working on the surrounding muscles, ligaments and facia, whereas chiropractic treats the problem joint directly, using high-velocity thrusts. Treatments vary according to the needs of the client.

The treatment will include an in-depth discussion about your medical details, lifestyle and symptoms, and your posture will be assessed. Any pain you are feeling will be talked about and you will need to discuss how this is affecting your movement. Your pulse and blood pressure may be taken and your reflexes checked. Your spine will be studied in detail and, while sitting, it will be palpated to test the muscles, bones, joints and connective tissue.

The actual treatment used may include, for example, manipulation of a painful lower lumbar joint, while the patient lies on one side. The chiropractor will then manually rotate the upper spine one way and the lower spine in the opposite direction. This movement will partially lock the joint which needs adjusting. Often the patient's uppermost leg will be flexed to assist the locking. The chiropractor will then feel the vertebra either above or below the joint. At this point the chiropractor will apply slight pressure and it is this, combined with the patient's position, that frees the joint to resume its normal position.

The chiropractor will then make a very rapid thrust to the vertebra which will move the joint just a little beyond its normal range. This will allow normal movement in the joint and a sudden

relaxing of the surrounding muscles, which helps the deep spinal muscles to relax around the affected joint. Normally four or five treatments will be necessary to ensure the joints maintain their correct positions. Advice will be given on correct posture to aid in the recovery process and to avoid further misalignment where possible.

Chiropractic, like osteopathy (page 274), is highly regarded by complementary and orthodox practitioners, including many doctors. Chiropractors may use X-rays to help with diagnosis. It is used to treat: musculo-skeletal problems; neck, shoulder and back pain; RSI; sports injuries; indigestion; sciatica; lumbago; slipped disc; asthma; arthritis; catarrh; constipation; migraine; period problems; stress.

Colonic irrigation

Colonic irrigation is an extremely effective way of cleansing the colon. The colonic irrigation equipment is far more elaborate than an enema, although it is based on the same hygienic principles.

Purified water at the same temperature as the body is flushed into the colon through the rectum. The water then flows out again through a two-way tube. The water reaches up through the descending colon, to the transverse and ascending colon as well, areas that are not within the reach of normal defecation. Repeatedly washing this water in and out allows for a deeper cleansing, loosening fecal matter stored in all areas of the ascending, transverse and descending colon.

A colonic irrigation treatment generally lasts about 45 minutes. Treatments are often conducted in conjunction with a dietary cleansing regime and/or a fast. Problems that can be effectively treated by means of colonic irrigation include bloating, constipation, wind, fatigue, headaches, PMT, skin problems and circulatory disturbances.

Colour therapy

The entire material world is a symphony of colour, and our bodies are not separate from this experience. From the subtle to the

overt, colours – and the vibrations with which they resonate – make up our world. It therefore makes sense that the body can be brought back to a state of wholeness by treating it with the spectrum of colour. Even the Ancients understood this and the temples of Ancient Greece and Egypt were deliberately painted with strong colours to induce different psychological states in initiates and worshippers.

A colour therapist can diagnose imbalances within the energetic field by assessing to which colours you are drawn, by asking you your likes and dislikes, and where possible, by sensing what colours are predominant in your aura. If there is an imbalance in the energy field, or it is compromised in any way, that will be directly reflected in the colour field of the aura. Colour therapy works by restoring the full harmonic resonance of colour to the body and redressing this balance.

It is best to work with a colour therapist, since all colours have both positive and negative attributes, and extremes of exposure to different colours can upset the balance towards which you need to work. Anxiety and depression respond well to colour therapy.

An interesting adjunct to this therapy is the Lüscher Colour Test. Developed by Dr. Max Lüscher, this self-administered test can uncover aspects of our psychological makeup, that in turn reflect in our personality, and our emotions of the moment.

Cranial osteopathy

In the 1930s, William Garner Sutherland, an American osteopathic student of Still (page 274), discovered that the dome of bone that protects the brain, the skull, is made up of eight separate parts, with an intricate joint system and minute gaps between them. Contrary to previous belief that the skull was one complete structure, it was now found that these separate parts move very slightly. William Garner Sutherland felt that if this were true, that the bones move, then dysfunction could also occur. He experimented by compressing his own skull, which caused grave physical and mental problems, and then took to finding out why.

The brains and the spinal column and nerves are surrounded by cerebrospinal fluid. This fluid has a perceptible rhythm that could be affected by breathing and any disturbance in the cranial bone system. Sutherland's research demonstrated that, by applying a series of gentle manipulations to the skull, the rhythms could be adjusted, thus reducing tension in the tissues.

If the rhythm is imbalanced, this can cause pressure on parts of the brain or affect other parts of the body via nerves originating in the brain. Any injury to the head, or dental work that misplaces the jaw – even temporarily – will affect this delicate system of movement of fluid and displaced bones.

After making a thorough assessment of your medical history, treatment will commence involving movements that include gentle manipulation, tapping, moulding and holding the bones to encourage them into correct alignment.

Cranial osteopathy is a wonderfully relaxing and healing therapy. Although the movements are barely perceptible, they are incredibly powerful and induce a profound sense of healing and balance throughout the entire body and all its systems. Mentally, one can expect to feel calm and peaceful. As with any powerful therapy, stuff may – and often can – come up. Anything that has been held within may resurface. This is part of the redressing and balancing process and will lead to a more relaxed and healthier you.

After treatment be aware of your needs and if possible, take time to relax to allow the full effects of the treatment to instil themselves within you. These are some of the advantages you will experience, along with profound benefits to your physical being.

Craniosacral therapy can treat: migraine, neuralgia and headaches; sinusitis; dizziness; general aches and pains; stress-related asthma; digestive complaints and irritable bowel syndrome: stomach ulcers; discomfort after blows to the head, including whiplash and dental work; high blood pressure; breathing problems generally.

Crystal healing

Precious and semi-precious stones have been appreciated for their beauty and value for thousands of years. They have also long been recognized as possessing healing and balancing properties. In China, jade has been used for centuries to treat bladder and kidney problems. The recent resurgence of power bracelets makes a more fashionable use of gemstones and their therapeutic properties.

The therapeutic powers of crystals can form the basis for a complete healing session, or be used to intensify a different modality of healing work. Quartz crystals act as intensifiers for other gemstones and can also be used as a focal point for the dynamic energy of any healing session. Different gemstones resonate with different energy spectra. Since we are all different packages of energy, gems are useful in reflecting back to us individual or multiple parts of the energy wave that we might lack.

In a crystal healing session the therapist will ask questions about your current emotional and physical state, determining what needs to be rebalanced, and then place appropriate stones on different energy centres of the body. The subtle vibrations of the human energy field are balanced through the subtle vibrations of the gemstones, as they, in turn, resonate with the energy centres.

After it has been determined what crystals will work best for you at that time, there are many ways of linking with that energy at other times during the day. You can carry the stones with you, or place them prominently about your home or work environment. Some crystal therapists may even suggest that you leave a stone you are working with in a glass of water from which you drink: since the water will then be charged with energy vibrating at the frequency of that particular crystal.

While there are many types of crystals with which to work, the following is a brief list of the healing properties of some of the more common gemstones:

Amethyst is excellent for calming the mind and is therefore useful in meditation.

Rose quartz, with its dusky pink colour, is a gentle but powerful cleanser of the heart.

Citrine is generally a vibrant golden orange in colour and is used both for energizing the body and stimulating the mind.

Smoky quartz ranges from dark brown to black in colour, and is excellent for cleansing and grounding.

Green aventurine is useful for stimulating healing in the heart chakra.

Jasper is generally brick-red in colour and works as an all-round grounding and protector stone.

Tiger's eye in polished form is dynamic in appearance and its properties are also dynamic: being energetic and, at the same time, stabilizing.

Detoxification

In working with detoxification, one can make use of many of the other therapies mentioned in this section as a means of cleansing the system. Looking therapeutically at the wellness of the body as a whole, it is important not just to treat the symptoms, but to move to the root cause of the disorder that creates the imbalance and realign that body system accordingly. Since our wellness depends on the proper functioning of the body, it is vital that the waste from the environment around us, as well as waste products from our organs and body systems, are safely excreted. See more on pages 83–87.

Fasting

Fasting involves abstaining from solid foods for a period of time as well as drinking plenty of pure liquids, including water and fruit juices. It allows for the body to focus resources on enhancing the immune system functions, as well as cleansing the body of accumulated environmental and food toxins. The entire physical organism has less stress placed on it by not having to work digesting foods, thereby allowing the digestive system a well-deserved rest.

Stimulated emotional responses are not uncommon during a fast, as the body now has extra reserves of energy to focus elsewhere. Suppressed emotional states can be brought to the foreground, in which case working with a rebirther or body therapist can help you to clear these states.

As a preventative measure, regular fasting for one or two days a month is often recommended by naturopaths. Fasting is also recommended in cases of digestive complaints as well as during acute cases of rash or skin problems. There are many types of fasts recommended for different conditions, such as fruit fasts, juice and saline fasts, all of which should be undertaken with the guidance of a naturopath, nutritionist or physician.

The initial side-effects of fasting can be extremely unpleasant, and include diarrhoea, headaches, vomiting, dizziness and bad breath. Fortunately, the frequency of these experiences diminishes as the fast progresses. Extended fasts are best undertaken in retreat or in residential clinic situations, since one can retreat from the stresses of city life as well.

Controlled fasting should be strictly under the supervision of a naturopath. Fasting is not to be used for weight loss and should not be practised if you are pregnant or have diabetes, heart conditions or ulcers. Consult your doctor or naturopath for advice on starting or finishing a fast.

Feldenkrais therapy

Feldenkrais work aims to develop new pathways within the brain, enabling the body to move consistently in ways which do not cause it pain or damage. Moshe Feldenkrais, its founder, was plagued with an old knee injury, which he theorized was compounded by an improper pattern of movement. The ultimate goal of Feldenkrais work is to have the body organized to move with minimum effort and maximum efficiency. This pragmatic approach to movement stems from Feldenkrais's own training as an engineer and applied physicist.

The Feldenkrais method comprises two separate elements: Functional Integration, and Awareness through Movement. Functional Integration is a one-on-one therapeutic session in which the practitioner uses manipulation techniques to retrain the body/mind into more efficient pathways of movement. People with strenuous, or physically active, jobs find that Feldenkrais work increases their physical efficiency and improves their performance levels as well.

Awareness through Movement is taught in classes, where students are given apparently minor physical exercises to perform. The aim is to bring as much consciousness as possible to each activity. Recognizing how many extraneous muscles are often involved in simple movements is a fundamental step along the path to relaxing the body and making it more efficient.

Functional Integration and Awareness through Movement work are both useful for patients recuperating from strokes, and for those with spinal disorders, chronic pain, arthritis and muscular injuries.

Flotation therapy

A truly modern-age form of water therapy, flotation therapy allows for the complete relaxation of the body and provides the ultimate new way to reduce stress. Flotation therapy effortlessly relaxes the body by floating the client in a dense mineral salt solution. This induces a sensation similar to the weightlessness achieved while bathing in the waters of the Dead Sea. The water in a flotation tank is kept at an even body temperature, and all external stimuli are screened out.

The combination of the water's buoyancy and the lack of external stimuli allows the client to turn their attention completely inwards. Once the attention is so directed, if desired, one can work powerfully to achieving deep and resonant states of meditative awareness. In addition, one can also work at regulating blood pressure and heartbeat through mental techniques.

Flotation therapy can be used to alleviate problems associated with stress, such as anxiety and insomnia, and can be used to help stop addictive cycles of behaviour. Speakers located inside the tank can play hypnosis or meditation tapes to assist you in your journey along the road to complete wellness.

Healing

The aim of healing, or spiritual healing as it is often called, is to restore the physical, spiritual and emotional bodies back to a peaceful yet dynamic state of balance. Almost every culture in history has acknowledged the power of healing and prayer, and tests have proved that healing works even in cases where the patient does not believe in a higher power or consciousness.

In a healing session, the therapist actively surrenders his/her will to an energy flow greater than their own. They surrender their perceptions of limitation and ask, while in a meditative state, that the powers of divine mind or universal flow be channelled through them. The healer will act as a receiving vessel and subsequently as an instrument for the transmission of this energy through to the patient. This process allows for the patient to be reintroduced gently to a state of harmonic balance, restoring them back to their own unique energetic dance with the divine.

Find a healer who resonates with you, in whose presence you feel comfortable. In a session, the healer will have you either sit or lie down, depending on their particular preference for working. You will remain clothed as the healer either places their hands on your body, or simply holds them in your energy field. You may feel warmth or a tingling sensation as the energy being channelled through to you passes into your energetic field and thence into your body.

Although they do sometimes happen, miracle or instant cures are the exception rather than the norm. Most people feel the benefits building up over a period of a few sessions, but one can also feel the effects of balance and a resurgence of energy virtually instantly. How you experience each session is not only individual to you, but also to each time you see your healer.

Some healers will also provide what is called 'absent healing', in which healing thoughts are sent to the person without their actually being present. Some healers choose to do this at certain fixed times, and most will require a full name, as well as some information about the area in which the patient requires healing. Spiritual healing works extremely well with small children and animals, and experiments show that controlled healing has a positive effect on plant and seed growth, as well as a strongly mitigating effect on cancer cells.

Herbalism

Herbal medicine, in its broadest sense, is as old as eating. Throughout history people gradually accumulated a knowledge of the healing power of plants. Those who prepared the food and tended the sick, usually the women, came to know and understand what plant to use when particular problems were encountered. This knowledge was passed on through the generations and has become the basis of herbal medicine throughout Europe.

It is still possible to find communities where people rely heavily on the wild herbs of the countryside for both prevention and healing. Traditionally the herbs were gathered, often at specific times of day or on certain days of the lunar months. They were made into soups, into drinks or dried and used in powdered form.

The origins of herbalism are rooted in antiquity. There is evidence of the use of herbs for medicine as well as food in every ancient culture, and herbalism still forms the basis for the medicines of most modern-day cultures. Records of the use of herbal medicine date back several millennia before Christ in China, Egypt and India, to name only a few places. If you could visit an apothecary a few centuries ago you would find herbal everything – tinctures, creams, poultices, elixirs, syrups, plasters, cordials.

Herbalism teaches the art and science of using plant remedies to maintain natural optimum strength and well-being, to prevent degenerative conditions or to accelerate healing and restore health. Regular drinking of well-chosen organic herbal teas makes positive use of plants in their most natural state, extracting all their nourishing qualities and medicinal properties to redress and restore bodily balance. (See more on pages 106–108.)

A herb is defined as 'a plant... used for food, medicine, scent, flavour...' However, in therapeutic usage the term 'herbs' has developed a broader meaning and 'herbal medicine' has come to mean a form of therapy that involves plant extracts, be they from true herbs or from other plants. Herbal remedies are also made from other parts of the plant as well as the leaves. Hawthorn berries come from a perennial woody bush, and rose hips, used for treating colds and 'flu, come from a persistent woody briar. When red clover is the remedy the flower head is used, when celery is used for the urinary system the seeds are used and when dandelion is given for liver problems it is the root that is used.

Herbs can be used for culinary as well as medicinal purposes and often are. There are, indeed, only very fine distinctions between food, nutritional medicine and herbal medicine. Many times the purposes overlap. Caraway will help to relieve the flatulence that may be caused by cooked cabbage. Cardamom and cumin seeds chewed after a spicy meal help to relieve flatulence and settle the stomach. The same result is achieved by peppermint. Rose hips make a pleasant tea and also add to the intake of vitamin C and help to ward off colds; alfalfa tea is refreshing and provides some alkaline minerals for help in acidic conditions such as arthritis.

It is now common to use the term 'herbal medicine' to cover the use of the active physical ingredients in any part of the plant. This distinguishes herbal medicine from homoeopathy and the Bach flower remedies, which make use of the subtly extracted energy of the plant rather than its physical substance. Do not underestimate the efficacy of herbal remedies, simply because you may have been used to thinking of herbs as simple and delicate plants. Some very strong compounds are found in them (as those who use poppy and hemp can tell you), and some very potent drug medicines have been made by extracting, concentrating and sometimes modifying the active ingredients.

Herbs can be used for treating a variety of simple health problems, ranging from colds to headaches, as well as more serious conditions and illnesses under the guidance of a qualified practitioner. When self-administering, always remember that herbs are powerful substances. Eat or drink them as normal if they come as culinary herbs and spices, or as herbal teas. When you buy and use them in tablet form or as tinctures or extracts, you must stick to the recommended dosages given with the product. It is all too easy to think that just because it is a herb it can do no harm.

Holistic massage

As discussed in detail on page 223, the benefits of massage go far beyond the simple 'feel-good' factor. Holistic massage is a tangent therapy of therapeutic massage (page 280), and is more concerned with focusing on the wellness of the whole person, rather than just the physical body. A holistic massage therapist will often incorporate moves from therapeutic massage, but will mainly focus on using effleurage (page 222), or long connected strokes, that act to soothe the body and emotional states. The aim is to induce a sense of peace and well-being within the body.

On your first visit, a holistic massage therapist will ask questions about your medical history. Generally treatments begin with the client lying face downwards, and covered. The parts of the body that are not immediately being worked on remain covered and warm, while the therapist works with long connected strokes to soothe away tensions and bring back a state of peace to the physical body. Once induced in the physical body, this is then gently able to spill out to the emotional body, restoring peace and balance to mind, body and spirit.

Homoeopathy

Homoeopathic treatment has been in existence since the fifth century BC, when it was developed by the father of medicine, Hippocrates, the famous Greek physician who proclaimed 'like cures like'. The word homoeopathy comes from two Greek words: homos, meaning like, and pathos, meaning suffering, literally meaning 'like suffering'.

In the late eighteenth century, Dr Samuel Hahnemann, a German physician, rediscovered this highly effective natural form of medicine after becoming disillusioned with the harsh medical practices of his day. He had been working on a translation of W. Cullen's *Materia Medica* and noticed that the symptoms quinine produced on a healthy body were the same as the symptoms it was used to alleviate. This gave Hahnemann the idea for his theory, 'similia, simillibus curantur' or 'like is healed by like', published in 1796.

Dr Hahnemann experimented for some years on himself, family and friends, applying the principles he had discovered, with considerable success. Hahnemann put forward the theory that instead of using drugs that opposed and suppressed the symptoms of an illness, a medicinal substance should be used that, in its undiluted form, would cause the illness. By diluting substances to the point that none of the original substance could be detected, Hahnemann began putting into practice the theory of treating 'like with like'.

These principles continue to be employed in homoeopathic practice to this day. Homoeopaths believe that the more the remedy is diluted, the more effective it is. The most commonly available remedies are usually diluted to 1/1,000,000 of the strength of the original active substance. On the label this strength is described as '6x'. However, practitioners often prescribe remedies of 30x and some even greater. The numbers and letters refer to the homoeopathic potency; the higher the number, the more dilute and the more effective the substance is thought. As can be expected, this theory has caused an enormous amount of controversy in conventional medical circles.

A homoeopath will treat the person as a whole, not a list of symptoms. A holistic approach is adhered to, following the belief that all the symptoms, as well as the patient's character, lifestyle, habits and medical history must be considered before a remedy can be prescribed. All these aspects are thought to be closely interconnected and their relationships and patterns must be traced.

The client may find the questions asked by their homoeopath extraordinary, or even bizarre, particularly in the initial consultation. Due to this holistic approach to treatment, two patients presenting with the same illness will often be prescribed entirely different remedies.

Another principle of homoeopathy that has caused much consternation and controversy is the belief that the healing process is thought to start inside the body and work towards the outside, with symptoms moving in the same direction. Consequently, as one internal symptom improves, another external symptom may develop. This may mean that a patient feels worse before feeling better.

Many, many people have responded so positively to homoeopathic treatment. It continues to grow in popularity, despite no one being absolutely certain how it works. We do know, however, that potentized homoeopathic remedies have the power to catalyze a healing response in the patient. It is without doubt a gentle approach to helping the body maintain and restore health and balance, and is especially suited to the elderly, the very young and those with allergies. It is completely safe, non-toxic and free of serious side-effects.

Remedies are made from a variety of sources, animal, vegetable, mineral and human. They are first dissolved in alcohol and water for a few weeks, during which time they are shaken regularly. This liquid is then strained and becomes the 'mother' tincture, which is then diluted to make the various potencies. These are then measured on the decimal (x) or centesimal (c) scale. To make a 1c dilution, one drop of tincture is added to 99 drops of alcohol and water and shaken vigorously. For a common, more diluted, 6c remedy, this would be repeated six times, each time taking a drop from the previous solution.

Dr Hahnemann was a firm believer in prevention rather than cure, and in the ability of a healthy body with an efficient immune system to fight off invading infection. He particularly stressed the importance of personal hygiene in combination with a healthy diet and lifestyle to help limit the chances of contracting day-to-day viruses like colds, 'flus and so on.

Furthermore, Dr Hahnemann argued that the treatment of such minor ailments helps in preventing the development of more serious disease. In accordance with this theory, homoeopaths will impress upon the patient the importance of dealing with these minor ills, prescribing arnica following an injury to reduce bruising, for example, which in turn limits blood loss and infection of the wound.

You may receive treatment for just one day, or over an extended period of time. A patient can expect to revisit their homoeopath about two weeks after first treatment, to assess their reaction and progress, at which time continued treatment may be discussed. Homoeopathic remedies are widely available from chemists, health food shops and speciality natural medicine outlets, and you and your pets may benefit from many simple homoeopathic first-aid remedies. However, always consult a professional homoeopath for advice on more serious conditions.

Hydrotherapy

For hundreds of years, the wealthy have retreated to water spas throughout Europe to alleviate and heal numerous illnesses. Ancient Rome and Turkey built spas over naturally occurring mineral hot springs, knowing that water in many forms helped restore balance to the body. A renaissance in hydrotherapy occurred in the 19th century, with its great proponent, Father Sebastian

Kneipp, a Roman Catholic priest from Bavaria, at the forefront of this movement.

Hydrotherapy – literally 'water therapy' – is often used to alleviate circulatory problems as well as chronic pain, through the application of water in its many forms, from liquid to steam and ice treatments, often alternating.

Internal hydrotherapy, like colonic irrigation and enemas, is sometimes recommended by practitioners for cleansing, detoxification, and clearing digestive problems, as well as for stimulating the immune system.

Today hydrotherapy is widely accepted by the medical establishment; many hydrotherapy pools are located in hospitals and prescribed by doctors, particularly in cases of recuperation from physical accidents and for rehabilitating damaged cartilage and musculature. Various applications of hot and/or cold water treatments can alleviate pain, reduce inflammation and strengthen muscles after an injury. Controlled immersion in increasingly warm pools of water also acts to stimulate the responses of the sweat glands, in order more efficiently to remove the body's waste products.

Many forms of hydrotherapy can be undertaken at home, including cold compresses and alternating hot and cold showers, which are prescribed to stimulate the circulatory system. Inhalation therapy utilizes the medium of water vapour to allow for herbs or oils with medicinal properties to be carried to the particularly receptive respiratory membranes.

Of course, a whirlpool tub at home is a dream for home hydrotherapy, but more rigorous treatments should be undertaken at a hospital's or clinic's spa, with a trained therapist. With home treatments, please consult a physician before starting if you have diabetes, arteriosclerosis or are pregnant.

Hypnotherapy

We all have access to a naturally occurring trance state in which the consciousness is equally balanced between sleeping and waking. This state of equilibrium provides the working space for clinical hypnotherapy, a widely recognized and medically established complementary therapy.

In a hypnotherapy session the client is helped to reach this state through guided imagery techniques. Clear vocal modulations help the client relax deeper into this natural trance, where the consciousness is simultaneously poised and alert, yet deeply relaxed.

In this trance state both halves of the brain are equally receptive and both process suggestions made. The client remains fully aware of all that is being suggested and, because of this state of equipoise, the subconscious easily receives these suggestions, which are generally made for therapeutic choices the client and practitioner have discussed before the treatment begins. The hypnotherapy trance state can easily be left, either through the simple suggestions made by the therapist or by the client, if they should choose to end the session at any time.

Hypnotherapy can be successfully used for a number of beneficial outcomes – from stopping addictive patterns to reprogramming emotional states of imbalance. A good therapist will clearly help you to navigate the waters of the subconscious and allow for new and more life-affirming values to replace old negative and limiting beliefs. The root cause of the imbalance can also be examined and addressed while in this state.

Hypnotherapy helps to guide the choices of the subconscious and assists the client with automatically making the right life-supporting future choices. It is particularly effective in treating the causes of panic and anxiety, depression and low self-esteem, as well as assisting the body in coping with stress factors in positive and dynamic ways. (See also Self-Hypnosis, page 279.)

Iridology

To an iridologist, a map of the imbalances within the physical body can be found by studying the markings on the iris of the eye, as well as tracking how these markings change and evolve. Iridology can therefore act as a diagnostic tool as well as an easily accessible method of monitoring the progress that a course of healing treatments has on rebalancing the internal organs.

In 1881, the father of iridology, Dr. Ignatiz von Peckzely, published his findings, claiming that illnesses in the body can be linked to abnormal flecks, white lines, spots or dark streaks in the iris. In the 1950s, Dr. Bernard Jansen published an eye map, precisely pinpointing the exact location linked to each of the organs in the body, which revolutionized the use of iridology as a diagnostic tool.

The left iris reflects the left side of the body, the right reflects the right side. The eye is then divided into six zones or rings around the pupils, each of which link to systems within the body. The zone or ring closest to the pupil links with the stomach, the health of the intestines can be studied by examining the second zone or ring, the third reflects the lymphatic system, the fourth ring relates to the state of the internal organs and glands, the fifth to the muscular and skeletal system, and finally the outer ring links to the elimination of waste and the skin. In general, top parts of the body are reflected in the upper half of the iris, and the lower organs in the lower part of the iris. In addition there are 10 physical constitutional types within the framework of iridology, corresponding to the ten fibre pattern types found in the iris.

Since iridology is such an effective diagnostic tool, it can be used to identify early signs of imbalance or illness, and a skilled iridologist can recommend a course of healing to prevent problems before they occur.

Kinesiology

Kinesiology takes its name from the Greek word kinesis, meaning 'motion'. Kinesiologists believe that each group of muscles is related energetically to other parts of the body, such as the organs, glands, circulatory system, bones and digestive system. Kinesiologists diagnose by muscle

natural therapies

testing, that is applying light pressure to muscles to ascertain whether or not there are imbalances in the areas of the body.

For example, the pectoral muscle relates to the stomach meridian and reveals the condition of digestive health. Another example is the hamstring muscles, which relate to the large intestines. If a muscle is strong, that is, it does not give way when pressure is applied, then health is good. If a muscle is weak and so does give way under pressure then that will indicate an imbalance that needs to be addressed. Kinesiologists, rather than diagnosing for illness, look for imbalances or deficiencies in nutrition and energy.

This system was developed in 1964 by an American chiropractor called George Goodheart. While working on a patient who had severe leg pains he discovered that when he was massaging a muscle called the fascia lata, which runs from the outside of the leg from the hip to just below the knee, the patient experienced relief from the pain. Through this the muscle had been strengthened, whereas massage of other muscles did not produce similar results. Goodheart remembered research undertaken by osteopath Dr Frank Chapman at the turn of the century which showed that massaging pressure points could improve the flow of lymph fluid throughout the body.

Light therapy

Light therapy makes use of natural and artificial light to create a state of balance and wellness within the patient. In a naturally balanced state, our bodies are exposed to all the wavelengths in the spectrum of sunlight, from ultraviolet to infrared. While taking in the right amount of full-spectrum light is important for balance, taking in the wrong kinds of light on a consistent basis can create hyperactivity in children and stress in adults.

Full-spectrum light therapy will activate the pineal gland via light entering the eyes. This, in turn, induces a healing within the parasympathetic system. Serotonin levels are raised, which in turn increases calactonin, thyroid and growth hormones in the bloodstream. In addition, because the patient is in a meditative state while receiving light therapy, the intake of oxygen is automatically increased.

The recent rise in Seasonal Affective Disorder (SAD) cases that have been effectively treated by light therapy has brought this practice more into the foreground. In addition, light therapy is used successfully in treating cases of high blood pressure, depression, sleep disorders, skin problems, PMS, jaundice in infants and even migraines.

Sunlight is like food, and a minimum adequate amount of light is necessary for the complete functioning of the human body. For example, not only does artificial full-spectrum light increase the absorption of calcium in the body, but the circadian rhythms that regulate the body's sleep patterns are also directly affected by the amount of light we absorb.

One of the obvious benefits of light therapy is that it can be self-administered once you have purchased the equipment. Getting a full spectrum of light indoors can be as simple as replacing fluorescent light bulbs (which only emit a small portion of the light spectrum) with full-spectrum light bulbs.

Bright light therapy boxes can be purchased and require that you sit before them every morning for about 30 minutes. Coloured light therapy can be used to bathe the body in filtered floodlights, or through beams of light specifically directed over the area of the body that needs healing.

The biological rhythm of the body is affected by light, and various forms of light therapy aim to keep these rhythms in a normal flow, thereby maintaining both physical and mental well-being. Light therapy can easily be used in conjunction with other forms of therapy. If, however, you have any eye problems, do consult with your optometrist first to be safe.

Magnetic therapy

Our entire physical organism is dependent for life on the constant influences of magnetic energy. Most human organs have a magnetic functional vibratory rate of approximately 7.96 cycles per second. Working with either the static or electronically pulsed energies of magnets can increase the efficiency of all internal organs, as well as stimulate the blood flow.

Magnetic or oxygen deficiencies in an internal organ can precipitate the degeneration of cell structures, eventually leading to a lack of operational efficiency within that organ. The application of negative magnetic fields allows for the oxygenation of tissues by creating a high-energy field, directly leading to an increased number of electrons within that organ.

Research currently being carried out in the USA suggests that negative magnetic energy is a primary-force healer. Treatments involving positive and negative magnetic force therapy are useful in the rehabilitation of injuries. In addition, magnetic forces can act as a controlling agent against the formation of free radical cells – precursors to many known illnesses. Magnetic therapy is also useful in the treatment of pain and injury, and with conditions such as tendonitis, fibrositis, rheumatism and neuralgia.

Treatment with magnets takes place by means of either static or pulsed techniques. Working with static magnetic energy simply involves the positioning of magnets over various parts of the body, wearing belts or bandages with magnets sewn into them or sleeping on a mattress that can be purchased with magnets already placed inside it. With pulsed magnetic therapy, an electronic device directs alternating positive and negative magnetic fields at the affected area.

Magnetic and electromagnetic therapy are also useful in prolonging the beneficial effects of many other alternative and complementary therapies, and work well as an adjunct to many holistic therapies.

Manual lymphatic drainage

Manual lymphatic drainage (or MLD) is a gentle form of massage that actively works to stimulate the lymphatic system of the body. Movements are deep, rhythmic and methodical, and stretch the tissues in the direction of the lymphatic flow.

Since the lymphatic system has a directly regulatory effect on the immune system, MLD can assist in protecting the body against the development of serious illnesses and infections. In addition to stimulating these vital immune defences, manual lymphatic drainage is useful in the detoxification of the body.

The lymphatic system is responsible for the production of antibodies as well as the transportation of fats, hormones and proteins. If the body is overloaded with toxins the lymphatic receptors are tender to touch. This acts as an alarm for the body, signalling that a detoxification is in order, which is where MLD is useful.

As a beauty treatment, MLD is a successful adjunct to a weight-loss regime, as it helps eliminate excess fluid. Facial appearance can also be dramatically altered as MLD improves the quality of the skin and reduces swelling and puffiness. (See more on pages 223–224.)

Naturopathy

The history of naturopathy, which is really a collage of natural therapies, is rich and long. Botany, the study of plants, and herbalism, the application of plants and herbs for medicinal purposes, reaches down the ages to the beginning of time. The great Chinese herbal, *The Pentsao,* dates from around 3000 BC and presents a detailed analysis of herbal treatments. Until the birth of 'Modern Medicine' in the last 100 years, doctors always prescribed herbal and natural remedies as a matter of course. Indeed, the orthodox drugs of today are synthetic versions of the natural medicines of the past – from those of the very early Greeks, Egyptians, Chinese, Native Americans, any culture you can think of. Each has some sort of herbal natural tradition, often passed down as part of oral teachings, through medicine men and wise women.

Hippocrates, who was born in 460 BC, created one of the very early written herbal pharmacopoeias. There are,

however, much earlier ones, such as the Chinese one mentioned earlier and the Ebers Papyrus dated about 1500 BC, which lists about 900 herbal remedies/treatments.

Hippocrates is not only considered the 'father of medicine' but the father of naturopathic medicine as well. His was a holistic school, which taught how to prevent and cure disease by releasing inner vitality and allowing the body to heal itself. In the Hippocratic school, preventative medicine was practised and diseases treated by means of diet, herbs, fasting, exercise, spinal manipulations, cleansing and relaxing with hydrotherapy. They believed in the body's ability to heal itself if given half a chance; their basic philosophy is summed up in the language of their time – '*medicatrix naturae*' or 'only nature heals'.

In internationally renowned naturopath Ross Trattler's book, *Better Health Through Natural Healing*, he describes the Philosophy of Naturopathic Medicine: 'The natural therapeutic approach maintains that the constant effort of the body's life-force is always in the direction of self-cleansing, self-repairing and positive health. The philosophy maintains that even acute disease is a manifestation of the body's efforts in the direction of self-cure. Disease, or downgraded health, may be eliminated only by removing the real cause and by raising the body's general vitality so that its natural and inherent ability to sustain health is allowed to dominate. Natural therapeutic philosophy also maintains that chronic diseases are frequently the result of mistaken efforts to cure or attempted suppression of the physiological efforts of the body to cleanse itself.'

Negative ion therapy

The atmosphere contains both positive and negative electrical emissions, known as positive and negatively charged ions. An excess of positive ions can drain the body of energetic reserves, while negatively charged ions are energizing. These negative ions act beneficially to improve a person's health and mental well-being.

Negatively charged ions are mainly the direct result of cosmic radiation from space and electromagnetic radiation from our sun. Air near waterfalls or by ocean waves as well as high up in the mountains and around lightning is also highly negatively charged. We can all feel the charge that is released directly following a thunderstorm, when the air is dynamic and electrically charged with negative ions. Being in such places has a direct beneficial effect on the metabolism, the central nervous system, and the respiratory system. Simply standing in a shower can act to charge the electrical current around us with negatively charged ions, enabling us to feel more spontaneously alert and uplifted.

For the most part, air particles are electrically neutral. Other particles acquire either a positive or negative electrical charge. Unfortunately, aspects of modern living directly contribute to the positive charging of particles: pollution and central heating each contribute to removing the negative charge from the air. Many electronic devices, including televisions and computers, favour positive ions. In places where there are too few negative ions many people experience headaches, depression, lethargy and general irritability.

Negative ion machines are available that charge the ions in the air negatively. These machines can be used in the home or office and directly act to reduce such problems as hay fever, allergies and headaches, as well as increase wellness within the respiratory system. Such machines are often used in conjunction with Light Therapy in treating cases of Seasonal Affective Disorder.

Nutritional therapy

Food is the most natural medicine there is; it has powerful restorative and healing powers. By understanding the nature of food, we can use it to treat specific deficiencies which lead to an under-functioning body or, more seriously, illness. More importantly, by being aware of what you eat and paying attention to breaking bad habits, and implementing good new eating habits, you can prevent many health problems that are the result of poor nutrition.

It makes good health sense to discover your own optimum diet. It is not the same for everyone. Many people have food sensitivities or more serious allergic reactions or natural dislikes to certain foods. There are a few ways you can determine food intolerances. You could have a food intolerance test, but you can find some obvious sensitivities by reducing to the simplest diet and then starting to add foods one by one and noting how you feel after each one. Food sensitivity increases if you are run down, stressed or ingesting toxins like pesticides in your food.

Regardless of your individual preferences and sensitivities, there are certain basic guidelines you can follow to achieve a better healthier level of nutrition. Most of these are covered in the chapter on Healthy Eating on pages 36–87.

Diet is the most direct way to treat all manner of common ailments and illnesses. For example, few people realize conditions such as allergy, asthma, alcoholism, arthritis, dry skin, eczema, inflammatory conditions, learning difficulties, poor memory, schizophrenia and many others all relate to deficiencies or imbalances of fatty acids (pages 41–42). The huge changes to our diet this century mean that almost everyone has a deficiency of these essential nutrients, or an unbalanced consumption of them, which can also cause chaos in our chemistry.

Understanding how to correct these imbalances could be life saving. It could also help to heal long-standing symptoms and delay the progress of degenerative disease. Mothers-to-be need to know the facts before conception because brain growth, intelligence, eyesight and many other functions need the correct supply of fatty acids for optimum development.

Discover your own optimum diet by consulting a qualified nutritionist, who will help you create an eating plan that will bring you the greatest benefit and may

even cure an ailment or two. A detailed consultation with a nutrition consultant could help put your health on a better course for life.

You will be asked to fill in a detailed health questionnaire before your first consultation and, depending on your answers, it may be suggested that you also have food intolerance tests. The nutritionist will adjust your diet to your body ailments and symptoms: one person may need more raw food, another more warm cooked food.

Even if you are very disciplined and every day eat a diet of brilliant, fresh healthy foods, you might still need a top-up with a good supplement. There are many reasons for taking supplements. Very few people eat a diet with maximum nutrients every day. Most people compromise along the way – often there seems no choice; many foods are now grown on soils depleted in some trace minerals and picked before they have ripened and been able to develop their full vitamin content. Many foods lose their freshness and some nutrients because they have been transported and stored for varying lengths of time before they are purchased. Although experts agree that a healthy balanced diet has to be your priority, as pills do not contain the fibre, protein and carbohydrates – as well as the wide range of phytochemicals (see pages 27 and 93) – that are essential for a healthy body, many experts now agree supplements are not only a good thing, but are essential to your health and well-being. For more advice, see Supplements, Herbs and Tonics, pages 88–125.

Osteopathy

Osteopathy was founded in 1874 by Andrew Taylor Still, an American doctor who had become dissatisfied with orthodox medicine. As well as being a doctor, he was an accomplished engineer and this combined knowledge gave him an interesting slant on the human body, viewing it like a machine.

His disillusionment with the methods of orthodox medicine, including the over-prescribing of sometimes dangerous drugs

with side-effects, furthered his desire and research into other methods of healing. He became certain that much illness is caused by misalignment in the body and devised a system of manipulation which could bring the body back into balance. Osteopathy rapidly became accepted by the orthodox world and is now a highly regarded and established medicine.

Osteopathy treats the body's large framework of bones, joints, muscles and ligaments. The body is meant to have a full range of motion, allowing it to run, walk, jump, twist, dance, speak, write, play sports, drive and perform any task that requires even the slightest movement. Problems in the framework of the body, the musculo-skeletal system, that may have come on through habitual poor posture, injury or accident, repetitive strain, disease, abuse or misuse of the body, can be successfully treated with osteopathy.

Stress alone can cause problems in the framework of the body, when muscles tighten and therefore restrict blood supply to the muscle tissues and surrounding areas, causing defects in the bones that the muscles surround or to which they are attached. Dr Still believed that the body should run like a well-tuned engine, with the minimum of wear and tear. Like an engine, a body may require maintenance and certainly taking care of oneself and adopting a healthy lifestyle will help to keep that engine running smoothly.

Treatment will commence with questions about your symptoms, when is the 'problem' worse or better... morning, evening, after walking, when sitting? Your medical history will be taken, along with details of any other treatments you are receiving, followed by a thorough physical examination. You will be observed performing a normal range of movements and adopting various normal positions, including sitting, lying down, standing and bending forwards, backwards and sideways.

Particular joints will be assessed and the osteopath will apply pressure to various areas of soft tissue to ascertain whether they are overly tired, tense or stressed. Reflexes may be tested with a small hammer, as a doctor might do, and in some cases an X-ray may be necessary, especially if your visit to the osteopath follows an accident or serious injury. An assessment will then be made as to appropriate treatment. In acute and long-term conditions, treatment may continue for several months. Other problems could be cleared up with a few sessions.

Each session will last about half an hour and most people find the release of tension and following relaxation in the surrounding muscles a very soothing and enjoyable experience. The osteopath may use a variety of techniques, including massage, soft tissue manipulation and gentle repetitive movement of certain joints to aid their mobility. In the case of fixed joints where there is a problem, the joint could be released by guiding the joint rapidly through its normal range of movement. This will produce the clicking sound that is often associated with osteopathic treatment. An immediate release of tension will be experienced, almost like a drug-induced high, with instant relief of pain.

The osteopath will advise his/her patient on postural correction. In order for the condition not to recur or become permanent, it is important that the patient continues to practise postural correction and generally take care of themselves according to any advice given.

Osteopathy can treat: arthritis; asthma; athletic injuries; back problems; bronchitis; bursitis; carpal tunnel syndrome; constipation; earache; endometriosis; 'flu; headache; hearing problems; heartburn; haemorrhoids; menstrual problems; muscle cramps; pain both chronic and acute; prostate problems; sinusitis; varicose veins.

Polarity therapy

Polarity therapy draws from a wide range of both Eastern and Western healing techniques. The main belief of this system is that all illness is caused by blockages of the body's vital energy. By freeing up the blockages and allowing energy to flow naturally, illness can be alleviated and further illness prevented or recurrence of the same condition prohibited.

This therapy was developed by Austrian-born Dr Randolph Stone, who lived from 1890 to 1983. Over a period of 50 years, Dr Stone utilized knowledge he had gained from a vast range of training, which included chiropractic, osteopathy and naturopathy, as well as Eastern systems such as acupuncture, yoga and ayurvedic medicine. His main training, where he used manipulation, often brought good results and relief from symptoms, but he discovered that illness often recurred and that there was often an underlying, residual condition that had perhaps been hidden by the acute symptoms of the moment, and so illness returned.

His therapy draws greatly from the Chinese belief in chi (vital energy), called prana in India. He found that good health is wholly dependent on 'polarity relationship', that is between positive, negative and neutral. Achieving balance between these polarities is essential to good health and well-being, including spiritual well-being, and so the aim of polarity therapy is to bring about balance in all areas. The techniques used include manipulation and touch; stretching postures; correct diet and healthy mental attitude through counselling. Negative thoughts and attitudes can bring about illness in the body as reliably as a poor diet.

Polarity therapy does not generally deal with specific symptoms but concentrates on achieving and creating balance throughout. Anyone who suffers from any kind of illness will benefit from taking responsibility through addressing diet, correcting their posture and stretching regularly, as well as addressing any issues through counselling. With the help of a polarity therapist to see this process through, the benefits can be magnificent. It is important that the patient is able fully to commit to their own health-care and is not simply wanting someone else to 'do it for them', i.e. handing over responsibility.

The polarity therapist will take a full medical history. Then your energy patterns will be assessed and any blocks within your system will be found by testing the pressure points and reflexes. You will be encouraged to be aware of the body's own healing processes throughout; for example, if you have an unrelenting headache, you will asked to focus your attention, concentrate on the affected area and then to note any thoughts, mental images and emotions that come up for you. This process will then be repeated throughout so a complete picture of your physical, emotional and mental health can be drawn up.

You may be asked to make changes to your diet at this point and if there are valid reasons you may be given a cleansing diet, devised by Dr Stone himself, for an appointed period. If necessary, counselling may be advised also, if there are significant issues that need more focused attention and support in dealing with them.

The benefits of this form of therapy cannot be overstated. Anyone who is willing to incorporate regular attendance at a practitioner's and to take responsibility for themselves can only grow enormously in self-awareness. With the therapist's support throughout, this process is hugely enhanced.

Psychological therapies

While most of the therapies in this section take a holistic, mind/body approach, it is important to remember that the brain is a very complex organ and, as such, deserves a section of its own! Therapy has become an increasingly popular form of self-discovery and new theories are emerging all the time. Descriptions of some of the most important therapies in the field of psychology follow.

Behavioural therapy

This seeks to predict and control behaviour in a scientific way. Based on learning theories, it began in the early years of the 20th century. In the 1960s cognitive therapy developed and this is concerned with belief systems and perception, helping the client change the way they view things and therefore changing their outcome.

Analytical therapy

This form of therapy began towards the end of the 19th century and includes many variations, such as psychoanalytical psychotherapy, psychodynamic psychotherapy and psychoanalysis. The theory behind analysis considers an individual's mindset as the outcome of conflict between internal forces, and looks for answers within the individual's unconscious. The aim is to analyse the effects of early experience and to discover how they may cause difficulties in the present day.

Freudian psychotherapy

Freudian psychotherapy is based on the theory that unconscious factors play a large part in determining behaviour. Its founder, Sigmund Freud, worked extensively with patients suffering from mental problems in the late 19th century and, while his theories were ridiculed at the time they still endure today, and are the foundation for many other types of therapy.

The relationship between therapist and patient is paramount in psychotherapy, as it is important to the process of recovery that the patient is able to trust and confide in their therapist. By analysing physical manifestations of the workings of the unconscious – dreams, emotions and thoughts – and re-experiencing key events with the therapist, repetitive patterns of behaviour and emotional blocks are revealed, which over time provide clues as to the source of the patient's problems.

Typically, psychotherapy is a long-term process; patients will often have several sessions a week over a period of six months or more, in order to work through their problems. Psychotherapy is thought to work particularly well for people who are physically strong, and may have achieved a lot, but who tend to be plagued by problems like depression and low self-esteem.

Jungian psychotherapy

Psychiatrist Carl Jung built upon Freudian psychoanalytic theory by extending the definition of the unconscious mind to include the 'collective unconscious'. This part of the mind contains elements that, unlike Freud's unconscious, are not dependent on personal experience and are instead inherited. The collective unconscious is made up of archetypes based on primitive images that shape our perception of the world, and are universally present, regardless of race, gender, etc.

Because of the close connection with Freudian theory, a typical Jungian psychotherapy session provides a very similar experience. Dream analysis and the open discussion of feelings and emotions are tools common to both disciplines; however, the methods of interpretation differ between the two. A Jungian therapist will analyse a dream, for instance, with reference to the symbolic imagery of the collective unconscious – ancient motifs that mirror and describe our external experiences. The therapist aims to help the patient become aware of patterns of behaviour and recurring themes in such dreams that highlight areas of difficulty in their life. Again, this is a long-term process and is suitable for people with specific problems – introversion, low self-esteem, etc. – and those who simply want to increase their self-awareness.

Gestalt therapy

The aim of this therapy is to achieve self-realization through here-and-now experiments in awareness. The feelings and emotions of the patient in the present moment are paramount, in contrast to psychotherapy which emphasizes the importance of past experiences and repressed desires in determining behaviour. This is because extensive discussion of emotions tends to result in a 'theorizing' of those feelings, which means that emotional honesty is hard to achieve.

Patients are encouraged to bring their feelings into the present using role-play and other methods of improvization to re-enact important situations in their lives. In this way, the patient feels spontaneous and genuine emotions about that particular situation and can recall past experiences with clarity, rather than playing out learned responses tainted by hindsight. The aim of gestalt therapy is to help the patient develop new reactions to stressful and emotional situations based on genuine, in-the-moment feelings.

Group therapy

There are many kinds of 'therapeutic groups' – group therapy, group counselling, encounter groups, awareness groups, support groups, self-help groups, T (training) groups, and personal awareness or sensitivity training groups all have many dynamics in common. Individuals in 'therapeutic' or 'growth' groups give themselves and the other participants an opportunity to explore feelings in a safe and confidential atmosphere (even if all the participants do not feel equally safe or up to the risk). Things we might never discuss regarding our personal or professional lives might find an outlet in the context of a group, which gives us permission – and, indeed, encourages us – to explore and share our individual agendas and the feedback thus provoked.

Group therapy and group counselling evolved during the Second World War, when there was a shortage of trained therapists available to provide individual therapy. At first the group therapist assumed a traditional, therapeutic role, frequently working with a small number of clients with a common problem. However, leaders gradually began to experiment with different roles. Many of them discovered that the group setting offered unique therapeutic possibilities, and began to take advantage of these. The dynamics of a group offered support, caring, confrontation and other qualities not found in the framework of individual therapy. Within the group context, members could practise new social skills and apply some of their new knowledge.

Group counselling is not aimed at stimulating major personality changes and is not concerned with treating neurotic or psychotic disorders in the way that group or individual therapy is. The counselling group seeks to resolve specific, usually short-term, issues and deals with more conscious problems than the 'therapy' group.

Integrative therapy

This form of therapy is holistic and many therapists working in this way have a humanistic background. Integrative therapy considers the whole person – mind, body and spirit – and seeks to achieve integration between the three aspects.

Transactional analysis

Transactional Analysis (TA) focuses on external behaviour patterns rather than internal psychological processes, by looking at our interpersonal interactions, and how these reveal toxic patterns of behaviour that prevent us from dealing honestly and openly with others.

The TA theory of the ego provides an easily understandable way of describing our relationships. The interplay of the three ego states, and the degree to which one dominates, determines the types of 'games' – devious strategies used to manipulate others into doing what we want – the individual plays. In theory, the 'child' is emotional and seeks approval and attention, the 'adult' is rational and logical and the 'parent' is disciplinary and moralistic. This translates into real life, for instance, as a dominating partner who acts out the 'parent' role in a relationship in order to get what they want. The 'games' we play make up the damaging patterns of behaviour or 'life scripts' that the individual follows and it is the aim of the TA therapist to expose these toxic games. In doing so, the therapist tries to encourage the individual to throw away their dysfunctional life script and replace it with honest and direct interactions.

Transpersonal therapies

See pages 256–257.

Psychosynthesis

The purpose of psychosynthesis is to unite the separate and conflicting elements of the mind to form a complete and comprehensive whole including, for example, those parts that determine personality, desires and impulses and values and morals. The aim of this integration is to increase self-awareness and to aid the mental and emotional growth process, in order to fulfil the massive human potential we all possess that too often goes unrecognized.

Psychosynthesis is based on the premise that life has meaning and purpose, which is to further the universal evolution of consciousness. Therefore, it represents a strongly holistic approach to psychology, with a heavy emphasis on the spiritual.

Radionics

As in so many other areas of natural medicine, every aspect of physical existence is seen to vibrate on multiple levels. Radionics is a method of working with the interface between the energetic realm and the psychical. Radionic practitioners recognize that all aspects of existence, including states of illness and wellness, vibrate at specific rates that are directly reflected through sound in the calibrated dials of radionic instruments, which look rather like sophisticated radio sets.

Someone seeking radionic treatment will send in a sample of hair or blood, which the practitioner uses to tune in to their frequency. Harnessing the energetic interface between the psychic realm and the physical, the treatment takes place in the more subtle realms of energetics. The patient need not even be present at the time diagnosis takes place.

A radionics practitioner uses the equipment to tune into the patient's energetic imbalances simply through the medium of the sample of the patient's hair or blood. In addition to the use of the radionic instrument, the practitioner uses what is a type of ESP or radiesthetic faculty to obtain answers to questions posed in the therapist's mind about the patient's health. The vibratory rate of the illness is subsequently reflected on the frequencies received through the radionic instrument.

Using the hair or blood spot as a direct link back to the patient, the radionic practitioner then finds the right frequency directly to counteract the frequency of the imbalance or illness of the patient. A supplementary healing effect can be added by placing a homoeopathic remedy, flower remedy, vitamin or mineral sample near to the hair or blood sample, while the practitioner is broadcasting the radionic treatment back to the patient.

Since radionics is such an effective diagnostic tool, other forms of alternative healing or dietary changes can be suggested once the nature of the imbalance has been determined. Radionic dowsing can help find other methods that would additionally facilitate wellness for the patient. Like so many other forms of alternative medicine, radionics can be used as an adjunct to other healing modalities.

Rebirthing

Mention the word 'rebirthing' and images crowd forward of reliving a moment of which your mother may often remind you. Since she was likely to have been in extreme discomfort at the time, why call a healing therapy after that moment?

The name rebirthing is taken because some therapists have felt that the strength of 'life-denying' and limiting choices can trail all the way back to the choices actually made at the moment of one's birth. The process of 'conscious connected breathing' allows one to go back and simply 'choose again' at the moment of birth – or, indeed, any other moment since – this time choosing instead thoughts that support the highest and most loving experience for the self. The activity of breathing safely in a conscious connected fashion means that the client is then able spontaneously and gently to bring up whatever choices are blocking the experience of joy that is our birthright.

This transformational breath-work allows for those memories by which you have not always lived to be gently accessed. The opportunity for forgiveness is then offered to you by your Rebirther, thereby facilitating the highest possible emotional healing in that moment. Rebirthers often work with body work and/or affirmations to support the client in making these most loving and highest choices in any session. However, it is not always necessary to relive the moment of birth in order to reap the numerous benefits.

Often people experiencing a series of sessions (12 is the usual recommended amount with which to start) find their lives improving dramatically as their previous choices to hold back their life force are renegotiated. One can be consciously aware of making the choice to live differently/more joyously/more peacefully, but these realizations can also happen subtly. People sometimes simply feel their life force and capacity for joy expanding, without consciously having to access the memories or the stuck patterns that have held them back.

The making of the highest choices in life is the most supportive dynamic tool in creating a more loving space for your relationship with yourself, your family and your friends. Rebirthing session-work is a profoundly life-altering tool, and working in a series of sessions can dynamically improve the quality of your life. Rebirthing allows for the expansive beauty of the soul to be experienced in the healing breath-work and loving choices made in the present moment.

Reflexology

Reflexology is a popular natural therapy that treats health problems or potential problems by means of massage of the feet, and sometimes the hands. This is an ancient healing art practised by the Chinese more than 5,000 years ago and by the ancient Egyptians, Greeks and native North Americans, like the Hopi.

Reflexology is based on the idea that the whole body and its systems are reflected in specific areas on the feet. These specific areas are called reflex zones and there are particular spots that link to a specific organ or function, that are called reflex points. The use of pressure therapies to clear energy blocks along the paths of energy is commonplace among the peoples of the East. Acupuncture, acupressure and shiatsu are other well-respected Oriental energy therapies.

A reflexologist gently and firmly massages the feet, pressing various reflex points to clear blockages and toxic build-up in the organs and various internal body systems that can lead to something more serious if unchecked. Although it does not hurt, you may experience a certain sensitivity and tenderness to pressure on certain points on the feet, ankles and, in some cases, the hands. Not all reflexologists use the hands in their treatment – but the feet are always treated.

Precisely where you feel the most tenderness or sensitivity reflects where in the body you may be experiencing congestion or imbalance.

According to practitioners, reflexology stimulates the body's immune system and recharges your personal powers for self-healing. It divides the body into 10 zones, each of which corresponds to an area on the foot. The left side of the body is linked to the left foot and the right side to the right foot. Perhaps this is why it was known as 'zone therapy' before it was called reflexology.

If you are treated specifically for migraine for instance, the reflexologist would massage and press the corresponding zone and point on your feet, in this case the top of your big toes. It is a simple principle – for every important organ or body system there is a tiny area that corresponds to it on one or both of your feet.

Reflexology does seem to have many beneficial effects and is gaining recognition as more and more good testimony comes to light. Reflexology is an excellent complementary therapy to any orthodox treatment as it uses no drugs or devices and has a wonderful, soothing, relaxing benefit which seems to help eliminate stress build-up even after the first session. Increasingly, nurses are training in reflexology and/or aromatherapy, using these treatments in hospitals around the country and reporting excellent results.

Reflexology can help protect your health and prevent illness. An area of pain on a particular point may indicate a problem in the corresponding organ or body system – or it may just mean there is a potential weakness in that area that may lead to a more serious problem later if not addressed. In this way reflexology can be a very useful tool in your prevention programme. Always consult your doctor for any persistent or serious symptoms.

Reflexology can be used to treat: arthritis, asthma, bronchitis, constipation, depression, digestive disorders, irritable bowel syndrome, insomnia, migraine, muscular tension, PMS, sciatica, sinus problems and stress.

Reiki

Reiki, pronounced 'ray-kee', is Japanese for 'universal life energy'. This ancient healing art is believed to have originated thousands of years ago in Tibet via Tibetan Buddhism. It was rediscovered in the 19th century by Mikao Usui, a Japanese minister at a Christian seminary in Kyoto, Japan.

According to tradition, Usui spent 21 days fasting on a sacred mountain outside Kyoto, and it is there that he received a vision incorporating four symbols that could be used to enable healing to pass to others and revealed how the universal life energy described in ancient Sanskrit writings, Indian Sutra or sacred text, could be accessed and utilized to provide hands-on healing.

Dr Usui had spent 14 years seeking the ability to heal and it was his belief that he might achieve this by studying Buddhism and learning both Chinese and Sanskrit to promote his research. Tuning into the symbols creates the ability to channel healing power. Dr Usui died in the 1930s having initiated 16 other people into the secret of reiki, teaching them the master attunement. Thanks to Dr Chujiro Hayashi, one of Usui's students, reiki has remained with us. He established a reiki clinic in Tokyo after having noted all the sequences of hand movements in a reiki session and the results of healing sessions.

Now reiki is flourishing worldwide and is available to everyone. Reiki practitioners hold the belief that the body becomes ill only when the universal life energy is imbalanced. The treatments therefore aim to bring balance and harmony to the physical and treat any emotional or spiritual disorders at the same time. Anyone can train to be a reiki practitioner through a series of courses, although it is not actually taught but transferred from teacher to pupil.

A reiki treatment will promote emotional, spiritual and physical well-being. Clients will usually lie down, clothed, while the practitioner gently lays his or her hands over the energy centres of the body, thus allowing healing energy to flow into the body. The treatment usually starts with the head and ends with the feet, to promote grounding of energy. There are some reiki practitioners that do not make contact with the body but send healing energy into the aura, the energy field that surrounds the earthly body.

Reiki can successfully be used as a self-treatment and for those in training this is actively encouraged to promote their own wellness. Reiki energy can even be directed into the future or far away places. Animals and plant life also respond well to reiki healing.

Courses are a series of 'degrees', with the first usually lasting a weekend and then four further initiations by a reiki master. By the end of the first degree the trainees will be able to send healing energy to themselves and others. After completion of the second degree, the trainees will be able to give distant healing and those wishing to go into training others take the third degree, based around 'teaching' transferral.

The results of reiki treatment are often quite dramatic and sudden, and just as often they are gradual. The recipient of

reiki must seek to take responsibility for themselves as well as receiving treatments from a practitioner. The results of reiki can be long-lasting and can effect cures if the recipient makes the decision to foster a self-loving and self-caring attitude.

Reiki practitioners feel that daily self-treatment, together with taking active preventative measures in terms of physical health, also provides spiritual growth and emotional support and thus will work on themselves further to ensure their efficacy in treating others. Treatments normally last from 30 to 60 minutes and the format is usually four sessions over four consecutive days. However, depending on the individual, sessions may be spread out over two months, once a week or more.

Reiki can treat absolutely anything and has no contraindications. Anyone who feels they are experiencing serious illness of any type will benefit from reiki, but should always take the precaution of at least having a diagnosis from an orthodox doctor. Minor illnesses, including emotional disturbances, can be treated with this peaceful, loving therapy as successfully as more chronic or acute conditions.

The ever-growing popularity of this particular form of healing worldwide would indicate the vast numbers of people who have benefited from treatment in this way. Perhaps the disciplined manner of 'education' this healing therapy employs adds to its appeal amongst the Western populations, who increasingly look more to Eastern forms of healing.

Relaxation therapy
See page 252.

Self-hypnosis
Self-hypnosis, incorporating visualization techniques, can be used in conjunction with a course of hypnotherapy and is especially useful in cases where the patient requires on-the-spot treatment and the therapist cannot be around, such as with insomnia and asthma. Self-hypnosis makes use of the mind's own unconscious healing powers to

help alleviate pain, speed recovery and lessen depression, anxiety, phobias and addictions.

An excellent time to practise self-hypnosis is at night, just before falling asleep, and in the morning, just after waking up. The countdown to trance can be provided for you on a tape by the hypnotherapist with whom you are working. Otherwise you can make use of the natural trance-like state between sleeping and waking.

Self-hypnosis is particularly valuable in the alleviation of pain. One technique for this is called 'glove anaesthesia'. The person puts themselves into a trance or uses a tape to provide the countdown to trance. Their hand is placed over the painful area and the suggestion is that the sensation in the hand is one of heaviness and numbness in a completely relaxed state. That sensation is then transferred into the body part in pain, allowing for the pain to decrease and a comforting sensation of peace to ensue.

Shiatsu
Shiatsu is a Japanese holistic bodywork system that aims to achieve well-being through an efficient flow of energy around the body. The system is similar to acupuncture in that it involves stimulation of the body's meridians or energy paths, but uses a rhythmic series of massage techniques instead of needles – shiatsu literally means 'finger pressure'. These techniques aim to reduce muscle tension, release toxins such as lactic acid and carbon monoxide from the joints and relieve any general stiffness that can impair the body's energy flows and result in ill-health.

Although shiatsu is largely a preventative practice, aimed at maintaining the quality and quantity of the body's chi and its flow around the body, it is also believed to treat a range of specific complaints. Some of these complaints include stress, circulatory problems, fatigue, digestive conditions such as irritable bowel syndrome, constipation and diarrhoea, back pain, migraine, menstrual problems, paralysis, arthritis, allergies, asthma, insomnia and sexual problems.

A shiatsu practitioner will diagnose your state of health by asking you about your medical history and how you feel physically and emotionally. He or she may also use traditional Oriental methods of diagnosis, such as a pulse- or face-reading, to look for signs of fatigue or bloating, for example.

The shiatsu session takes place lying down, as correct body positioning and gravity play a large part in achieving effective results, and may begin with stretching and breathing exercises aimed at relaxing the muscles and creating a quiet and meditative atmosphere. After the initial general energy-balancing moves, the practitioner will concentrate on specific problem areas, holding each point for between three and five seconds to release blocked energy, and will end with calming techniques aimed at pacifying disturbed energy and restoring an efficient flow.

Sound therapy

The use of sound and music for healing and therapeutic purposes is now accepted in many academic circles (as well as artistic ones). Most of us have some first-hand experience of the depth of feeling evoked by a particular sound or song, but the concept of the healing power of sound is finally gaining recognition and respect.

More and more people have been awakened to their own natural voice and the power that comes from giving themselves permission to use it and not lose it. Our real natural voice is a gift and everyone has the right to treasure, explore and share the gift of their true voice to express themselves. Whether by sounding the 'om' or singing the song.

Music is one of the most ancient forms of expression and the recent rediscovery of sound healing is the current alternative rave. More and more complementary therapists are using chanting and singing to heal. Many believe that we made music before we made words and we are rewarded with increased vitality and self-esteem when we reclaim or discover our natural voice and give ourselves permission to use it.

Qualified music therapists now work at numerous NHS hospitals. As well as the numerous therapists available now, plus toning and choir masters and music teachers, there is also the simple therapy provided by bands, simple chanting or just plain singing in the shower. The journey through sound is so individual – what really moves you or stimulates a 'peak' experience might irritate or just grate on your partner. Respect that what makes your heart sing may make another weep – but it doesn't really matter as long as it's not your propensity to join the 'dawn chorus' unless you live on an isolated mountain top. Your natural voice is beautiful and you have the right to use it when and how it feels natural for you.

Thai massage

Like many Oriental systems of medicine, Thai massage aims to disperse energy blockages that are believed to be the cause of illness. Traditional Thai medicine takes a particularly holistic approach to well-being, aiming to restore equilibrium to the mind/body/spirit relationship. Drawing heavily on Buddhist philosophy, it has a strong tradition of practice within the family. Massage is only one component of the total Thai medicine system, the others being nutrition, herbal remedies and spiritual counselling, particularly meditation.

Thai massage is strongly influenced by yoga, evident in the passive stretching techniques that are its trademark, and also by traditional Chinese medicine, in the stimulation of the body's meridians. Thai massage may at first seem too vigorous to be relaxing, but it has the power to calm disturbed energies and emotions while simultaneously energizing the body. Other benefits include improved circulation, increased flexibility, realignment of the spine and bones, pain relief, release of muscle tension and stimulation of the internal organs and nervous system.

The typical Thai massage session lasts between one and two hours and is performed on a mat on the floor. It is important to wear loose, comfortable clothing that you can move around in easily. The masseur applies gentle pressure to various points of the body depending on the individual's needs, using fingers, thumbs, palms, elbows, knees and feet.

A key part of Thai massage is the passive stretching of the torso and limbs – the practitioner will support your body in various poses that encourage the opening up of the joints without straining the muscles, in order to release toxins and relieve stiffness. A Thai massage should leave you feeling balanced and energized.

Therapeutic massage

Sometimes called Swedish massage, therapeutic massage is a medically respected therapy, based on the oldest healing modality in the world. Hippocrates suggested a daily massage was the way to maintain optimum health, and therapeutic massage treatments are certainly one of the nicest ways to take your medicine.

Using a basis of five different moves, pressure is applied to the body either in small rhythmic motions, long connected strokes, deep kneading or cupping moves that stimulate the circulatory system and allow for the efficient removal of waste from the lymphatic and muscular systems.

The therapeutic massage therapist will first ask you questions about your medical history, ensuring that you do not have any contraindications to the treatment. Once this has been established, the patient lies down on the massage table, and the therapist usually starts the treatment on the back, using either talc or oil as the massage medium. Pressure is firm but gentle and the overall effect is one that simultaneously stimulates and soothes the body. See more on pages 220–229.

Tissue salts

Biochemical remedies are the result of the life's work of a German doctor, Wilhelm H. Schuessler, who lived from 1821 to 1898. Our bodies are made up of millions of cells and in order to function properly they require a constant supply of chemical substances, including some quite natural substances like mineral salts. Dr Schuessler believed an imbalance or deficiency of certain mineral substances in the cells could cause a disturbance of function and health. He isolated 12 mineral salts as essential cell nutrients and called them tissue salts and his form of treatment became known as nutritional biochemistry.

To support his findings, Schuessler put forward five main principles:

1 disease does not occur if cell activity is normal;

2 cell activity is normal if cell nutrition is normal;

3 the human body requires both the complex organic compounds and inorganic (mineral) substances as cell nutrients;

4 a mineral salt deficiency will impair the ability of cells to assimilate and utilize the organic compounds;

5 cell nutrition and metabolism can be revitalized by supplying the deficient mineral salts in a readily assimilable form.

Even with a balanced diet it is still possible to have a localized deficiency, due to fatigue or injury, that will respond well to tissue salts. The principle of assimilation is fundamental to Dr Schuessler's theory of biochemistry. Assimilation into the body can be achieved by the administration of a micro-dose of the tissue salts, which pass quickly into the bloodstream through the mucous lining of the mouth and throat.

The homoeopathic principle of trituration – a controlled mixing and grinding process – is used to incorporate the mineral salts in micro-dose amounts into a milk sugar base. Small moulded tablets are prepared from this mixture. When these are placed on the tongue, assimilation immediately begins.

Tissue salt therapy is suitable as a first-aid treatment for many minor, simple and easily recognized conditions. All the tissue salts are totally safe and quite free from side-effects.

Tui na

Tui na is a Chinese form of bodywork similar to physiotherapy in Western medicine and to shiatsu in Japanese medicine. By means of vigorous massage and bone manipulation, using a wide variety of hand movements, Tui Na stimulates the body's meridians – or paths of energy flow – and disperses the energy blockages that lead to illness and disease.

After a general question-and-answer session covering illnesses, allergies and other health problems, the practitioner will identify the important energy trigger points for your particular condition or surrounding the affected area for more specific complaints. Tui na is very much a collaborative effort – its effectiveness depends to some degree on the practitioner's ability to harness their own energy and redirect it into their hands, to encourage a revitalizing flow of energy between you.

Tui na translates literally into 'push grasp', a good indication of the hand movements used. Typical techniques include pressing and dragging, rolling, vibrating, twisting, shaking, patting and beating the skin and muscles, to stimulate blood flow and flexibility and relieve stiffness in the muscles and joints.

Tui Na is believed to be effective for a wide range of conditions, including bone misalignment, migraines and neck pain, digestive disorders and viral illnesses, as well as various paediatric complaints. You should, however, avoid Tui na if you are pregnant, if you have heart disease or cancer (particularly of the skin or lymphatic systems), if you suffer from brittle bones (osteoporosis) or if you have particularly sensitive skin.

Yoga therapy

Yoga therapy involves the patient working with specifically directed yoga asanas (see page 168) in conjunction with a yoga therapist. The yogic asanas work directly on toning the muscles, but they also have a profound effect on revitalizing the internal organs, since working yogically helps to realign the body properly. The life force of the body becomes more readily available, thereby allowing for the complete healing process to be speeded up in cases where there has been an injury or illness.

Yoga therapy has successfully helped millions with cases of chronic and acute pain, anxiety, menstrual problems or disorders, asthma and bronchitis. If you are considering undertaking directed yoga therapy for an injury or illness, do make sure that your condition is first properly diagnosed by your GP.

Zero balancing

Zero balancing is a type of bodywork that works directly at the interface points between the muscular and skeletal systems. Points where these structures meet are used as vital energetic pathways to access and rebalance the vibrational and physical bodies. In this respect, zero balancing works with both the physical and energetic structures of the body.

Created in the 1970s by the American Dr. Fritz Smith, zero balancing combines both Western and Eastern healing modalities. Applied specific finger pressures are combined with held stretches called fulcrums. This work allows for a still point through which old energetic and physical patterns that no longer serve the client can be released. The resulting effect is the release of deeply accumulated tensions that have been held in the physical body.

Zero balancing is so called because the work enables the client to reach a 'zero point', an energetically balanced state that feels clear and neutral. The client is able to experience a strong 'original state' of balance. This integrated state allows for a deep and profound sense of peace and relaxation, akin to that of intensive meditation.

The evaluation of the body by the therapist is performed through testing the range of motion around a joint. This work is a very effective and safe way of treating physical pains as well as integrating emotional stresses. The ensuing experience is one in which the client's overall sense of well-being is ultimately enhanced.

index

bibliography

Alexander, Jane, *Spirit of the Home* (Thorsons, 1998).

Appleton, Nancy, *Healthy Bones: What You Should Know About Osteoporosis* (Avery, 1997).

Atkins, Dr Robert, *Dr Atkins' Age-Defying Diet Revolution* (Vermilion, 2000).

Baker, Dr Sidney MacDonald and Baar, Karen, *The Body Clock Diet* (Vermilion, 2001).

Balch, Dr James F., *10 Natural Remedies That Can Save Your Life* (Doubleday, 1999).

Beeken, Jenny, *Yoga of the Heart* (White Eagle, 2000).

Borysenko, Joan, *Guilt is the Teacher and Love is the Lesson* (Warner, 1991).

Brownstein, Dr Art and Borysenko, Joan, *Healing Back Pain Naturally* (Harbor Press, 1999).

Cameron, Julia, *The Artist's Way* (Pan, 1995).

Campion, Kitty, *Holistic Family Herbal* (Bloomsbury, 1997).

Cochrane, Amanda, *Perfect Skin* (Piatkus, 2000).

Cochrane, Amanda, *Treat Your Child the Natural Way* (Thorsons, 2001).

Chopra, Deepak, *Ageless Body, Timeless Mind* (Rider, 1999).

Chrystyn, Julie, *Lifeforce* (Blake, 1998).

Clark, Susan, *The Sunday Times Vitality Cookbook* (HarperCollins, 2000).

Cousin, Pierre Jean, *Facelift at Your Fingertips* (Quadrille, 2001).

Crawford, Dr Michael and Marsh, David, *Nutrition and Evolution* (Keats, 1995).

D'Adamo, Dr Peter and Whitney, Catherine, *The Eat Right Diet* (Century, 1997).

Dean, Dr Ward and Morgenthaler, John, *Smart Drugs and Nutrients* (B&J, 1990).

Dossey, Dr Larry, *Meaning and Medicine: A Doctor's Tales of Breakthrough and Healing* (Bantam, 1992).

Edwards, Betty, *Drawing on the Right Side of the Brain* (Harper Collins, 1993).

Firshein, Dr Richard, *The Nutraceutical Revolution* (Vermilion, 1998).

Geffen, Dr Jeremy, *The Journey Through Cancer* (Vermilion, 2000).

Goodrich, Janet, *Natural Vision Improvement* (Celestial Arts, 1987).

Harris, Gail, *Body & Soul* (Kensington, 1999).

Heller, Dr Raechel F. & Dr Richard F., *The Carbohydrate Addict's Diet* (Vermilion, 2000).

Hoffman, David, *The New Holistic Herbal* (Element, 1983).

Holford, Patrick, *100% Health* (Piatkus, 1999).

Holford, Patrick, *The Optimum Nutrition Bible* (Piatkus, 1998).

Holford, Patrick and Ridgway, Judy, *The Optimum Nutrition Cookbook* (Piatkus, 1999).

Ivker, Robert S., Anderson, Robert A. & Trivieri, Larry, *The Complete Self-care Guide to Holistic Medicine* (Jeremy P. Tarcher, 1999).

Keating, Kathleen, *The Little Book of Hugs* (Doubleday, 1998).

Kenton, Leslie, *The Raw Energy Bible* (Vermilion, 1998).

Lee, Dr John R., *Natural Progesterone* (John Carpenter, 1999).

Mellor, Constance, *Natural Remedies for Common Ailments* (Beekman, 1981).

Peirce, Andrea, *The American Pharmaceutical Association Practical Guide to Natural Medicines* (William Morrow, 1999).

Plant, Jane, *Your Life in Your Hands* (Virgin, 2000).

Powell, Trevor, *Free Yourself from Harmful Stress* (Dorling Kindersley, 1997).

Reid, Daniel, *The Tao of Health, Sex and Longevity* (Simon & Schuster, 2000).

Richardson, Rosamond, *Natural Superwoman* (Kyle Cathie, 1999).

Robinson, Lynne and Thomas, Gordon, *Pilates: The Way Forward* (Pan, 1999).

Shapiro, Debbie, *Your Body Speaks Your Mind* (Piatkus, 1996).

Shapiro, Eddie & Debbie, *A Time for Healing* (Piatkus, 1994).

Shapiro, Eddie & Debbie, *Ultimate Relaxation* (Quadrille, 1999).

Spillane, Mary & McKee, Victoria, *Ultra Age* (Pan, 2000).

Sun, Howard and Dorothy, *Colour Your Life* (Piatkus, 1998).

Tisserand, Maggie, *Aromatherapy for Women* (Thorsons, 1985).

Trattler, Ross, *Better Health Through Natural Healing* (Thorsons, 1987).

Van Straten, Michael and Griggs, Barbara, *Superfoods* (Dorling Kindersley, 1990).

Washnis, George J., *Discovery of Magnetic Health* (Nova, 1993).

Weil, Dr Andrew, *8 Weeks to Optimum Health* (Warner, 1998).

Wellings, Nigel and Wilde McCormack, Elizabeth, *Transpersonal Psychology* (Continuum, 2000).

Whole Person Catalogue, ed. Mike Consadine (Brainwave, 1992; mail order only).

Williams, Xandria, *Fatique* (Ebury, 1996).

Williams, Xandria, *From Stress to Success* (Thorsons, 2000).

Williams, Xandria, *The Liver Detox Plan* (Ebury, 1998).

Wills, Judith, *The Food Bible* (Quadrille, 2000).

Yesudian, Selvarajan (trans. Stephenson, D.), *Yoga Week by Week* (Allen & Unwin, 1976).

addresses

Suppliers

(The) AcuMedic Centre
101–105 Camden High St,
London NW1 7JN
020 7388 6704
Mail order suppliers of Chinese herbal remedies.

Aromatherapy Associates Ltd
68 Maltings Pl, Bagley's Lane,
London SW6 2BY
020 7731 8129
Practitioners; a range of specialised oils.

G Baldwins & Co
173 Walworth Rd, London SE17
020 7703 5550
Herb suppliers.

Bioforce (UK) Ltd
2 Brewster Pl, Irvine, Ayrshire
KA11 5DD
0800 085 0821 for orders
Mail order suppliers of herbal remedies.

P J Cousin
Kensington Therapy Centre,
211–213 Kensington High St,
London W8 6DD
020 7376 1199
Acupuncturist & supplier of Chinese herbs.

Higher Nature Ltd
The Nutrition Centre, Burwash
Common, E Sussex TN19 7LX
01435 882 880
Free advice; mail order suppliers of vitamins, minerals and other supplements.

Neal's Yard Remedies
15 Neal's Yard, Covent Garden,
London WC2H 9DP
020 7379 7222
Suppliers of essential oils and herbal remedies.

Nelsons Homeopathic Pharmacy
73 Duke St, London W1M 6BY
020 7629 3118
Suppliers of homoeopathic first aid remedies.

Potters Ltd
Douglas Works, Leyland Mill
Lane, Wigan, Lancs WN1 2SB
01942 405 100

Suppliers of western herbal remedies.

Eddie and Debbie Shapiro
edshapiro@channelhealth.tv
Renowned meditation and consciousness teachers.

(The) Tisserand Institute
PO Box 746, Hove, E Sussex
BN3 3XA. 01273 206 640
Supplier of essential oils.

Weleda UK Ltd
Heanor Rd, Ilkeston, Derbyshire
DE7 8DR. 0115 944 8200
Supplier of homeopathic remedies

Organic Food

The Soil Association
Bristol House, 40–50 Victoria St,
Bristol BS1 6BY. 01179 290 661
www.soilassociation.org
For details on organic food manufacturers and distributors.

The Organic Food Market
Spitalfields Market, Brushfield
Street, London E1 6AA
Open Sundays. A broad range of organically produced foods.

Planet Organic
42 Westbourne Gr, London W2
020 7727 2227
A wide range of organic food; also, health and beauty products.

The Organic Marketing Company Ltd
Leighton Crt, Lower Eggleton,
Ledbury, Herefordshire HR8
2UN. 01531 640819
For details of suppliers of organic fruit and vegetables in any area.

Scragoak Organic Farm
Brightling Rd, Robertsbridge,
E Sussex TN32 5EY
01424 838420
www.scragoak.co.uk
Delivers organic vegetables.

USEFUL ADDRESSES

Acupuncture

Qualified acupuncturists use the initials MBAcC (Member of the British Acupuncture Council). A list of practitioners can be obtained from:

The British Acupuncture Council
63 Jeddo Rd, London W12 9HQ
020 8735 0400
www.acupuncture.org.uk

The British Medical Acupuncture Society
12 Marbury Hse, Higher Whitley,
Warrington, Ches WA4 4AW
01925 730 727
www.medical-acupuncture.co.uk

Alexander Technique

Qualified practitioners are members of STAT (Society of Teachers of the Alexander Technique), who can supply a list of qualified practitioners in your area on request.

The Society of Teachers of the Alexander Technique
20 London House, 266 Fulham
Rd, London SW10 9EL
020 7284 3338 *www.stat.org.uk*

Professional Association of Alexander Teachers
Rm 706, The Big Peg, 120 Vyse
St, The Jewellery Quarter,
Birmingham B18 6NF
0121 248 1133

Aromatherapy

Trained aromatherapists meet the standards outlined by the Aromatherapy Organisations Council which represent the various different aromatherapy organisations. A practitioner's list can be obtained from the IFA.

The International Federation of Aromatherapists (IFA)
182 Chiswick High Rd, London
W4 1TH. 020 8742 2605
www.int-fed-aromatherapy.co.uk

International Society of Professional Aromatherapists
82 Ashby Rd, Hinckley, Leics
LE10 1SN. 01455 637 987
www.the-ispa.org

Bach Flower Remedies

A list of trained practitioners can be obtained from:

The Bach Centre
Mt Vernon, Sotwell, Wallingford,
Oxon OX10 0PZ. 01491 834 678

Biochemic Tissue Salts

There is no specific training or

accreditation. Training is often given with homoeopathy courses (see also Homoeopathy).

Ainsworths Homoeopathic Pharmacy
36 New Cavendish St, London
W1M 7LH. 020 7935 5330
See also 'Nelsons' in Suppliers.

Chinese Herbalism

Practitioners must be registered with the RCHM, who can supply you with a list of practitioners in your area. Some practitioners of Chinese origin use the courtesy title of 'Dr', which is not recognised in the UK as a qualification for practising Chinese herbalism.

The Register of Chinese Herbal Medicine (RCHM)
PO Box 400 Wembley, Middlesex
HA9 9NZ

Chiropractic

Chiropractors have a range of titles, including: BSc (Bachelor of Science); BAppSC (Bachelor of Applied Science); and DC (Diploma in Chiropractic). A list of qualified practitioners can be obtained from:

British Chiropractic Association
Blagrave Hse, 17 Blagrave St,
Reading, Berks RG1 1QB
01189 505 950
www.chiropractic-uk.co.uk

Cranial Osteopathy

The General Osteopathic Council
176 Tower Bridge Rd, London
SE1 3LU. 020 7357 6655
www.osteopathy.org.uk

General

British Allergy Foundation
Deepdene House, 30 Bellgrove
Rd, Welling, Kent DA16 3PY
020 8303 8583 (Helpline)
www.allergyfoundation.com

(The) British Dietetic Association
7th Flr, Elizabeth Hse, 22 Suffolk
St, Queensway, Birmingham
B1 1LS. 0121 643 5443
www.bda.uk.com

Chartered Society of Physiotherapists
14 Bedford Row, London WC1R
4ED. 020 7306 6666
www.csp.org.uk

Digestive Disorders Foundation
3 St Andrew's Pl, Regents Park,
London NW1 4LB
020 7486 0341
www.digestivedisorders.org.uk

Eating Disorders Association
103 Prince of Wales Rd, Norwich
NR1 1DW. 01603 621414
www.edauk.com

Health Development Agency
Trevelyan Hse, 30 Great Peter
St, London SW1P 2HW
020 7222 5300
www.hda-online.org.uk

(The) Institute for Complementary Medicine
PO Box 194, London SE16 7QZ
020 7237 5165
www.icmedicine.co.uk

(The) National Back Pain Association
16 Elmtree Rd, Teddington,
Mddx TW11 8ST. 020 8977 5474
www.backpain.org

National Progesterone Information Service
PO Box 24, Buxton, Derbyshire
SK17 9FB

National Register of Personal Fitness Trainers
Thornton Hse, Thornton Rd,
London SW19 4NG
020 8944 6688

(The) Pesticide Action Network
Eurolink Centre, 49 Effra Rd,
London SW2 1BZ. 020 7274 8895
www.pan-uk.org

School of Meditation
158 Holland Park Ave, London
W11 4UH. 020 7603 6116
www.schoolofmeditation.org

Sport England
16 Upper Woburn Pl, London
WC1H 0QP. 020 7273 1500
www.english.sport.gov.uk

Transcendental Meditation
24 Linhope St, London NW1 6HT
020 7402 3451
www.tm-london.org.uk

World Health Organisation (WHO)
20 Avenue Appia, 1211, Geneva
27, Switzerland
0041 22 791 2111

Homoeopathy

Medical doctors who are also trained homoeopaths become members of the Faculty of Homoeopathy and use the letters
MFHom or FFHom. NHS
homeopathic hospitals exist in
London, Glasgow, Liverpool,
Bristol and Tunbridge Wells.
Details and a list of trained
practitioners from the BHT.

British Homeopathic Trust (BHT)
15 Clerkenwell Cl, London EC1R
0AA. 020 7566 7800
www.trusthomeopathy.org

British Homeopathic Association
27A Devonshire St, London W1N
1RJ. 020 7935 2163
Qualified non-medical homoeopaths use the letters RSHom or FSHom. A list of fully qualified homoeopaths may be obtained from:

The Society of Homeopaths
4A Artizan Rd, Northampton
NN1 4HU. 01604 621 400
www.homeopathy-soh.org

Massage

Massage practitioners use any of these: ITEC (International Therapies Examination Council); DipLCM (Diploma London College of Massage) or CHM (College of Holistic Medicine). For a list of therapists, call the British Massage Therapy Council.

British Massage Therapy Council
01865 774 123
www.bmtc.co.uk

The Register of the Massage Training Institute Practitioners Assoc
0117 914 3960

London College of Massage
5 Newman Passage, London W1P
3PF. 020 7323 3574
www.massagelondon.com

Naturopathy

Qualified naturopaths have a diploma in naturopathy and use the initials ND (Naturopathic Diploma). Those who use the initials MRN are registered with the General Council and Register of Naturopaths, who will supply a list of practitioners in your area upon request.

The General Council and Register of Naturopaths
Goswell Hse, 2 Goswell Rd,
Street, Somerset BA16 0JG
01458 840072
www.naturopathy.org.uk

British College of Naturopathy and Osteopathy
Frazer Hse, 6 Netherall Gdns,
London NW3 5RR
020 7435 6464 www.bcno.ac.uk

Nutrition

Many nutritionists have studied the subject to degree level and have BSc (Bachelor of Science) after their names. Others may use the initials SRD (State Registered Dietitian). Qualified nutritionists may also be medical doctors. For a list of qualified practitioners, contact the BNF.

British Nutrition Foundation (BNF)
High Holborn Hse, 52–54 High
Holborn, London WC1V 6RQ
020 7404 6504
www.nutrition.org.uk

Institute for Optimum Nutrition (and IoN Book Club)
12–3 Blades Crt, Deodar Rd,
London SW15 2NU
020 8877 9993 www.ion.ac.uk

Higher Nature (Nutrition Dept)
The Nutrition Centre, Burwash
Common, E Sussex TN19 7LX
01435 882 964

Osteopathy

Medical doctors who have trained in osteopathy at the London College of Osteopathic Medicine use the title MLCOM. Qualified osteopaths use the following initials: DO (Diploma of Osteopathy) and BSc(Ost) (Bachelor of Science in Osteopathy). A list of local practitioners can be obtained from the Osteopathic Council.

The General Osteopathic Council
See Cranial Osteopathy.

British College of Naturopathy and Osteopathy
See Naturopathy

The British School of Osteopathy
275 Borough High St, London
SE1 1JE. 020 7407 0222
www.bso.ac.uk

Psychotherapy
UK Council for Psychotherapy
167–169 Great Portland St,
London W1N 5FB
020 7436 3002

Centre for Transpersonal Psychology
86A Marylebone High St,
London W1U 4QT
020 7935 7350

British Association for Counselling
1 Regent Place, Rugby, Warwicks
CB21 2PJ. 01788 550 899
www.counselling.co.uk

Reflexology

Ensure you visit a reflexologist who has membership with a regulated federation such as the British Reflexology Association.

The British Reflexology Association
Monks Orchard, Whitbourne,
Worcester WR6 5RB
01886 821 207
www.britreflex.co.uk

The British School of Reflexology
92 Sheering Rd, Old Hollow,
Essex CM17 0JW. 01279 429 060
www.footreflexology.com

Shiatsu
The Shiatsu Society
Eastlands Court, St Peter's Rd,
Rugby, Warwicks CV21 3QP
01788 555 051

Yoga
British Wheel of Yoga
1 Hamilton Place, Boston Road
Sleaford, Lincs NG34 7ES
01529 306851 www.bwy.org.uk

Sivananda Yoga Vedanta Centre
49 Felsham Road, London
SW15 1AZ. 020 8780 0160

Western Herbalism

Degree courses in western Herbalism are available. A member or fellow of the National Institute of Medical Herbalists will have MNIMH or FNIMH after their name, having received training and accreditation by their governing body. Contact the institute for a list of practitioners.

The National Institute of Medical Herbalists
56 Longbrook St, Exeter EX4
6AH. 01392 426 022

The College of Phytotherapy (herbal medicine)
Bucksteep Manor, Bodle St
Green, Nr Hailsham, E Sussex
BN27 4RJ. 01323 834 800
www.collegeofphytotherapy.com

acknowledgements

1 Images Colour Library; 9 Gettyone Stone/Mark Davison; 10-11 Telegraph Colour Library/Antony Nagelmann; 12 Gettyone Stone/Bill Pogue; 16 Gettyone Stone/Steve Ragland; 18-19 Images Colour Library; 24 Image Bank/M Regine; 27 Images Colour Library; 28 Gettyone Stone/Mark Davison; 31 Gettyone Stone/D Young Riess MD; 33-36 Images Colour Library; 38 Lorry Eason; 39 Anthony Blake Photo Library/Martin Brigdale; 40 Anthony Blake Photo Library/Matthew May; 42 above Photonica/CSA Plastock; 42 centre Anthony Blake Photo Library /Maximilian Stock Ltd; 42 below Photonica/CSA Plastock; 43 Images Colour Library; 44 Gettyone Stone/Z & B Baran; 46 Marie Claire Maison /Manfred Seelow/stylists Jacqueline Saulnier & Eric Solal; 48-49 Images Colour Library; 51 Insight Picture Library/Michelle Garrett; 52 Stockbyte; 54 Special Photographers Library /Barbara & Zafer Baran; 56-59 Images Colour Library; 61 Anthony Blake Photo Library/Paola Zucchi; 62 Gettyone Stone/D Young Riess MD; 64-65 Images Colour Library; 67 Telegraph Colour Library/Stuart Hunter; 69 Gettyone Stone/Sheena Land; 70-71 Gettyone Stone; 72-73 Gettyone Stone /Sheena Land; 74-75 Stockbyte; 76 Telegraph Colour Library/Francesca Yorke; 78 Gettyone Stone/Deborah Davis; 79 Stockbyte; 80 Telegraph Colour Library/Andy Eaves; 82-83 Gus Filgate; 84 Stockbyte; 85-86 Images Colour Library; 87 Stockbyte; 88 Gettyone Stone/Moggy; 90 Gettyone Stone/Ray Massey; 92 Hémisphères /Stéphane Frances; 93-95 Images Colour Library; 96 Gettyone Stone /Spike Walker; 97 Images Colour Library; 98-99 Collections/John Wender; 99 Images Colour Library; 100 Photonica/CSA Plastock; 101 Martin Brigdale; 102 Gettyone Stone/Chris Craymer; 102-103 Telegraph Colour Library/Hugh Jones; 104 Gettyone Stone/Tony Stone Imaging; 104-105 Images Colour Library; 106 Gettyone Stone/Z & B Baran; 107 Images Colour Library; 108 robertharding.com/Lee Frost; 110 Gettyone Stone/Amy Nennsinger; 110-111 Gettyone Stone /Steve Taylor; 112-114 Images Colour Library; 115 Gettyone Stone/Anwell; 116 Food Features; 116-117 Images Colour Library; 118 Photonica/Patricia McDonough; 120 Gettyone Stone/Nick Vedros & Associates; 121 Gettyone Stone/Darryl Torckler; 122 left Stockbyte; 122 right Photonica/CSA Plastock; 124 Stockbyte; 126 Images Colour Library; 128 Gettyone Stone /Darryl Torckler; 129 Gettyone Stone /David Epperson; 130 Images Colour Library; 131 Gettyone Stone /Claudia Kunin; 132 Gettyone Stone /Stuart Miclymont; 134 Gettyone Stone/Sheena Land; 136-137 Gettyone Stone/Jack Ambrose; 138 Gettyone Stone/David Roth; 140 Gettyone Stone /Nicholas Devore; 141 Gettyone Stone /Gary Faye; 142-143 Gettyone Stone /Christopher Thomas; 143 Gettyone Stone/Paul Edmondson; 144-157 Vic Paris; 156 Gettyone Stone /David Ash; 158-159 Gettyone Stone /Aldo Torelli; 160-161 Gettyone Stone/A & L Sinbaldi; 162 Gettyone Stone/Gary Nolton; 162-163 Gettyone Stone /Sheena Land; 164-165 Photonica /Richard Seagraves; 166-167 Gettyone Stone/Bill Pogue; 169 Gettyone Stone/Michelangelo Gratton; 170-181 Vic Paris; 182 Gettyone Stone/Eric Larrayadien; 183 Gettyone Stone /Martin Barrand; 185 Contact Images /Michael Cole; 186 Image Bank/Juan Silva; 187 Photonica/Ann Cutting; 188 Encore; 190-191 Gettyone Stone /Hulton Getty; 192-193 Encore; 194 Gettyone Stone/Laurence Monneret; 196-199 Encore; 200 Gettyone Stone /Hulton Getty; 202 Gettyone Stone /David Chambers; 203 Gettyone Stone /Shaun Egan; 204-205 Encore; 206 Gettyone Stone/Ross Anania; 207 Gettyone Stone /Bob Torrez; 208 Image Bank/Rob van Petten; 211-213 Images Colour Library; 214-215 Encore; 216 Image Bank/Paolo Curto; 218 Gettyone Stone/Keren Su; 220 Image Bank/Marc Romanelli; 221 Gettyone Stone/Nina Rizzo; 223-225 Encore; 225 Gettyone Stone/Jack Ambrose; 226 Image Bank/Nino Mascardi; 228-229 Images Colour Library; 230 Gettyone Stone /Claire Hayden; 231 Gettyone Stone /Donna Day; 232 Powerstockzefa; 235 Gettyone Stone/Don Bousey; 238-239 Gettyone Stone/Chip Porter; 240-241 Gettyone Stone/Natalie Fobes; 242-243 Images Colour Library; 243 Gettyone Stone /Hulton Getty; 246 Gettyone Stone /Ebby May; 247 Gettyone Stone/Reza Estakhrian; 248 left Gettyone Stone/Stanley Brown; 248 right Gettyone Stone/Brandtner & Staedeli; 251 Impact/Mike McQueen; 253 Gettyone Stone/Giantstep; 254-255 Gettyone Stone/Giantstep; 256 Encore; 257 Gettyone Stone/Eric Larrayadien

Author Acknowledgements
My heartfelt thanks and deepest gratitude to Jennifer Dodd and Catharine Christof, whose continual support has made this project possible. I am also grateful to Lewis Esson, Emma Noble, Anne Furniss, Mary Evans, Françoise Dietrich, Rachel Gibson, Jo Barnes and all the team at Quadrille for their excellence and perseverance. Thank you also to Caroline Turner, Vic Paris, Amanda Clarke, Paul Bailey, Paul Walker, Carole Diplock, Michael Skipwith, Sue Beechey, Anne Harling, Michael Phillips, Joanne Sawicki, Alannah Tandy, Graham Wilson, Bridget Bodoano, Nick Parsons and Sophie Bracken. I am especially grateful to the generous contributions and support of many people who have inspired me and taught me much of the information that is included in this book.

Love and thanks to my family and friends for their support, especially Eleanor and Philip Schwartz, Zoe and Sean Wellband, Jane and Ron Silk, Peter Schwartz and family, Richard Shorr and family, Aron, Charlotte, Thea and Eve Wellband, John, Alex and Amanda Lowson, Oscar, Dreamy and Lily, Tina Fletcher, Jane Weldon, Barbara Freji and Mani Morice.

The author is grateful to these people for their permission to use extracts, as follows: Pierre Jean Cousin; Patrick Holford & Judy Ridgway; Eddie and Debbie Shapiro; Mary Spillane and Victoria McKee; Xandria Williams; Celia Wright.

Thank you to the following people for their permission to use their text:
Alison Belcourt; Sarah Bridgland; Jerome Burne; Catharine Christof; Pierre Jean Cousin; Jennifer Dodd; Lewis Esson; Emma Noble; Susie Perry; Caroline Turner.

We are grateful to the consultants listed at the front of this book for their valuable expert advice and recommendations.